Review of Radiologic Physics

Third Edition

Walter Huda, Ph.D.

Professor of Radiology
Medical University of South Carolina (MUSC)
Charleston, SC

Wolters Kluwer | Lippincott Williams & Wilkins
Health

Philadelphia • Baltimore • New York • London
Buenos Aires • Hong Kong • Sydney • Tokyo

Acquisitions Editor: Brian Brown
Managing Editor: Ryan Shaw
Marketing Manager: Angela Panetta
Production Editor: Beth Martz
Creative Director: Doug Smock
Compositor: Aptara, Inc.

Third Edition

Library of Congress Cataloging-in-Publication Data

Huda, Walter.
    Review of radiologic physics / Walter Huda.—3rd ed.
        p. ; cm.
    Includes bibliographical references and index.
    ISBN 978-0-7817-8569-3
    1. Radiology, Medical—Outlines, syllabi, etc.   2. Medical physics—Outlines, syllabi, etc.
I. Title.
    [DNLM: 1. Health Physics—Examination Questions.   WN 18.2 H883r 2010]
R896.5.H83 2010
616.07'54076—dc22
                                                        2009008871

DISCLAIMER

Care has been taken to confirm the accuracy of the information present and to describe generally accepted practices. However, the authors, editors, and publisher are not responsible for errors or omissions or for any consequences from application of the information in this book and make no warranty, expressed or implied, with respect to the currency, completeness, or accuracy of the contents of the publication. Application of this information in a particular situation remains the professional responsibility of the practitioner; the clinical treatments described and recommended may not be considered absolute and universal recommendations.

The authors, editors, and publisher have exerted every effort to ensure that drug selection and dosage set forth in this text are in accordance with the current recommendations and practice at the time of publication. However, in view of ongoing research, changes in government regulations, and the constant flow of information relating to drug therapy and drug reactions, the reader is urged to check the package insert for each drug for any change in indications and dosage and for added warnings and precautions. This is particularly important when the recommended agent is a new or infrequently employed drug.

Some drugs and medical devices presented in this publication have Food and Drug Administration (FDA) clearance for limited use in restricted research settings. It is the responsibility of the health care provider to ascertain the FDA status of each drug or device planned for use in their clinical practice.

To purchase additional copies of this book, call our customer service department at **(800) 638-3030** or fax orders to **(301) 223-2320**. International customers should call **(301) 223-2300**.

Visit Lippincott Williams & Wilkins on the Internet: http://www.lww.com. Lippincott Williams & Wilkins customer service representatives are available from 8:30 am to 6:00 pm, EST.

To my parents,
Stefan and Paraskevia Huda,
for their resolute support and encouragement

*Ordinary language is totally unsuited for expressing
what physics really asserts, since the words of everyday life
are not sufficiently abstract. Only mathematics and mathematical
logic can say as little as the physicist means to say.*

—BERTRAND RUSSELL

Contents

Six years have now passed since the second edition of *Review of Radiologic Physics* appeared. The focus of this book remains imaging using x-rays (i.e., projection radiography, fluoroscopy, and CT), as well as nuclear medicine, ultrasound, and magnetic resonance (MR). Only essential information is included to help radiology residents and radiologic technologists understand how images are created, as well as the corresponding risks of the radiation used to make these images. Basic physics topics relating to the production and interaction of x-rays have been kept to a minimum, while more important topics of radiation biology, radiation protection, and nuclear medicine have been expanded.

In this third edition, major changes have been made with respect to the organization as well as content of the text, tables, figures, and questions. The first two chapters deal with x-ray production and x-ray interactions. Three chapters address how x-rays can be used to generate projection and tomographic images. Image quality (i.e., contrast, resolution, and noise) is now comprehensively covered in one chapter, which describes both the basic concepts and the specific values of these parameters for all imaging modalities that use x-rays. Radiation biology and radiation protection are both very important topics that now merit their own chapters. Material on nuclear medicine, ultrasound, and MR has been updated, but these chapters continue to focus on basic physics. Accordingly, only minimal information is provided on the more advanced applications of nuclear medicine, ultrasound, and MR that are currently used in clinical practice.

One important theme in the revised books is to focus on the material that non-physicists need to understand to permit them to perform routine clinical duties. Selection of material has been guided by whether the material is necessary to really understand three issues: (a) the *essentials* (but not details) as to how any image is created; (b) the factors that impact on the image quality, and how this feature can be controlled and optimized; (c) the factors that impact on (any) imaging risks and other imaging costs, and how these characteristics can be minimized without adversely affecting diagnostic information. Another important goal has been to simplify the material by minimizing superfluous details as well as streamlining all tables and simplifying the figures to convey only the most important features. The author firmly believes that the provision of an approximate conceptual mental picture of image formation is much more valuable than detailed descriptions that may be technically accurate but are of minimal *didactic* value.

Most of the questions in the book have now been revised and, hopefully, improved. Each question relates to a specific piece of information that the author believes to be important for residents and technologists to know. In writing these questions, every effort has been made to ensure that they are clear and unambiguous; as such, the author would expect that *any* physics teacher would grasp why a particular question was being asked, as well as being able to *immediately* identify the correct answer. The two practice tests contain 10 questions from each chapter, and are designed to permit residents to assess how well they have assimilated the material presented in this review. As with previous editions, readers need to understand that this review book does not explain any topic in full detail. Accordingly, the material covered in this book should be read in conjunction with a more comprehensive textbook on the topic of medical imaging.

Acknowledgements

The author gratefully acknowledges the assistance of

S Balter, PhD
M Bilgen, PhD
SC Bushong, PhD
C Daniels, PhD
RG Dixon, MD
S Elojeimy, MD/PhD
GD Frey, PhD
C Gadsen, RT
EL Gingold, PhD
NA Gkantsios, PhD
K Green-Donnelly, MBA, RT
W He, MEng
KR Johnson, PhD
EM Leidholdt Jr, PhD
E Mah, MS
M Mahesh, PhD
PS Morgan, PhD
KM Ogden, PhD
RJ Pizzutiello, PhD
TL Pope Jr, MD
DW Rickey, PhD
DWO Rogers, PhD
ML Roskopf, RT
R Shaw
P Sprawls, PhD
NM Szeverenyi, PhD
L Theron
LK Wagner, PhD
AB Wolbarst, PhD
CE Willis, PhD
MV Yester, PhD

I. WHAT IS RADIOLOGIC PHYSICS?

Radiology is arguably the most technology-dependent specialty in medicine, and which has seen significant changes over the past decade. Computer integration with constant technical innovations have changed the workplace and influenced the role radiology plays in the diagnosis and treatment of disease. Radiologic physics is not an esoteric subject of abstract equations and memorized definitions, but rather the total process of creating and viewing a diagnostic image. A range of physical principles influence the process of image formation. Radiologists and technologists need to understand the technology and the physical principles that constitute the advantages, govern the limitations, and determine the risks of the equipment they use.

Radiologic physics covers the important medical imaging modalities of radiographic and fluoroscopic x-ray imaging, computed tomography, magnetic resonance, nuclear medicine, and ultrasound. Radiologic physics provides an understanding of the factors that improve or degrade image quality. Selection of the most appropriate way of generating a medical image is the responsibility of the radiologic imaging team, consisting of the radiologist, technologist, medical physicist, and equipment manufacturer. Optimizing medical imaging performance requires a solid understanding of how these images are generated, as well as the most important determinants of image quality.

All imaging modalities have a cost associated with their use. For modalities that use ionizing radiations, one of the costs is the radiation dose to the patient and staff working with these systems. Accordingly, radiation protection principles are important. Radiologists and technologists should understand the magnitude of the radiation dose to the patient and personnel exposed, and ensure that radiation levels are kept as low as reasonably achievable (ALARA principle) as well as within any relevant regulatory limits. MR and ultrasound do not have any specific risks, and the cost is generally the time required to perform the study.

II. WHY STUDY RADIOLOGIC PHYSICS?

Radiologists and technologists need to acquire an understanding of the underlying imaging science for each diagnostic modality and be able to pass their respective radiologic physics exams. However, neither will actually practice physics and there is no need to learn how to generate modulation transfer functions in radiographic imaging, write programs to perform filtered back projection algorithms in CT, or design RF pulses in MRI.

It is important for well-rounded radiologists and technologists to have a basic understanding of the following: (i) image quality parameters, such as mottle, spatial resolution, and contrast; (ii) how image quality is affected by radiographic techniques; (iii) how to evaluate commercial imaging equipment in terms of its ability to perform the required patient examinations; (iv) the radiation dose and risks associated with radiographic exposure; and (v) how to communicate with medical physicists and service personnel regarding imaging problems.

The focus of the text and allied questions is the essential physics underlying the creation of clinical images. Special emphasis has been given to the factors impacting on image quality, notably image contrast, spatial resolution, and mottle. Radiologists and technologists understand the achievable performance of any imaging equipment and how this equipment should best be used to solve patient imaging problems.

III. REVIEW BOOK STRUCTURE

This review book is designed to help prepare residents and technologists for the radiologic physics portion of their board and registry exams. It provides a source for comprehensive self-study in the area of diagnostic radiologic physics. The text assumes a background of instruction in radiologic physics and is *not* intended to replace the standard radiologic physics texts. This book is designed, rather, to provide a concise yet complete source of review to refresh and reinforce the concepts of radiologic physics expected of residents and technologists.

The text is divided into 11 chapters, each with approximately six subsections, covering everything from basic physics to image quality. Each chapter begins with a summary of the key information in point form pertaining to the area under review. This is followed by 30 questions designed to provide a self-test of the reader's knowledge and comprehension in each area. The philosophy adopted by the author is that material comprehension, rather than rote memorization, will guarantee success in the exam. The review book also contains two practice examinations with questions that range over the topics covered in this book. At the end of the book is a glossary of key terms commonly used in radiologic physics.

Radiation quantities are generally provided using SI units. Use of *roentgen* to specify radiation exposure is problematic, and use of the correct conversion factor (i.e., $1\,R = 2.58 \times 10^{-4}\,C/kg$) would be inappropriate given current practice in medical imaging literature. In diagnostic radiology, an exposure of 1 R can be taken to be equal to an air kerma of 8.76 mGy. In the text that follows, exposures have been replaced by air kerma, with an air kerma of 10 mGy taken to be *approximately* equivalent to an exposure of 1 R. In nuclear medicine, non-SI units predominate in clinical practice in the United States, whereas SI units are prevalent outside of the United States and in the scientific literature. In this book use is made of SI units (i.e., MBq), with the non-SI equivalent (i.e., mCi) provided in parenthesis. Magnetic fields are generally expressed in teslas, with recognition given to the fact that MR personnel are much more likely to refer to the 5-gauss line than a 0.5-mT line.

IV. RADIOLOGY RESIDENTS AND THE ABR EXAM

The physics portion of the American Board of Radiology (ABR) examination is administered in the fall of each year and taken on a computer. Board-eligible residents may register 1 year in advance to take the examination in September of their second, third or fourth year of training. The 4-hour examination contains about 130 multiple-choice questions, similar to the format used in this book. Calculators are not allowed, but one is available on the PC. Most residents comfortably finish the exam in the allowed time, with no need to perform any calculations beyond trivial additions, multiplications, or divisions.

About 60% of the questions cover x-ray-based imaging, image quality, ultrasound, and MR. *Approximately 20% of the questions relate to nuclear medicine, and the remaining 20% to issues relating to radiation biology and protection.* Results in the form of quartiles are provided to candidates who have taken the physics examination and pertain to each of these three syllabus categories. Further information regarding the American Board of Radiology and the written physics examination can be obtained at the ABR web site (theabr.org).

V. RADIOLOGY TECHNOLOGISTS AND THE ARRT EXAM

The American Registry of Radiologic Technologists (ARRT) administers credentialing examinations and provides continuing registration for radiologic technologists within the United States. A multiple-choice test format, consisting of approximately 200 questions, is used to assess the following categories: (i) radiation protection, (ii) equipment operation and maintenance, (iii) image production and evaluation, (iv) radiographic procedures, and (v) patient care. Examinees are given 3.5 hours to complete the exam, and testing centers provide an erasable board and pen (no scratch paper is allowed). A scientific calculator is available on the computer, or one will be provided if requested. Each version of the ARRT exam is score scaled, based on the overall difficulty accounting for slight variations in exam versions. A scaled test score of 75 is required to pass the ARRT exam. Further information on the American Registry of Radiologic Technologists can be obtained at the ARRT web site (www.arrt.org).

Chapter 1

X-RAY PRODUCTION

I. BASIC PHYSICS

A. Forces
- –The **mass** of a body is a measure of its **resistance** to **acceleration.**
  - –**Mass** is measured in **kilograms (kg).**
- –**Velocity** is the speed of a body moving in a given direction.
  - –Velocity is measured in **meters per second (m/s).**
- –**Acceleration** is the rate of change of velocity.
  - –Acceleration is measured in **meters per second squared (m/s^2).**
- –A **force** causes a body to deviate from a state of rest or constant velocity (**push or pull**).
  - –**Force = mass × acceleration,** measured in **newtons (N).**
- –The four physical forces in the universe are **gravitational, electrostatic, strong,** and **weak.**
  - –Relative strengths of these four forces are listed in Table 1.1.
- –**Gravity** pulls objects to the Earth, and is important in cosmology.
  - –At the atomic level, effects of gravity are extremely small and are ignored.
- –The **electrostatic** force causes protons and electrons to attract each other.
  - –Electrostatic forces **hold atoms together.**
- –**Strong** forces hold the **nucleus** together.
- –**Weak** forces are involved in **beta decay.**

B. Energy
- –**Energy** is the ability to **do work.**
  - –**Energy** is measured in **joules (J).**
- –**Energy** takes on various forms including **electrical, nuclear, chemical,** and **thermal.**
- –One common form of energy is **kinetic energy (KE)** caused by motion.
  - –A bullet with mass **m** and velocity **v** has a kinetic energy of $\frac{1}{2}$ **mv^2**.
- –Another form of energy is **potential energy (PE),** which is the energy of position.
  - –A raised ball has potential energy.
- –**Energy** *cannot* be **created** or **destroyed.**
  - –When a ball is released at a height, potential energy is converted into kinetic energy as the ball's velocity increases.
- –Einstein showed that **mass** and **energy** are **interchangeable.**
  - –**E = mc^2** where E is energy, m is mass, and c is the velocity of light.
- –**Rest mass energy** is the energy equivalence of a particle.
- –In diagnostic radiology, the **electron volt (eV)** is a convenient unit of energy.
  - –**1 eV = 1.6 × 10^{-19} J**
- –One electron volt (**1 eV**) is the kinetic energy gained by an electron when it is accelerated across an electric potential of 1 volt (V) as depicted in Figure 1.1.
- –An electron gains 1,000 eV (**1 keV**) when accelerated across an electric potential of 1,000 V.
- –An electron gains **1 MeV** (1,000 keV) when accelerated across an electric potential of 1,000,000 V.
  - –1 MeV = 10^3 keV = 10^6 eV

C. Electricity
- –**Electrons** are **negatively charged** and **protons** are **positively charged.**
  - –Electric charge of an electron (or proton) is 1.6 × 10^{-19} coulomb (C).

TABLE 1.1 · Relative Strength of Physical Forces

Type of Force	Relative Strength	Description
Gravitational	1	Binds earth to the sun
Weak	$\sim 10^{24}$	Involved in beta decay
Electrostatic	$\sim 10^{35}$	Binds electrons and protons in atoms
Strong	$\sim 10^{38}$	Binds protons and neutrons in the nucleus

–Applying a voltage in an electrical circuit causes electrons to move.
  –The **positive** region of an electrical circuit is called the **anode.**
  –The **negative** region is called the **cathode.**
–Electrons are repelled from the cathode and attracted to the anode.
–Any **voltage source** in a complete circuit results in a **flow** of **electrons** in the circuit.
–**Electric current,** measured in **amperes (A),** is the flow of electrons through a circuit.
–An **ampere** is the amount of **charge** that flows **divided** by **time.**
  –**1 ampere = 1 coulomb per second**
–Power supplies in any domestic home have a minimum of two wires and are **single phase.**
  –Single-phase power supplies have **one wire** that has an **oscillating voltage,** with the other carrying no voltage.
  –If there is a third wire, this is an "earth connection" for safety.
–In the **United States,** the electric power supply from utility companies is normally **110 volts (V).**
–U.S. electricity is an **alternating current (AC)** that oscillates at a frequency of **60 cycles per second (60 Hz).**
  –In Britain, AC voltage is 220 V and oscillates at a frequency of 50 cycles per second (50 Hz).
–**Three-phase** power supplies have **three lines** of voltage, each 120 degrees out of phase with the others.
  –Three-phase power supplies provide *much more* power than single phase.

D. Power
  –**Power** is the **rate** of performing **work.**
  –**Power** is the **energy** used **divided by time,** measured in **watts (W).**
    –**1 watt = 1 joule per second**
  –Table 1.2 lists the power and energies of a range of sources.
    –**1 horsepower (HP)** corresponds to **750 W.**
  –In electric circuits, the power (P) dissipated is the product of electric current (I) and voltage (V).
    –**Power (watt) = current (ampere) × voltage (volt)**
  –If the voltage is 100,000 V (**100 kV**) and the current is 1 A **(1,000 mA),** the power dissipated is 100,000 W (**100 kW**).
  –A typical household in North America uses a few kW of electrical power.
    –**X-ray generators** use up to **100 kW** of electrical power, or the power required for ~ 30 U.S. households.

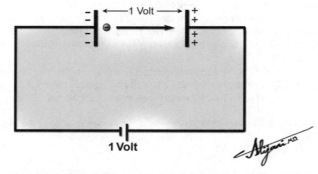

FIGURE 1.1   At the negatively charged plate, the electron has potential energy of 1 eV, which is converted into a kinetic energy of 1 eV as the electron is accelerated from the cathode to the anode.

TABLE 1.2   Common Power Sources

Source	Power (W)	Energy Used per Second (J)
Flashlight	2	2
Domestic light bulb	50	50
Microwave	500	500
Average U.S. home	3,000	3,000
X-ray generator	100,000	100,000

–The total energy generated is the product of power and time.
  –**Energy (joule) = power (watt) × time (second)**
–X-ray generators are only switched on for short periods of time.
  –A typical exposure time for a chest x-ray examination is 10 ms.
–**Energy utilization** in **making x-rays** is therefore **low** because of the very short exposure times that are used.

II. ELECTROMAGNETIC RADIATION

A. Waves
  –A **wave** is an entity that varies in space and time.
    –A common example of a wave is the variation of the water level in the ocean.
  –Waves are characterized by a **wavelength, frequency,** and **velocity.**
  –**Wavelength (λ)** is the distance between successive crests of waves.
    –Wavelengths are measured in **meters (m).**
  –**Frequency (f)** is the number of wave oscillations per unit of time.
    –Frequencies are measured in **cycles per second,** where one cycle per second is equal to one **hertz (Hz).**
  –The wave period is the time required for one wavelength to pass.
    –**Wave period** is **1/f.**
  –The **wave velocity (v)** is the product of the wavelength and frequency, and measured in **meters per second (m/s).**
    –**Velocity (m/s) = frequency (Hz) × wavelength (m)**
  –**Electromagnetic radiation** is a wave that is associated with oscillating **electric** and **magnetic fields.**
  –**Visible light** is a form of electromagnetic radiation.
  –The sun emits (loses) the energy that it generates in nuclear processes by radiating visible light.
B. X-rays
  –**X-rays** are a form of **electromagnetic radiation.**
  –Electromagnetic radiation represents a **transverse wave,** in which the electric and magnetic fields oscillate perpendicular to the direction of the wave motion.
  –Electromagnetic radiation travels in a straight line at the **speed** of **light (c).**
    –The value of c is 3×10^8 m/s in a vacuum.
  –The product of the wavelength (λ) and frequency (f) of electromagnetic radiation is equal to the speed of light **(c = fλ).**
    –**Low-frequency** electromagnetic radiation has a **long wavelength.**
    –**High-frequency** electromagnetic radiation has a **short wavelength.**
  –Figure 1.2 shows the electromagnetic spectrum that ranges from radio waves to gamma rays.
C. Photons
  –**Electromagnetic radiation** is **quantized,** meaning that it exists in **discrete** quantities called photons.
  –**Photons** may behave as **waves** or **particles** but have **no mass.**
  –**Photon energy (E)** is directly **proportional** to **frequency.**
    –Photon energy is inversely proportional to wavelength.
  –Photon energy is $E = hf = h\,(c/\lambda)$, where h is Plank's constant.
  –A **10-keV photon** has a wavelength of **0.1 nm,** comparable to the size of a small **atom.**
    –A 100-keV photon has a wavelength of 0.01 nm.

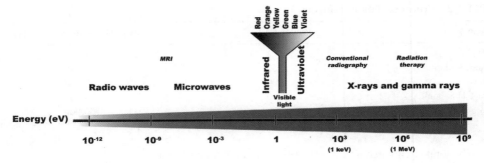

FIGURE 1.2   Electromagnetic spectrum ranging from radio waves to gamma rays showing that the photon energy is directly proportional to frequency.

   –**Radio waves** have low frequencies (low photon energies) and **gamma waves** have high frequencies (high photon energies) as depicted in Figure 1.2.
   –High energy photons are called **x-rays** if produced by **electron** interactions but **gamma rays** if produced in a **nuclear** process.
      –There are *no physical differences* between x-rays and gamma rays of the same energy.
D. Inverse square law
   –The **intensity** of an x-ray beam is proportional to the **number** of **photons** crossing a given **area** (e.g., square millimeter).
   –X-ray beam intensity **decreases** with **distance** from the x-ray tube because of the divergence of the x-ray beam.
   –The **decrease in intensity** is proportional to the **square** of the **distance** from the source. This nonlinear falloff in intensity with distance is called the **inverse square law.**
   –**Doubling** the **distance** from the x-ray source **decreases** the x-ray beam **intensity by** a **factor** of **4.**
      –Halving the distance *increases* the x-ray beam intensity by a factor of 4.
   –Table 1.3 shows how increasing and decreasing the distance from a source of radiation changes the radiation intensity.
   –In general, if the distance from the x-ray source is changed from x_1 to x_2, then the x-ray beam intensity changes by $(x_1/x_2)^2$.

III. X-RAY GENERATORS

A. Generator role
   –**X-ray generators** provide electrical power to the x-ray tube.
      –A small fraction of this power ($\sim$1%) is converted into x-rays.
   –Virtually all current x-ray generators in Radiology departments use **three-phase** power supplies.

TABLE 1.3   Relative Radiation Intensity as a Function of Distance from the Radiation Source (Inverse Square Law)

Distance from Radiation Source (m)	Intensity (Relative to Intensity at 1 m)
0.1	100
0.25	16
0.5	4
1	1
2	1/4
4	1/16
10	1/100

The intensity at 1 m has been arbitrarily set to 1.0.

–A generator uses a **transformer** to increase the voltage that is applied *across* the x-ray tube.

–The generator also **rectifies** the waveform **from AC** to **direct current (DC).**

–Generators permit x-ray operators to control three key parameters of x-ray operation.

  –The **tube voltage (kV)** that is applied **across** the **x-ray tube.**

  –The **current (mA)** that flows **through** the **x-ray tube.**

  –The total **exposure time (seconds)** for which the tube current flows.

–The **power** dissipated equals the product of tube voltage (V) in volt and current (I) in amps, or **VI,** and is measured in watts (kW).

–Typical transformer ratings in x-ray departments are **100 kV** and **1,000 mA,** which correspond to a power of **100 kW.**

B. Generator types

–**Generators** consist of an input **power supply, transformer,** and **rectification circuit.**

–**Single-phase** generators use a single-phase power supply.

–Single-phase generators use a **bridge rectifier circuit** that directs the alternating flow of high-voltage electrons so that flow is always from cathode to anode.

–**Single-phase** generators have been **replaced by three-phase generators** for use in diagnostic radiology.

  –**Single-phase** generators are common for **dental radiography** where teeth are relatively thin and longer exposure times are tolerable (no moving parts).

–**Three-phase** generators use a three-phase power supply.

–**High-frequency inverter** generators transform an AC input into low-voltage DC, then into high-frequency AC, and finally into high-frequency AC waveforms that are rectified to yield a nearly constant voltage waveform.

  –High-frequency generators are smaller and more efficient than three-phase generators.

–**Constant potential generators** provide a nearly constant voltage across the x-ray tube.

–Constant potential generators are expensive, require more space, and are used in interventional radiology.

C. Transformers

–A **transformer** changes the size of the input voltage and is capable of producing high and low voltages.

–**Step-up transformers increase** the **voltage.**

  –A step-down transformer decreases the voltage.

–If two wire coils are wrapped around a common iron core, current in the **primary** coil produces a current in the **secondary** coil by **electromagnetic induction.**

–The voltages in the two circuits (V_p and V_s) are proportional to the number of turns in the two coils (N_p and N_s)

  –$N_p/N_s = V_p/V_s$, where p refers to the primary and s to the secondary coils

–For an ideal transformer, the power in the primary and secondary circuits will be equal.

  –$V_p I_p = V_s I_s$

–The step-up transformers used in x-ray generators have a secondary coil with **many more turns (500:1)** to produce a high voltage, which is applied across the tube.

–Generators also have a **step-down transformer** with fewer turns in the secondary coil.

  –The step-down transformer produces a **low voltage (10 V),** which is applied across the **x-ray tube filament** circuit.

–An **autotransformer** permits adjustment of the output voltage using movable contacts to change the number of windings in the circuit.

D. Rectification

–The electric current from an **AC** power supply flows alternately in both directions, resulting in a voltage waveform shaped like a sine wave.

–**Rectification** changes the **AC voltage** into a **DC voltage** across the x-ray tube.

–Rectification is achieved using **diodes,** which permit current to flow in only one direction.

–Rectification for single-phase power supply normally uses four diodes and is called **full-wave rectification.**

–In full-wave rectification, there are **two pulses per cycle** of **1/60 second.**

  –AC electricity oscillation is 60 cycles per second.

–Each pulse ranges **from zero volts** to a **peak (maximum) voltage.**

  –The maximum voltage is known as the kV_p **(p stands for peak).**

–Rectification circuits in three-phase power supplies use a large number of diodes.

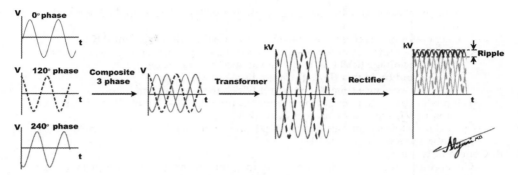

FIGURE 1.3   A three-phase generator (left) transforms and rectifies the input voltage to produce a high output voltage.

–Three-phase rectification circuits are arranged in combinations of **delta** and **wye** circuits.
  –Many **three-phase** power supplies generate waveforms that have either **6** or **12 pulses per cycle** of **1/60 second.**
E. **Voltage waveform**
  –**Voltage waveform** is a **plot** of **voltage over time.**
  –A **constant** high voltage is desired across the x-ray tube for x-ray production.
    –In practice, there is some variation in the voltage called **ripple.**
  –The **peak voltage** or **kilovolt peak (kV_p)** is the **maximum** voltage that crosses the x-ray tube during a complete waveform cycle.
  –The **voltage waveform ripple** is the maximum voltage minus the minimum voltage per cycle expressed as a percentage of the maximum voltage.
  –**Single-phase** systems have **100% ripple.**
    –**Three-phase 6-pulse** systems have ~**13% ripple.**
    –**Three-phase 12-pulse** systems have ~**4% ripple.**
  –**High-frequency** generators have ripple comparable to 12-pulse systems.
  –Figure 1.3 shows how the waveform is created for a three-phase generator, and the corresponding ripple.
  –The **average** (or effective) voltage will be *slightly lower* than the **peak voltage.**
  –Most ripples in diagnostic radiology are relatively small (<10%).
    –Nowadays in diagnostic radiology, **kV** and **kV_p** are **numerically similar.** (For this reason, kV rather than technically correct kV_p is used throughout this book.)
  –When the ripple is high (e.g., 100%), it is important to differentiate the peak voltage from the average value, as the latter will be *much lower* than the applied kV_p.

IV. MAKING X-RAYS

A. **Energetic electrons**
  –X-ray tubes produce x-rays by **accelerating electrons** to **high energies.**
  –The x-ray **tube filament** is heated to a high temperature, which then **emits electrons.**
  –A high voltage (V) is applied between the **filament (cathode)** and the **target (anode).**
  –Electrons from the filament are accelerated away from the negatively charged filament and attracted by the positive voltage on the target.
  –The **flow** of **electrons** from the filament to the target constitutes the **tube current (mA).**
  –When the electrons reach the target, they have a kinetic energy of **V eV,** which is determined solely by the value of the voltage (V) applied between the filament and target.
  –X-rays are produced when energetic electrons are stopped in the target.
  –Targets in most x-ray tubes are **tungsten (W).**
    –Most mammography targets are **molybdenum (Mo)** or **rhodium (Rh).**
  –When the electrons strike the target material, electron **kinetic energy** is transformed into **heat** and **x-rays.**
  –An energetic electron transfers most of its kinetic energy (~99%) to **atomic electrons** in the target.
    –**Excitation** occurs when atomic electrons are energized to higher energy states.
    –**Ionization** occurs when an atomic electron is removed from an atom.

−Electrons only penetrate a very short distance (<1 mm) into the anode before losing all of their kinetic energy.

−The **target** is embedded in an **anode material** that temporarily stores the **heat** produced in the target.

B. Bremsstrahlung radiation

−**Bremsstrahlung** x-rays are produced when energetic electrons interact with **nuclear electric fields.**

−*Bremsstrahlung* means **braking radiation** in German.

−The **maximum kinetic energy** of electrons incident on the target is determined by the **x-ray tube voltage.**

−A **voltage** of **100 kV** will produce electrons with **100 keV** of **kinetic energy.**

−Energetic electrons are **decelerated** by the nuclear electric field and change their direction of travel.

−The **energy lost** when the energetic electron decelerates **appears as** an **x-ray photon.**

−Figure 1.4A shows a bremsstrahlung process where a fraction of the initial electron kinetic energy is emitted as an x-ray photon.

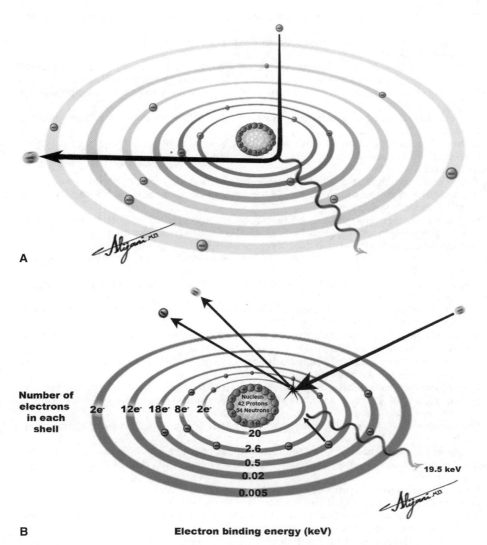

FIGURE 1.4   X-ray production for a molybdenum target showing **(A)** bremsstrahlung x-ray production and **(B)** characteristic x-ray production.

–Bremsstrahlung produces a **continuous range** of **x-ray energies** up to a maximum energy.

–An energetic electron **can lose** all of its **kinetic energy** in a bremsstrahlung interaction.

  –The **maximum bremsstrahlung** photon energy equals the kinetic energy gained by electrons accelerated across the x-ray tube (i.e., **V eV**).

–**Bremsstrahlung** x-ray production increases with increases in both the **accelerating voltage (kV)** and the **atomic number (Z)** of the **target.**

–**Most x-rays** produced in radiographic, fluoroscopic, and computed tomography (CT) imaging are via **bremsstrahlung** processes.

C. Characteristic radiation

–**Characteristic radiation** is produced when target electrons are ejected by the incident energetic electrons.

  –Only K-shell characteristic x-rays are important in diagnostic radiology.

–To eject a **K-shell electron,** the incident electron must have energy greater than the binding energy.

–The resultant **vacancy** is filled by an outer shell electron, and the energy difference emitted as **characteristic radiation.**

  –K-shell x-rays result from vacancies in the K shell, L-shell x-rays from vacancies in the L shell, and so on.

–**Characteristic x-rays** occur only at **discrete** energy levels, unlike the **continuous energy spectrum** of bremsstrahlung.

–For tungsten, K-shell characteristic x-rays are produced only when the applied voltage exceeds 70 kV.

  –A voltage of >70 kV will produce electrons with kinetic energy >70 keV, which is sufficient to eject K-shell electrons that have a binding energy of 70 keV.

–Following the ejection of a K-shell electron, the excess energy may also be emitted as an **Auger electron.**

–**K-shell characteristic x-ray energies** are always *slightly lower* than the K-shell binding energy.

–**L-shell** characteristic x-rays always accompany K-shell x-rays, but these have very low energies and are absorbed by the x-ray tube glass envelope.

D. X-ray spectra

–X-ray beams in diagnostic radiology generally have a wide **range** of **photon energies.**

–A graph of **x-ray tube output** showing the number of photons at each x-ray energy is called an **x-ray spectrum.**

–For most radiologic imaging (e.g., radiography, fluoroscopy, and CT), the **effective photon energy** is between **one third** and **one half** of the **maximum photon energy.**

  –**Effective energy** is also called the **average energy.**

–Each target material emits characteristic x-rays of *specific discrete energies* as shown in Figure 1.4B.

  –**Tungsten (Z = 74; K-shell binding energy 70 keV) has characteristic x-ray energies** of **58 to 67 keV.**

  –**Molybdenum (Z = 42; K-shell binding energy 20 keV) has characteristic x-ray energies** of **17 to 19 keV** (Fig. 1.4B).

–In Figure 1.4B, if the K-shell vacancy is filled by an electron in the L shell, the characteristic x-ray has an energy of 17.4 keV.

  –When the K-shell vacancy is filled by an electron in the M shell, the characteristic x-ray energy is 19.5 keV.

–**K-shell characteristic x-rays** contribute **less than 10%** of the whole spectrum **at 100 kV.**

–For **voltages <70 kV,** there are **no K-shell characteristic x-rays** in the x-ray spectrum.

E. X-ray intensity and mAs

–The number of x-rays produced by the x-ray beam is related to the **x-ray beam intensity.**

  –Doubling the number of x-ray photons will double the x-ray intensity.

–X-ray beam intensities are measured in terms of **air kerma (mGy)** (see Chapter 2, Section VI).

–X-ray **beam intensity** is proportional to the **x-ray tube current.**

  –Doubling the tube current will double the x-ray beam intensity.

–X-ray **beam intensity** is proportional to the **exposure time,** which is the total time during which a beam current flows across the x-ray tube.

  –Doubling the exposure time will double the x-ray beam intensity.

–The product of the **tube current (mA)** and **exposure time (s)** is known as the **mAs.**

–The **x-ray beam intensity** is always **proportional** to the **mAs.**

TABLE 1.4   Representative X-ray Tube Outputs at 100 cm

Voltage (kV)	Output (mGy/mAs)
80	0.08
100	0.12
120	0.17

–Doubling the current at constant exposure time has the same effect as doubling the exposure time at constant tube current.
–mAs affects x-ray beam intensity, but *does not change the energy spectrum.*
    –Changes in mAs have no effect on the **average x-ray photon energy.**
    –mAs has no affect on the **maximum x-ray photon energy.**
    –**Maximum** x-ray photon **energy** is determined by x-ray tube **voltage.**
F. **X-ray intensity and kV**
    –Increasing the **x-ray tube voltage (kV)** increases the x-ray tube output intensity.
    –For **three-phase generators,** the x-ray beam intensity is approximately proportional to the **square** of the **tube voltage.**
        –**Relative x-ray beam intensity is proportional to $\sim kV^2$.**
    –Table 1.4 shows the typical x-ray tube output in mGy/mAs for a range of kV.
    –Increasing the x-ray tube voltage from **80** to **120 kV** more than **doubles** the x-ray **beam intensity.**
    –Changing the x-ray tube voltage changes the *shape* of the x-ray spectrum.
    –Increasing the **x-ray tube voltage** increases the **maximum x-ray photon energy.**
        –**Average** x-ray photon **energy** also **increases** when raising **kV.**
    –In radiographic imaging, **increasing** the **kV by 15%** has the same effect on the radiation incident on the image receptor as **doubling** the **mAs.**
        –Increasing tube voltage by 10 kV (from **65** to **75 kV**) normally has the same effect on the **film density** as **doubling** the **mAs.**

V. X-RAY TUBES

A. **Tube design**
    –The **x-ray tube** converts the **electric power** from the generator into **x-ray photons.**
    –Figure 1.5 is a diagram of a radiographic x-ray tube.
    –X-ray tubes contain a **negatively charged cathode** containing the **filament** that serves as an electron source.
    –The **anode** is **positively charged** and includes the **target** where x-rays are produced.
        –Anodes may be stationary or rotating.
    –Rotating anodes work in a **vacuum** by use of a **rotor** and **stator.**
    –The anode and cathode are contained in an **evacuated envelope** to prevent the electrons from colliding with gas molecules and losing their kinetic energy.
    –The envelope is contained in a **tube housing** that protects and insulates the tube and provides shielding to prevent **leakage radiation.**
    –The housing contains an **oil bath** to provide electrical **insulation** and help **cool** the tube.
    –**Primary x-rays** exit through a **window** in the tube housing.
    –The x-ray window may be a thinner area in the glass.
        –Windows used in **mammography** are made of **beryllium,** which absorbs fewer low-energy x-rays.
B. **Filament**
    –The **filament** is the source of electrons that are accelerated toward the anode to produce x-rays.
    –The filament is usually made of **coiled tungsten wire,** with modern x-ray tubes having **two filaments** to allow a choice of **two focal spot sizes.**
    –A **focusing cup** surrounds the filament and helps direct the electrons toward the target.
    –**Voltages** across the x-ray tube **filament** are $\sim$**10 V,** and **currents** through the cathode **filament** are $\sim$**4 A.**
        –**Power** dissipated in the filament ($I \times V$) is $\sim$**40 W.**
    –The high resistance in the filament causes temperature to rise ($>2,200^\circ$C), resulting in the **thermionic emission** of **electrons.**

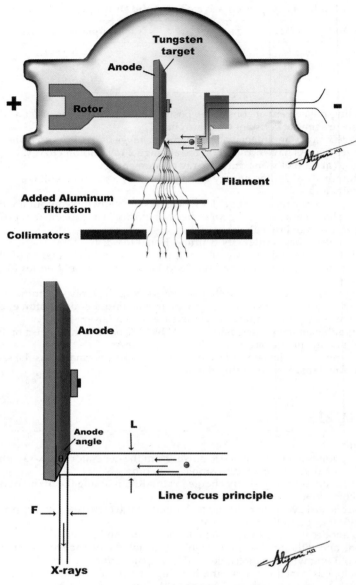

FIGURE 1.5   Major components of an x-ray tube. The inset shows a magnified view of the target and illustrates the line focus principle, whereby the focal spot size (F) is smaller than the electron beam (L) because of the anode angle (θ°).

C. Tube current

-Electrons emitted from a heated filament form a **negative cloud** around the filament called a **space charge,** which *prevents* further emission of electrons.

-The **tube current** is the flow of **electrons** from the **filament** to the **target** embedded in the **anode.**

-Electrons flow *from* the negative filament toward the positive anode.

-At **low voltages,** the potential is insufficient to cause all the electrons to be pulled away from the filament, and a residual space charge remains **(space charge limited).**

-At the **saturation voltage,** all electrons are immediately pulled away from the filament, and the x-ray **tube current** is **maximized.**

-Above **40 kV,** the filament current is proportional to and determines the tube current **(emission limited).**

TABLE 1.5   Nominal Focal Spot Sizes in Mammography and Radiography

Focal Spot Size (mm)	Clinical Application
0.1	Magnification mammography
0.3	Mammography; magnification radiography
0.6	Fluoroscopy; extremity radiography (<25 kW)
1.2	Radiography ($>95\%$ of all radiographs)

-Tube currents are normally increased by increasing the filament heating (i.e., increasing the filament current).
-**Tube currents** range between **1 mA** and **1,200 mA.**
-Tube currents of a **few mA** are used in **fluoroscopy** and a **few hundred mA** in **radiography** and **CT.**

D. **Focal spots**
   -The area of the target struck by the electrons is determined by the **filament size** and **focusing cup.**
   -The **focal spot** is the **size** of the **source** of **x-rays** as viewed by the patient (Fig. 1.5).
   -The **line focus principle** is used to permit larger heat loading while minimizing the size of the focal spot (see inset in Fig. 1.5).
      -Note that in Figure 1.5 inset, the **length** of the **target** that is irradiated (L) is **much larger** than the **focal spot size (F).**
   -The **anode angle** (θ° in Fig. 1.5 inset) is an important factor in determining the **focal spot size.**
      -The anode angle is the angle between the target surface and the central beam.
   -Typical **anode angles** range from **7 degrees** to **20 degrees.**
      -**Radiation field coverage increases** with **increasing target angle.**
   -Focal spots need to be **small** to **produce sharp images.**
      -Focal spots need to be **large** to **tolerate** a **high heat loading.**
   -The choice of the focal spot size is achieved by **balancing** the conflicting need for sharp images, and being able to tolerate high heat loadings.
      -**Large focal spots** are favored when a **short exposure** time is important, and **small focal spots** are needed to obtain the best **spatial resolution.**
   -Focal spot sizes, as quoted by manufacturers of x-ray tubes, range from about **0.1 mm** to $\sim$**1.2 mm.**
      -Focal spot sizes can be measured using **pinhole cameras, star** or **bar test patterns,** or **slit cameras.**
   -**Measured focal spot** sizes may be up to **50% larger** than the nominal values listed in Table 1.5.

E. **Anodes**
   -Electrons striking the target produce **heat** and **x-rays.**
   -The target is embedded in an **anode material,** which temporarily stores the heat energy deposited into the target.
   -A stationary anode usually consists of a tungsten target embedded in a **copper block.**
   -Although **copper** is a **good heat conductor,** heat dissipation is limited.
   -**Stationary anodes** are used in **portable x-ray units.**
   -A **rotating anode** greatly increases the **effective target area** used during an exposure and therefore **raises** the **heat capacity.**
   -To maintain the vacuum required inside the x-ray tube, **rotating anodes** employ an **electric induction motor.**
      -The **rotor** (inside the envelope) turns in response to the changing electric current in the **stator electric windings** (outside the envelope).

VI. X-RAY TUBE PERFORMANCE

A. **X-ray techniques**
   -In **manual** mode, the operator selects the **kV,** x-ray **tube current,** and exposure **time** on the control panel.
      -In **automatic exposure** mode, the operator chooses a kV while the generator circuit controls the tube current and exposure time.

TABLE 1.6   Representative Techniques (kV/mA), Power Loadings, and Energy Deposition in X-ray Imaging

Type of Examination	Techniques	Exposure Time	Power (kW)	Energy (kJ)
Chest x-ray	140 kV/500 mA	5 ms	70	0.35
Abdominal x-ray	80 kV/1,000 mA	50 ms	80	4
Fluoroscopy	80 kV/3 mA	Continuous	0.24	0.24 per second
CT	120 kV/750 mA	0.5 s rotation	90	45 per x-ray tube rotation

–**Tube current** in **radiography** ranges between **100** and **1,000 mA.**
–**Radiographic exposure times** range between **tens** and **hundreds** of **milliseconds.**
–**Fluoroscopy** tube currents range between **1** and **5 mA.**
–For small body parts, such as the **extremities,** x-ray tube voltages are **55** to **65 kV.**
–Most **radiographic** and **fluoroscopy** imaging is performed at x-ray tube voltages between **70** and **90 kV.**
   –Higher voltages may be used to penetrate excessively larger patients.
–**Chest radiography** is often performed at higher x-ray tube voltages of about **120 kV.**
–High voltages (>**100 kV**) are also used in some fluoroscopy performed with **barium contrast** agents to provide sufficient **penetration.**
–Table 1.6 shows typical radiographic techniques used for a range of x-ray imaging modalities.
B. **Energy deposition**
   –Only about **1%** of the **electric energy** supplied to the x-ray tube is converted to **x-rays.**
   –Approximately **99%** of the electrical energy supplied to an x-ray tube is converted to **heat.**
   –**Heat energy** deposited during an x-ray exposure is known as **tube loading.**
   –**X-ray tube loading** depends on the **peak kV,** voltage **waveform, tube current,** and **exposure time.**
      –The total energy deposited in the anode also depends on the number of exposures.
   –For a constant x-ray tube voltage (V) and current (I), the energy deposited during an x-ray exposure is **V × I × t joules,** where t is the exposure time measured in seconds.
   –Table 1.6 shows typical energy deposition rates for common radiologic examinations.
   –This energy is **temporarily stored** in the **anode,** which has a heat capacity of **several hundred thousand joules.**
      –**Anodes** in CT x-ray tubes have a capacity of **several million joules.**
   –When the tube voltage is not constant, calculation of energy deposition is complicated.
   –For systems with **single-phase** power supplies and full-wave rectification, the quantity (kV$_p$) × (mA) × (time) is **given in terms of heat units.**
      –**One heat unit** is ∼**0.7 J.**
   –Single-phase generators are no longer used in Radiology departments and **heat units** are an **anachronism.**
   –Energy deposition in the focal spot, anode, and x-ray tube housing must be considered to ensure none of these components overheat.
C. **Tube rating**
   –The **rating** of an x-ray tube is based on **maximum allowable kilowatts (kW)** at an exposure time of **0.1 second.**
   –For example, a tube with a rating of **100 kW** (100,000 W) tolerates a maximum exposure of **100 kV** and **1,000 mA** for an exposure lasting **0.1 second.**
   –Typical x-ray tube **ratings** are between 5 and 100 kW and depend on focal spot size.
   –In radiography, power loading is ∼**100 kW** for a **large focal spot size.**
      –Power loading is ∼**25 kW** for the **small focal spot.**
   –Increasing the exposure time or using a larger focal spot size may be required to achieve the required x-ray tube output without overheating.
   –In **fluoroscopy, power** loadings are very low, and typically between **100** and **500 W.**
   –Table 1.6 shows power loadings for x-ray imaging modalities encountered in diagnostic radiology.
D. **X-ray tube heat dissipation**
   –**X-ray tubes** are designed to efficiently **dissipate heat.**
   –Modern anodes are circular and rotate at high speeds (**3,000** to **10,000 rpm**) to spread heat loading over a large area.

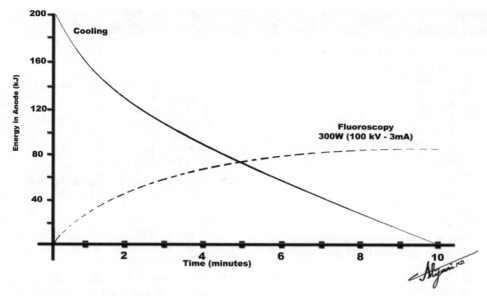

FIGURE 1.6 The *solid curve* shows how heat energy stored in the anode is reduced when starting at the maximum anode capacity (i.e., 200 kJ); the *dashed line* shows the increase of heat energy in the anode when 300 W (300 J/s) is *continuously* being added during fluoroscopy.

–Heat is transferred from the **focal spot by radiation** to the **tube housing** and by **conduction** into the **anode.**
–**Radiation** is the primary way that **anodes transfer heat** to the housing.
  –**Anodes** get **white hot** during the x-ray exposure and lose their acquired energy by emitting light photons.
–X-ray tubes are usually immersed in **oil,** which aids heat dissipation by convection.
–**Air fans** are sometimes used to increase the rate of heat loss.
–Taking a large number of radiographs, or performing long CT scans can saturate the anode heat capacity.
–When the **anode heat capacity** is **reached,** anodes must **cool down** before additional exposures are allowed.
–Figure 1.6 shows the cooling/heating curve.
  –It takes **several** minutes for a **hot x-ray tube anode to cool.**
–In **fluoroscopy, power** deposition in the anode is only a **few hundred watts,** which is dissipated *without reaching the maximum anode capacity* (Fig. 1.6).
  –The **low power loading in fluoroscopy** permits the use of the **small (0.6 mm) focal spot** size.
E. **Radiation from x-ray tubes**
  –X-rays produced in an x-ray tube are emitted **isotropically.**
    –*Isotropic* means that the intensity is equal in *all* directions.
  –The **primary** x-ray beam goes through the x-ray tube window, which is directed toward the patient.
    –The radiation that is incident on the patient is also known as the **useful** x-ray beam.
  –Primary beams produce radiographic and fluoroscopic images.
  –X-ray tubes are surrounded by lead to absorb **unwanted radiation.**
  –**Leakage radiation** is radiation that is transmitted through the x-ray tube housing.
  –**Leakage radiation** should not exceed **1 mGy per hour** at a distance of 1 m from the x-ray tube.
  –Leakage radiation is measured with the x-ray tube operated at the maximum techniques (kV and mA) and the collimators fully *closed.*
  –**Scattered radiation** has been deviated in direction after leaving the tube.
  –**Secondary radiation** is the sum of the **leakage** and **scattered** radiation.
  –Secondary radiation contributes no useful information, but will result in unnecessary exposure to any personnel in the x-ray room (radiologists, technologists, etc.).
  –Operators working within an x-ray room need to wear protective apparel to minimize their exposure to secondary radiation (see Chapter 8, Section III).

REVIEW TEST

1.1 Which of the following is *not* considered a force?
a. Electrostatic
b. Weak
c. Strong
d. Gravity
e. Electricity

1.2 Which of the following is *not* a unit of energy?
a. Erg
b. Joule
c. Watt
d. Calorie
e. eV

1.3 Which of the following would most likely be attracted to an anode?
a. Proton
b. Neutron
c. Electron
d. Positron
e. Alpha particle

1.4 Which quantity is the best measure of power?
a. Joule
b. Tesla
c. Watt
d. Coulomb
e. Newton

1.5 Which of the following is/are likely to have the longest wavelength?
a. Gamma rays
b. Microwaves
c. Radio waves
d. Ultraviolet
e. Visible light

1.6 For electromagnetic radiation, which increases with increasing photon energy?
a. Wavelength
b. Frequency
c. Velocity
d. Charge
e. Mass

1.7 If the distance from a radiation source is halved, the radiation intensity increases by a factor of:
a. 2^{-2}
b. 2^{-1}
c. 2^{0}
d. 2^{+1}
e. 2^{+2}

1.8 X-ray generators have a power level (kW) of approximately:
a. 0.1
b. 1
c. 10
d. 100
e. 1,000

1.9 Which of the following is *not* a type of x-ray generator?
a. Single phase
b. Double phase
c. Six pulse
d. Twelve pulse
e. High frequency

1.10 The purpose of x-ray transformers is most likely to change the:
a. magnetic field
b. electrical voltage
c. power level
d. waveform frequency
e. current intensity

1.11 When a secondary coil has 500 more turns than a primary coil, the ratio of the secondary voltage to the primary voltage is most likely:
a. 500
b. $500^{0.5}$
c. 1/500
d. $1/500^{0.5}$
e. Depends on AC frequency

1.12 Which of the following generators is likely to have the largest waveform ripple?
a. Constant potential
b. High frequency
c. Single phase
d. Six pulse
e. Twelve pulse

1.13 Electrons passing through matter lose energy primarily by producing:
a. bremsstrahlung
b. characteristic x-rays
c. atomic ionizations
d. Compton electrons
e. photoelectrons

1.14 Tungsten is most likely used as an x-ray target because it has a high:
a. physical density
b. electron density
c. electrical resistance
d. melting point
e. ionization potential

1.15 The maximum photon energy in x-ray beams is determined by the x-ray tube:
a. current
b. exposure time
c. target material
d. anode–cathode voltage
e. total filtration

1.16 The most likely characteristic x-ray energy (keV) from x-ray tubes used in chest radiography is:
   a. 19
   b. 33
   c. 65
   d. 75
   e. 140

1.17 At 65 kV and with a tungsten target, the percentage (%) of K-shell x-rays in the x-ray beam is most likely:
   a. 0
   b. 1
   c. 10
   d. 50
   e. 99

1.18 The average photon energy of an x-ray beam is least likely to be affected by changes in the:
   a. tube current
   b. tube voltage
   c. voltage waveform
   d. target composition
   e. beam filtration

1.19 The number of electrons accelerated across an x-ray tube is most strongly influenced by:
   a. anode speed
   b. focus size
   c. filament current
   d. tube filtration
   e. tube voltage

1.20 The most likely x-ray tube filament current (mA) is:
   a. 0.4
   b. 4
   c. 40
   d. 400
   e. 4,000

1.21 Changing x-ray tube current (mA) most likely changes the x-ray:
   a. field of view
   b. maximum energy
   c. average energy
   d. anode angle
   e. beam intensity

1.22 The large focus dimension is most likely larger (%) than that of the small focus by:
   a. 10
   b. 25
   c. 50
   d. 75
   e. 100

1.23 The anode angle (degrees) in an x-ray tube used for chest radiography is most likely:
   a. 15
   b. 30

c. 45
d. 60
e. 75

1.24 X-ray tube output would likely increase the most when increasing the x-ray tube:
   a. voltage
   b. anode angle
   c. target Z
   d. current
   e. exposure time

1.25 A chest x-ray examination on a dedicated chest unit would be least likely to use:
   a. 60-kV voltage
   b. 800-mA tube current
   c. 10-ms exposure time
   d. 1-mm focus
   e. 5-mm Al filtration

1.26 For specification of anode heat capacities, one heat unit corresponds to energy (J) of:
   a. 0.9
   b. 0.8
   c. 0.7
   d. 0.5
   e. 0.3

1.27 At the *same peak voltage,* which generator likely deposits most energy into an anode?
   a. Constant potential
   b. High frequency
   c. Three phase (12 pulse)
   d. Three phase (6 pulse)
   e. Single phase

1.28 Heat stored in x-ray tube anodes is most likely dissipated by:
   a. convection
   b. conduction
   c. radiation
   d. air cooling
   e. oil cooling

1.29 In a standard x-ray tube, the maximum power loading (kW) on the 0.6 mm focal spot is most likely:
   a. 1
   b. 2
   c. 5
   d. 10
   e. 25

1.30 Radiation transmitted through the x-ray tube housing is referred to as:
   a. useful
   b. secondary
   c. stray
   d. leakage
   e. scattered

ANSWERS AND EXPLANATIONS

1.1e. Electricity is the flow of charge, and is measured in amps (C/s).

1.2c. The watt is a unit of power, measured in J/s.

1.3c. Electron, since it has a negative charge that is attracted to the positive anode.

1.4c. Watt is a unit of power, where 1 W = 1 J/s.

1.5c. Radio waves have the lowest frequencies and longest wavelengths.

1.6b. Frequency, which is directly proportional to the photon energy

1.7e. 2^2 (i.e., 4). Halving the distance quadruples the radiation intensity (inverse square law).

1.8d. 100 kW is typical of the power of x-ray generators in radiography and CT.

1.9b. There are no double-phase generators.

1.10b. Transformers change (increase or decrease) voltages.

1.11a. 500. The increase in voltage is directly proportional to the increase in the number of turns.

1.12c. The ripple on a single-phase generator is 100%.

1.13c. Electrons lose most of their kinetic energy by knocking out (or exciting) outer shell electrons.

1.14d. Tungsten can tolerate very high temperatures, which makes it an attractive target material in x-ray tubes.

1.15d. The voltage across the x-ray tube determines the kinetic energy imparted to the electrons that are accelerated from the cathode (filament) to the anode (target), and thereby the maximum x-ray photon energy.

1.16c. The chest x-ray unit will use a W target; the characteristic x-ray energy is therefore ~65 keV.

1.17a. There will be no characteristic x-rays, as the electron kinetic energy (65 keV) is insufficient to eject W K-shell electrons that have a binding energy of 70 keV.

1.18a. The tube current does not affect the average (or maximum) photon energy in x-ray beams.

1.19c. The filament current affects the temperature of the filament and thereby how many electrons the filament "bubbles off".

1.20e. X-ray tube filaments are about 4 A, or 4,000 mA.

1.21e. Tube current controls the x-ray beam intensity, or the total number of x-ray photons produced.

1.22e. The large focal spot is typically 1.2 mm, and the small focal spot is 0.6 mm (i.e., 100% larger).

1.23a. 15 degrees is a typical anode angle.

1.24a. The x-ray tube output is (approximately) proportional to the square of the x-ray tube voltage.

1.25a. Chest x-rays are performed at high voltage (120 kV).

1.26c. The heat unit is 0.7 joule, and is an anachronism in modern radiology.

1.27a. Constant potential, since it has negligible ripple and the voltage across the x-ray tube is always the maximum possible value.

1.28c. Anodes get to be white hot and lose energy by radiation (light) to the tube housing.

1.29e. The small focal spot can tolerate power levels of 25 kW (higher power would require the large focal spot).

1.30d. Leakage radiation escapes through a fully closed collimator (the regulatory limit in the United States is <1 mGy/hr at 1 m).

Chapter 2

X-RAY INTERACTIONS

I. MATTER

A. Atoms
  –**Matter** is made up of **atoms,** which are composed of **protons, neutrons,** and **electrons.**
  –**Protons** have a **positive** charge and are found in the nucleus of atoms.
  –**Neutrons** are electrically **neutral** and are also found in the nucleus.
  –**Electrons** have a **negative** charge and are found outside the nucleus.
  –The **atomic number (Z)** is the number of protons in the nucleus of an atom and is **unique** for **each element.**
  –The **mass number (A)** is the total number of protons and neutrons in the nucleus.
    –**Protons** and **neutrons** are called **nucleons** because they are found in nuclei.
  –In the notation ^{A}X, **X** is the unique letter(s) designating the element and **A** is the **mass number.**
  –Electrically **neutral atoms** have equal numbers of electrons and protons (i.e., Z).
    –^{12}C is an **atom** of **carbon** that has **6 protons, 6 neutrons,** and **6 electrons** for an electrically neutral atom.
  –Mass on the atomic scale is measured in **atomic mass units (amu).**
  –One atomic mass unit is one-twelfth the mass of a carbon atom (^{12}C).
  –Protons and neutrons have a mass of $\sim$1 amu.
  –**Electrons** have a much smaller **mass** that is about **1,800 times less** than **protons** and **neutrons.**
  –Table 2.1 shows the relative mass and charge of atomic constituents.

B. Atomic structure
  –The nucleus of an atom is made up of **protons** and **neutrons** and contains **most** of the **atomic mass.**
  –In the **Bohr model** of an atom, electrons surround the nucleus in **shells** (e.g., K shell, L shell) as shown for tungsten in Figure 2.1.
  –Each shell is assigned a **principal quantum number (n)** beginning with **1** for the **K shell, 2** for the **L shell,** and so on.
    –The number of electrons each shell can contain is $2n^2$.
  –The K shell in tungsten (n = 1) has 2 electrons and the L shell (n = 2) has 8 electrons.
  –The number of electrons in the outer shell **(valence electrons)** determines the atom's **chemical properties.**
  –The **electron density** of a substance is $\rho\,N_0(Z/A)$ **electrons/cm³,** where ρ is the density measured in grams per cubic centimeter (g/cm³) and N_0 is Avogadro's number.
  –For most atoms making up tissues (e.g., oxygen, carbon, nitrogen, calcium), **Z/A** is equal to **0.5.**
  –For most patient tissues, **electron density** is **proportional** to the **physical density** ρ.

C. Electron binding energy
  –**Atomic electrons** are held in place by the **electrostatic pull** of the positively charged **nucleus.**
  –The energy required to completely remove an electron from an atom is called the **electron binding energy.**

TABLE 2.1   Characteristics of Atomic Constituents

Particle	Relative Mass	Electric Charge
Electron	1*	−1
Proton	1,836	+1
Neutron	1,839	0

*Rest mass energy is 511 keV.

–Binding energies are *unique* for **each electron shell** of **each element.**
   –Atomic binding energy values are available in reference books.
–The **binding energy** of **outer shell electrons** is **small.**
   –Outer shell electron binding energies are only a **few electron volts.**
–The **binding energy** of **inner shell electrons** is **large.**
   –For most elements, the binding energy of inner shell electrons is measured in **thousands** of **electron volts (i.e., keV).**
–**K-shell binding energies** increase with **atomic number (Z)** as listed in Table 2.2.
–Energetic particles can knock out inner shell electrons *only if* their energy is greater than the electron binding energy.
   –A **50 keV electron** *cannot* eject a **tungsten K-shell electron (K-shell binding energy is 70 keV)** whereas a **100 keV electron can.**
–A **vacancy** in the K shell will be filled by an **electron** from a **higher shell.**
–Electrons moving from an outer shell to an inner shell may emit excess energy as electromagnetic radiation (i.e., characteristic x-ray).
–The excess energy may be transferred to an **Auger electron,** which then leaves the atom.
   –Auger electron energy is the characteristic x-ray energy minus the binding energy of the outer shell electron.
–A **K-shell vacancy** results in either a **characteristic x-ray** or an **Auger electron** being emitted from the atom.

D. Ionization
   –**Ionization** occurs when an **electron** is **ejected** from a **neutral atom,** leaving behind a **positive ion.**
   –Electromagnetic radiation with sufficient energy to eject atomic electrons is called **ionizing radiation.**
   –**X-rays** are a form of **ionizing radiation.**
      –**Gamma rays** and **ultraviolet** radiation are also ionizing radiations.
   –Ionizing radiation is categorized as either **directly** or **indirectly ionizing.**
   –Radiation is **directly ionizing** when it is in the form of **charged particles.**
      –**Electrons** and **protons** are both **directly ionizing** radiations.

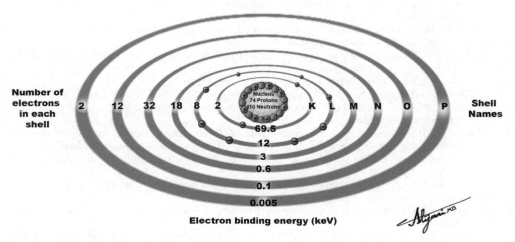

FIGURE 2.1   Shell model of the Tungsten atom, which consists of 74 protons, 74 electrons, and 110 neutrons.

TABLE 2.2   **Atomic Number and K-shell Binding Energy of Selected Elements**

Element	Atomic Number (Z)	K-shell Binding Energy (keV)
Oxygen	8	0.5
Calcium	20	4.0
Molybdenum	42	20
Iodine	53	33
Barium	56	37
Tungsten	74	70
Lead	82	88

–The loss of energy by a charged particle increases with increasing **charge** and decreasing particle **velocity.**
–Energy lost from energetic particles can **eject electrons** from atoms or **raise atomic electrons** to **more distant atomic shells** (excitations).
–**Uncharged particles** are **indirectly ionizing.**
  –**Neutrons** are **indirectly ionizing** radiations that interact with matter by first transferring energy to protons.
–**Indirectly** ionizing radiations include **x-rays,** and **gamma rays.**
  –**X-rays** and **gamma rays transfer energy** to **electrons.**
–When an electron is removed from a (neutral) atom, it leaves behind a **positive ion,** and thus results in **one electron-ion pair.**
–The **average** amount of **energy** needed to generate **one electron-ion pair** in air is ∼30 eV.
–A single **30 keV electron** that is slowed down in matter thus *produces ∼1,000 ionizations.*
–**30-keV electrons** travel a **distance** of ∼30 μm in soft tissue, comparable to the size of a very large cell.
–The **energy transferred** to electrons from x-rays is deposited *locally.*

II. X-RAYS AND MATTER

A. X-ray absorption and scattering
  –Three possible fates of x-rays incident on matter are **penetration, absorption,** and **scattering.**
  –X-ray photons that pass through matter **unaffected** are said to penetrate an object.
    –Very few x-rays **(∼1%) penetrate** through an average-sized patient.
  –When **x-ray** photons **interact** with matter, they **transfer energy** to **electrons.**
  –Interactions of x-rays occur with the individual electrons in atoms.
    –Interactions of x-ray photons with an **oxygen atom** are the **same** when the oxygen is bound to two hydrogen atoms as in a **water molecule.**
  –X-rays may be **absorbed** and transfer their energy to electrons.
  –X-rays may be **scattered,** resulting in a **change** of **direction,** and may lose energy to a scattered electron.
  –These **energetic electrons,** in turn, lose energy by interacting with the electrons in adjacent atoms, thereby **producing additional ionizations.**
  –An **energetic electron** may produce **hundreds** or **thousands** of **additional ion pairs.**
  –Three ways that diagnostic energy x-rays interact with matter are (i) **coherent scatter,** (ii) **photoelectric (PE)** effect, and (iii) **Compton scatter.**
  –**Compton scatter** and the **photoelectric effect** are **important** interactions in diagnostic radiology.
B. Coherent scatter
  –**Coherent scatter** occurs when a low-energy x-ray photon is **scattered** from an **atom** without any energy loss.
  –The **wavelength** of the **scattered** photon is the **same** as the wavelength of the incident photon.
    –**Coherent scatter** is sometimes referred to as **Rayleigh** or **classical scatter.**

          –Coherent scatter does not result in any **energy deposition** in the patient.
             –Coherently scattered photons travel in a **forward direction.**
          –Coherent scatter accounts for **less than 5%** of all photon **interactions** and is of **minor concern** in diagnostic radiology.
             –Scattered photons will **degrade image quality** if they reach the image receptor.

C. Photoelectric effect
          –The **photoelectric (PE) effect** occurs between **tightly bound (inner shell) electrons** and incident x-ray photons.
          –In a PE interaction, the **x-ray photon** is *totally* **absorbed** (photoelectric absorption) by an inner shell electron and that **electron** is **ejected** from the atom.
             –X-ray photons absorbed in **PE interaction** therefore **"disappear".**
          –As a result of the photoelectric interaction, a **photoelectron** is **emitted** and a **positive atomic ion** is left behind.
          –The energy of the emitted **photoelectron** equals the **difference** between the **incident photon energy** and the **electron binding energy.**
             –The photoelectron loses energy by **ionizing** other atoms in the tissue and contributes to patient dose.
          –Outer shell electrons fill the inner shell electron **vacancies,** with the excess energy emitted as a **characteristic x-ray** or **Auger electron.**
             –Auger electron energy is **slightly lower** than the **characteristic x-ray energy.**
          –Figure 2.2A shows a photoelectric interaction.

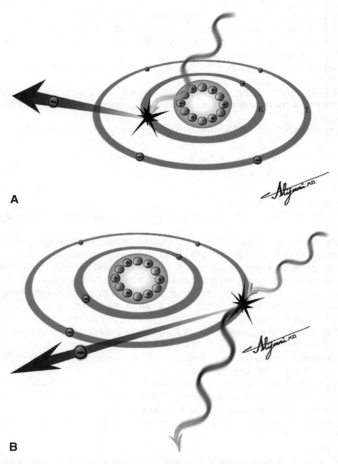

A

B

FIGURE 2.2   A: Photoelectric effect showing the total absorption of the incident x-ray photon and the ejection of a K-shell electron. **B:** Compton scatter showing the incident photon transferring kinetic energy to an outer shell electron and being scattered with a longer wavelength (i.e., lower photon energy).

D. Photoelectric effect probability
- –For the PE effect to occur with a K-shell electron, the incident x-ray must have an energy greater than the **binding energy** of the **K-shell electron.**
- –The absorption of photons **increases markedly** when the x-ray photon energy increases from **below** to **above** the binding energy of the K-shell electrons **(K edge).**
- –The binding energy of the K-shell electrons (K edge) in iodine is 33 keV, and a **sharp increase** in the interaction of photons occurs at this energy.
- –The probability of photoelectric absorption decreases rapidly as the photon energy (E) further increases above the K edge.
  - –Above the K-edge, **photoelectric** interactions are proportional to $1/E^3$.
- –The more tightly bound an electron is, the greater is the probability of the PE effect if E is greater than the electron binding energy.
- –The probability of **photoelectric** absorption increases with atomic number and is proportional to Z^3.
- –The **PE effect** is important when the **atomic number (Z)** is **high** and the **photon energy** is **just above** the **K edge.**
- –Important K-shell binding energies are shown in Table 2.2.

E. Compton scatter
- –In **Compton scatter,** incident photons interact with **outer shell** electrons.
- –A Compton interaction results in a **scattered photon** that has **less energy** than the incident photon and generally travels in a **different direction.**
- –A scattered **(ejected** or **recoil) electron** carries the **energy lost** by the **incident photon** as kinetic energy.
  - –This electron loses this kinetic energy by **excitation** and **ionizing** other atoms in the tissue, thereby contributing to the patient dose.
- –Figure 2.2B shows a Compton interaction.
- –As a result of the Compton interaction, a **positive atomic ion,** which has lost an outer shell electron, remains.
- –**Compton scattering** can be modeled as occurring with **free electrons,** since the binding energy of outer shell electrons is so low.
- –**Compton** interactions account for **most scattered radiation** encountered in diagnostic radiology.
- –The scattered photon may undergo *additional* tissue interactions.
- –**Scattered photons** may also reach the image receptor and **degrade image quality.**

F. Compton interaction probability
- –The **probability** of a **Compton** interaction is proportional to the number of outer shell electrons available in the medium (i.e., **electron density**).
- –**Electron density** of soft tissues is directly **proportional** to the **physical density.**
- –The probability of Compton interactions is inversely proportional to the photon energy (1/E).
- –**Scattered photons** may travel in **any direction,** including **180 degrees** from the direction of the incident photon **(backscattered).**
- –As the **angle** of **deflection decreases,** the **energy** retained by the **scattered x-ray increases** and the energy transferred to the recoil electron decreases.
- –**Energy transfer** to the electron is a **maximum** when the photon is **backscattered.**
- –The incident and Compton scattered x-ray energies at different scatter angles are listed in Table 2.3.
  - –A **backscattered 60 keV photon will transfer 11 keV** (18%) to the Compton electron.
  - –A **backscattered 120 keV photon will transfer 38 keV** (32%) to the Compton electron.

TABLE 2.3   Energies of Compton Scattered Photons

Incident Photon Energy (keV)	Scattered Photon Energy (keV)	
	Scattered 90 Degrees	Scattered 180 Degrees
60	54	49
80	69	61
100	84	72
120	97	82

The energy difference between incident and scattered photons is transferred to the Compton-scattered electron.

–For **soft tissue,** the **PE** and **Compton** effects are **equal** at **25 keV.**
  –In tissue, PE dominates at energies lower than 25 keV and Compton scatter dominates at energies greater than 25 keV.
–For **bone,** the **PE** and **Compton effects** are **equal** at **40 keV.**

III. ATTENUATION OF RADIATION

A. Linear attenuation coefficient
  –The **linear attenuation coefficient** (μ) is the fraction of incident photons removed from the beam in traveling unit distance.
  –Linear **attenuation** coefficients are expressed in **inverse centimeters (cm^{-1}).**
  –The **attenuation coefficient** accounts for *all* x-ray interactions, including **coherent** scatter, the **PE** effect, and **Compton** scatter.
  –The linear attenuation coefficient increases with increasing **physical density.**
  –Linear attenuation coefficients generally **increase** with **increasing atomic number.**
  –In diagnostic radiology, **attenuation decreases** with increasing **photon energy.**
    –An **exception** is at a **K edge,** where an increase in photon energy *markedly increases attenuation.*
  –**Monoenergetic** x-rays are absorbed according to the exponential formula **N = N$_0$e$^{-\mu t}$.**
    –N$_0$ is the initial number of photons incident on an absorber of thickness t (cm), N is the number of photons transmitted, and μ (cm^{-1}) is the attenuation coefficient.
    –Monoenergetic is sometimes referred to as **monochromatic.**
B. Quantitative transmission
  –When the value of μ is small, the numerical value of μ **represents** the **fractional loss** of **photons.**
    –A μ of **0.01 cm^{-1}** means that **1%** of the incident photons are **lost** (i.e., absorbed or scattered) in 1 cm.
    –A μ of 0.01 also means the remaining 99% of x-ray photons are transmitted.
  –When the value of μ is **not small,** the fraction of transmitted photons can be determined from the expression **e$^{-\mu t}$.**
    –If μ is 0.5 cm^{-1}, the fraction transmitted through 1 cm is e$^{-0.5}$, or 0.61 (61%) and the fraction lost is 0.39 (39%).
  –The value of soft tissue μ is 0.38 cm^{-1} at 30 keV, so the fraction of 30 keV photons transmitted through 1 cm of soft tissue is e$^{-0.38}$ or 0.68 (68%).
    –The value of soft tissue μ decreases to 0.21 cm^{-1} at 60 keV, with 81% transmitted through 1 cm.
  –The value of bone μ is 1.6 cm^{-1} at 30 keV so the fraction of 30 keV photons transmitted through 1 cm of bone is e$^{-1.6}$ or 0.20 (20%).
    –The value of bone μ decreases to 0.45 cm^{-1} at 60 keV, with 64% transmitted through 1 cm.
  –**Transmission** of the primary beam through an average patient is $\sim$**10%** for **chest radiographs,** $\sim$**1%** for **skull radiographs,** and $\sim$**0.5%** for **abdominal radiographs.**
C. Mass attenuation (theory)
  –The probability of an **x-ray photon interacting** with matter depends on the **number** of **atoms** encountered.
  –If the **density doubles,** there are **twice** as many atoms and the **linear attenuation coefficient** μ also **doubles.**
  –**Linear attenuation** μ is directly **proportional** to the **physical density.**
  –Attenuation would be the same with only half the thickness but double the density.
  –Compression of lung does *not* change photon transmission since total number of atoms in the path of the x-ray beam remains the same.
  –The **attenuation coefficient** (μ) and **density** (ρ) change as the lungs are expanded or compressed.
  –The **mass attenuation coefficient** is the **linear attenuation coefficient** (μ) **divided** by the **density** (ρ).
  –Since linear attenuation coefficient is proportional to density, dividing linear attenuation coefficient (μ) by density (ρ) provides a density-independent attenuation coefficient.
  –*Mass attenuation coefficient* (μ/ρ) *is independent of physical density.*

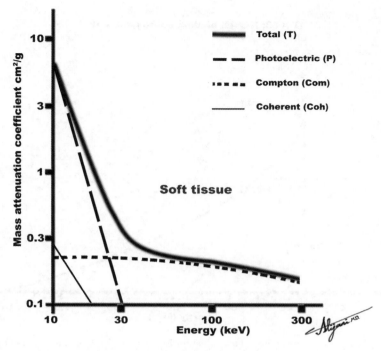

FIGURE 2.3   Tissue mass attenuation coefficient as a function of photon energy, showing contributions of coherent, Compton scatter, and photoelectric effects.

D. Mass attenuation (practice)
- Use of the mass attenuation coefficient allows attenuation to be described as a function of the mass of the material traversed.
- The **thickness** of the absorbing medium must be specified using the **mass thickness** **g/cm²**, or $\rho \times t$.
- X-ray attenuation is determined by the product of the mass thickness and mass attenuation coefficient, that is, $(\rho \times t) \times (\mu/\rho)$.
- This product equals $\mu \times t$, giving the attenuation factor $e^{-\mu t}$ because the densities (ρ) cancel out.
- Figure 2.3 shows the mass attenuation coefficient for soft tissues.
    - At the **lowest energies,** most of the attenuation is due to **PE effect.**
    - At **higher energies,** most attenuation is due to **Compton scatter.**
- Figure 2.4 shows the mass attenuation coefficient for iodine as a function of x-ray energy.
    - **Mass attenuation** coefficient shows a discontinuous increase at **33 keV** because this is the K-shell binding energy of iodine.
- To maximize absorption by iodine, the **average photon energy** needs to be **slightly higher** than 33 keV.

E. Half-Value Layer
- The **half-value layer (HVL)** quantifies the ability of an x-ray beam to **penetrate** tissue.
- The **HVL** is the thickness of material that **attenuates** an **x-ray beam** by **50%.**
- The thickness of material that attenuates an x-ray beam by 90% is called the **tenth-value layer (TVL)** because it transmits only one tenth of the incident intensity.
    - **One TVL equals** ~3 HVL.
- At average diagnostic x-ray beam energies, the **HVL** for **soft tissue** typically ranges from **2.5 to 3.0 cm.**
- At the low energies (28 kV spectra) used in **mammography,** the **HVL** for **soft tissue** is ~1 cm.
- The relation between the linear attenuation coefficient (μ) and HVL is **HVL = 0.693/μ.**
- Table 2.4 shows typical HVLs for monoenergetic x-ray photons.

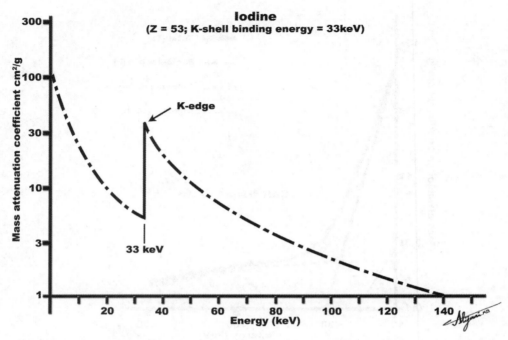

FIGURE 2.4 Variation of the photoelectric effect for iodine (Z = 53) as a function of photon energy, depicting a discontinuity at the K-shell binding energy (33 keV).

–HVL increases with increasing photon energy and decreases with increasing atomic number.
  –At **50 keV,** half the photons will be attenuated by **30 mm** of **tissue, 12 mm** of **bone,** or **0.08 mm** of **lead.**

IV. X-RAY FILTRATION EFFECTS

A. Filters
  –Very low-energy x-rays are stopped as they exit the **x-ray tube** by the **glass window,** which acts as an **inherent x-ray beam filter.**
  –The x-ray beam emerging from the x-ray tube may contain relatively low-energy photons.
  –**Low-energy photons** have a negligible chance of getting through the patient.
    –Low-energy photons irradiate the **patient** but add nothing to the image.
  –Filters are added to the x-ray tube window to **preferentially absorb low-energy photons.**
  –A typical filter for most x-ray tubes is a **few mm** of **aluminum (e.g., ~3 mm).**
    –Chest radiography, performed at higher x-ray tube voltages, may use increased filtration including **copper (Cu)** and **tin (Sn).**
  –Filtration does not affect the **maximum energy** of the x-ray beam spectrum.
  –**Filtration always reduces** the **x-ray tube output.**
  –Figure 2.5 shows the effect of filtration on an x-ray spectrum.

TABLE 2.4   Half-Value Layers for Monoenergetic Photons (mm)

Energy (keV)	Soft Tissue (Z ~7.6)	Bone (Z ~12.3)	Lead (Z = 82)
30	18	4	0.02
50	30	12	0.08
100	39	23	0.11
150	45	28	0.31

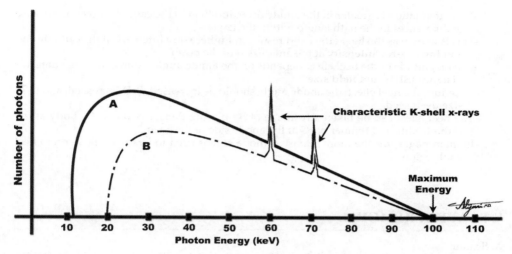

FIGURE 2.5   Representative spectrum emitted from an x-ray tube as filtered by the exit window **(A)** and with added filtration **(B)**.

B. **Beam hardening**
   –**Beam hardening** refers to the effect of a filter on a polychromatic x-ray beam containing a range of x-ray photon energies.
   –Adding **filters changes** the **x-ray spectrum.**
   –The **x-ray beam intensity (i.e., output)** is **decreased** with increased filtration, but the **average x-ray energy** is **increased.**
   –Beam hardening is the **preferential loss** of **lower-energy photons.**
      –Higher-energy photons are more likely to be transmitted through a filter.
   –The **x-ray beam becomes more penetrating** as the mean photon energy increases.
   –**Filtered beams** with higher mean photon energies are called **harder** x-ray beams.
   –Beam hardening does *not* occur with **monochromatic x-ray beams** because there is no differential energy filtration.
   –**Hard beams** are produced at **high voltages** using **heavy filtration.**
      –**Soft beams** are produced at **low voltages** using **less filtration.**
C. **X-ray beam quality**
   –**Quality** refers to the ability of an x-ray beam to **penetrate** the patient.
      –**X-ray beam quality** is directly related to the **average x-ray beam energy.**
   –Increasing beam quality increases the x-ray beam penetrating power because the average photon energy is higher.
   –**Increasing** the **x-ray tube voltage (kV)** is the most direct way to **increase** the **x-ray beam quality.**
   –**Reducing** the **voltage waveform ripple** increases the average photon energy and x-ray beam quality.
   –**Increasing x-ray tube filtration** also increases the beam quality, as low-energy photons are preferentially removed from the x-ray beam (beam hardening).
   –The **quality** of an x-ray beam can be specified as the **thickness** of **aluminum (mm)** that reduces the x-ray **beam intensity** by 50% **(i.e., HVL).**
   –At **80 kV,** the *legal minimum* x-ray beam HVL in many states is ~**2.5 mm** of **aluminum.**
   –A lower HVL means that the beam has too many low-energy photons.
   –A **typical HVL** is **3 mm** of **aluminum** for conventional radiography at 80 kV, including **internal** and **added beam filtration.**
   –After filtration by one HVL, the x-ray beam becomes more penetrating (harder).
   –For polychromatic x-ray beams, the **second HVL** is **always greater** than the **first HVL.**
D. **Heel effect**
   –X-rays produced within the **anode** travel equally in all directions **(isotropic).**
   –X-rays produced within the anode must pass through a portion of the target and are therefore **attenuated** *on their way out* of the **target.**
      –The target is normally **tungsten (Z = 74),** which has attenuation properties similar to those of **lead (Z = 82).**

–This attenuation is **greater** in the **anode direction** than in the cathode direction because of differences in the path length within the target.

–This is known as the **heel effect** and results in **higher x-ray intensity at** the **cathode** end and **lower x-ray intensity** at the **anode** end of the beam.

–The magnitude of the heel effect depends on the **anode angle, source to image detector distance (SID),** and **field size.**

–To **reduce** the **heel** effect, the **anode angle** should be **increased, SID increased,** and **field size decreased.**

–The heel effect can be taken advantage of by placing **denser parts** of the **body** at the **cathode side** and thinner parts at the anode side of the beam.

–In **mammography,** the more intense **cathode side** is used to **irradiate** the denser **chest wall** region.

V. SCATTER REMOVAL

A. Scatter
–**Scattered radiation** is undesirable in diagnostic radiology because it **reduces contrast.**
–Of paramount significance are the scattered photons resulting from **Compton scatter.**
–The **ratio of scatter** to **primary** radiation exiting a patient can be **5:1** or **even greater.**
–**Scatter increases** with increased **field size** (i.e., area of x-ray beam) and increased **patient thickness.**
–**Collimation reduces** the total patient mass irradiated and, therefore, reduces **scatter.**
–At **low voltage (kV),** there is **more absorption** due to the photoelectric effect and **less** Compton scatter.
–Lowering the x-ray tube voltage reduces patient penetration and also increases dose.
  –**Varying** the **kV** is **not** a *practical* method for reducing scatter.
–As voltage increases, the proportion of scatter interactions increases.
–Scatter is of **less concern** in **extremity radiography** because the patient thickness is small.
  –In **extremity** radiography, most interactions with **bone** are **photoelectric.**
B. Air gaps
–**Air gaps** between the patient and cassette **reduce scatter.**
–Scattered photons are less likely to reach the image receptor when there is an air gap.
  –**Primary photons** will reach the image receptor but result in **additional magnification.**
  –**Moving image receptors away** from **patients** to introduce an air gap is **not practical** for most radiographic examinations.
    –**Image receptors** in contact chest radiography are typically **43 cm × 43 cm** and would be too small to capture the patient anatomy with magnification.
    –**Larger x-ray tube output** is required when increasing the **focus** to the **image receptor distance (FID).**
–A major **drawback** of **magnification imaging** is the additional **focal spot blurring.**
–Magnification imaging is sometimes used in mammography and neuroradiology.
  –When **magnification** is used, an **air gap** is **introduced.**
–With **air gaps,** scatter is generally low, and **no additional scatter removal steps** are **required.**
C. Grids
–**Antiscatter grids** are made up of many **narrow parallel bars** of **lead** or other highly attenuating material.
–**Antiscatter grids** are used to **removing scatter** in diagnostic radiology.
–**X-rays pass between** the **strips,** which are filled with low-attenuation material such as aluminum or graphite.
–**Grids** are placed between the **patient** and the **image receptor.**
–Figure 2.6 shows how grids reduce the amount of scatter radiation reaching the screen–film combination.
–The **grid ratio** is the ratio of the **strip height (h)** along the x-ray beam direction to the **gap (D)** between the lead strips, so the **grid ratio** is **h/D.**
–**Grid ratios** typically range from **4 to 16.**
  –The typical radiographic **grid ratio** used clinically is **~10.**

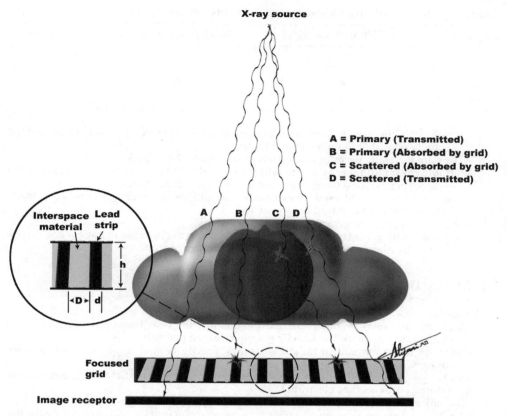

FIGURE 2.6   Grids reduce the amount of scattered radiation that reaches the film. The lead strips of a focused grid are designed to be parallel to the incoming beam.

- –The **strip line density** is **1/(D + d) lines per unit length,** where d is the strip thickness.
  - –Strip line densities range from **25** to **60 lines per centimeter.**
- –**Focused grids** have diverging strips and must be used at specified focal distances.
- –Most grids are **reciprocating grids,** where the **grid moves** during the exposure, spreading the image of the grid lines over the film and rendering them invisible.
- –The device that moves the grid is called a **Bucky,** named after its inventor.

D. **Grid performance**
- –**Primary transmission** is the percentage of incident primary radiation (i.e., not scattered) that passes through the grid.
- –The **Bucky factor** is the ratio of radiation incident on the grid to the transmitted radiation.
- –The **Bucky factor** is the **increase** in **patient dose** due to the use of a grid.
  - –Typical values for the **Bucky factor** range between **2** and **6.**
- –The **contrast improvement factor** is the ratio of contrast with a grid to contrast without a grid.
  - –**Contrast improvement factors** are ∼**2.**
- –**Artifacts** such as **grid cutoff** may be caused by **improper alignment,** the wrong **focal spot** to **film distance** for focused grids, and **inverted grids.**
- –**Increasing** the **grid ratio** *increases* **image contrast.**
  - –Grid ratios may be increased either by increasing the height of the lead strips or reducing the space between the lead strips.
- –**Increasing** the **grid ratio** increases **x-ray tube loading** and **patient exposure.**
- –Table 2.5 lists the characteristics of a range of common grids.
  - –Actual values will depend on the x-ray spectrum used and patient characteristics.

E. **Clinical applications**
- –A **12:1 (30 lines/cm)** ratio is common in a reciprocating grid.
- –**Stationary grids** with low ratios (∼6:1) are used with mobile x-ray units because a low grid ratio tolerates beam misalignments.

TABLE 2.5   Representative Characteristics of Scatter Removal Grids

Grid Ratio	Scatter Transmission (%)	Primary Transmission (%)	Bucky Factor
5:1	18	75	2
6:1	14	72	3
8:1	10	70	4
12:1	5	68	5

–A high strip line density (~45 lines per cm) is used for stationary grids to reduce the visibility of grid lines on resultant radiographs.

–**Grids** are generally used for body parts **greater than 12 cm thick.**

–**Portable chest radiography** is generally performed at lower x-ray tube voltages to minimize scatter, because using grids at the bedside is very difficult.

–**Grids** are generally **not used** for **extremity radiographs** in which scatter is negligible.

–Grid ratios up to **8:1** are **used below** ~**90 kV.**

–Higher ratio grids are generally used above ~90 kV.

–**Very high ratio grids (16:1)** are **seldom used** because the increase in patient dose is not justified by a corresponding improvement in image contrast.

VI. MEASURING RADIATION

A. Air kerma

–**Air kerma** is a *source-related* term used to quantify the **x-ray beam intensity.**

   –**Air kerma** stands for the <u>K</u>inetic <u>e</u>nergy <u>r</u>eleased per unit <u>m</u>ass.

–**Intensity** is the amount of radiation, and is directly related to the **number** of **x-ray photons.**

–Air kerma is the **kinetic energy transferred** from **uncharged particles (e.g., photons)** to **charged particles (i.e., electrons).**

–The unit of air kerma is **joules per kilogram (J/kg),** where **1 J/kg** is **1 gray (Gy).**

–Air kerma from an x-ray source obeys the **inverse square law** and decreases with the square of the distance from a source.

–**Entrance air kerma** is a measure of the amount of x-ray radiation that is **incident** on the patient undergoing an x-ray examination.

–**Air kerma** has recently **replaced exposure** as the quantity that measures the amount of radiation in any x-ray beam.

B. Exposure

–**Exposure** is the total charge of **electrons liberated** per **unit mass** of **air** by the x-ray photons.

–**Exposure** is measured in **coulombs per kilogram (C/kg)** in the SI system or in **roentgens (R)** in non-SI units.

   –**1 R = 2.58 × 10⁻⁴ C/kg**

–An exposure of 1 R corresponds to an air kerma of 8.7 mGy (i.e., 1 R = 8.7 mGy air kerma). (In this book, 10 mGy air kerma is taken as an exposure of ~1 R, and an exposure of 1 R is taken as an air kerma of ~10 mGy.)

   –**1 R = ~10 mGy air kerma,** and **10 mGy air kerma = ~1 R.**

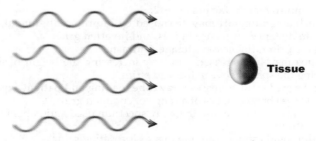

FIGURE 2.7   An x-ray beam with an air kerma K incident on a small tissue volume (i.e., no backscatter) results in an absorbed dose to the tissue of K R (R values are listed in Table 2.6).

TABLE 2.6   Values of R That Convert Air Kerma (mGy) to Absorbed Dose (mGy) in a Specified Tissue (i.e., Dose = R × Air Kerma) when Irradiated as Shown in Figure 2.7 (No Backscatter)

Photon Energy (keV)	Fat (Z ~6.5)	Soft Tissue (Z ~7.6)	Bone (Z ~12.3)
30	0.60	1.1	5.1
50	0.75	1.1	4.2
100	1.1	1.1	1.7
150	1.1	1.1	1.2

C. Absorbed dose

- –**Absorbed dose (D)** measures the amount of radiation **energy (E) absorbed per unit mass (M)** of a **medium: D = E/M.**
- –Absorbed dose is specified in gray (Gy) in the SI system.
- –**One gray** is equal to **1 J** of energy deposited **per kilogram.**
- –The rad was the unit of absorbed dose in non-SI units (rad stands for radiation absorbed dose).
  - –**1 Gy = 100 rad; 1 rad = 10 mGy**
- –For the same air kerma (intensity), the **absorbed dose** depends on the **material** or tissue that is placed into the x-ray beam.
- –The **absorbing medium** (e.g., air, soft tissue, bone) always needs to be **specified** for dose assessment.
- –The **location** of the **absorbing medium** (e.g., entrance skin, thyroid, spleen) also needs to be **specified.**
  - –For example, the risk to a pregnant patient will require an estimate of the absorbed dose to the conceptus.
- –**Absorbed dose** is the preferred dose quantity in **radiobiology.**

D. Air kerma and absorbed dose

- –Figure 2.7 shows an x-ray beam incident with an intensity (air kerma) of K Gy that is incident on an absorbing medium (e.g., soft tissue).
- –The amount of **radiation absorbed** by a **medium** depends on the physical characteristics of the absorber (**density, atomic number,** etc.), as well as the average **x-ray beam energy.**
- –For the **irradiation geometry** shown in Figure 2.7 (i.e., **no backscatter**), the relation between absorbed dose (D) and air kerma (K) is **D = R × K.**
  - –**R** depends on the characteristics of the medium irradiated, primarily the **atomic number (Z)** of the absorbing medium.
- –R can be calculated by dividing the medium attenuation coefficient by the air attenuation coefficient.
  - –The value of **R** depends on the **photon energy** of the x-rays.
- –Table 2.6 lists the values of R for a range of photon energies and absorbing media.
- –An **air kerma** of **1 mGy** results in an absorbed dose of ~**1.1 mGy** in **soft tissue.**
- –An **air kerma** of **1 mGy** (50 keV photons) results in a **bone dose** of **4.2 mGy.**
  - –Increasing the x-ray beam energy to 100 keV reduces the bone dose to 1.7 mGy.
- –An **air kerma** of **1 mGy** (50 keV photons) results in a **fat dose** of **0.75 mGy.**
  - –Increasing the x-ray beam energy to 100 keV increases the fat dose to 1.1 mGy.
- –In computing **skin doses** in radiology, it is also necessary to account for **backscatter** (see Chapter 7, Section V).

2.1 Which of the following refers to the number of nucleons in a nucleus?
a. Mass number
b. Atomic number
c. Avogadro's number
d. Atomic mass unit
e. Nuclear density

2.2 Which element has an atomic number of 56 and a K-shell binding energy of 37 keV?
a. Calcium
b. Selenium
c. Molybdenum
d. Barium
e. Tungsten

2.3 The outer shell electrons most likely have binding energies (keV) of approximately:
a. 0.001
b. 0.005
c. 0.025
d. 0.1
e. 0.5

2.4 Ionizing radiations are least likely to include:
a. x-ray photons
b. energetic electrons
c. infrared radiation
d. alpha particles
e. fast neutrons

2.5 The total number of atomic ionizations produced following absorption of a 30 keV photon is most likely:
a. 10
b. 100
c. 1,000
d. 10,000
e. 100,000

2.6 The most likely percentage (%) of coherent scatter photons in an x-ray beam emerging from a patient having a chest x-ray is:
a. <5
b. 5
c. 10
d. 20
e. >20

2.7 The energy (E) dependence of photoelectric absorption above the K edge varies as:
a. $1/E^3$
b. $1/E^2$
c. $1/E$
d. E^2
e. E^3

2.8 After an x-ray undergoes photoelectric absorption by a K-shell electron, which emission is *least* likely?
a. Photoelectron
b. Scattered photon
c. K-shell x-ray
d. L-shell x-ray
e. Auger electron

2.9 The likelihood of Compton interactions is best quantified using:
a. physical density
b. electron density
c. atomic number
d. K-shell energy
e. outer shell energy

2.10 For a given absorber, if the Compton attenuation coefficient at 50 keV is 0.1 cm^{-1}, its value at 100 keV (cm^{-1}) is most likely:
a. 0.01
b. 0.025
c. 0.05
d. 0.1
e. 0.2

2.11 In bone, at what photon energy are photoelectric and Compton effects approximately equal?
a. 4.0
b. 25
c. 40
d. 70
e. 88

2.12 If the linear attenuation coefficient is 0.1 cm^{-1}, how many x-ray photons (%) are lost in 1 mm?
a. 0.1
b. 1
c. 10
d. e^{-1}
e. $e^{-0.01}$

2.13 If the attenuation of bone is 0.5 cm^{-1}, the fraction of x-ray photons transmitted through 1 cm is most likely:
a. 0.05
b. 0.5
c. $e^{-0.5}$
d. $e^{+0.5}$
e. $(1 - e^{-0.5})$

2.14 The mass attenuation coefficient is least likely to depend on absorber:
a. composition
b. K-shell energy
c. physical density
d. electron density
e. atomic number

2.15 An x-ray beam, attenuated by three half-value layers, is reduced by a factor of:
a. 3
b. 4
c. 6
d. 8
e. 9

2.16 Increasing the filtration of an x-ray beam most likely reduces the:
a. exposure time
b. average energy
c. maximum energy
d. half-value layer
e. beam intensity

2.17 The x-ray tube output most likely increases when reducing the:
a. mA
b. exposure time
c. kV
d. filtration
e. focal spot

2.18 Adding Aluminum filters to an x-ray beam is most likely to increase x-ray:
a. intensity (air kerma)
b. air kerma–area product
c. maximum energy
d. beam hardening
e. leakage radiation

2.19 The adequacy of the filtration of an x-ray tube is best determined by measuring the:
a. tube voltage
b. air kerma
c. field size
d. half-value layer
e. leakage radiation

2.20 The heel effect most likely increases when reducing the:
a. tube voltage
b. tube current
c. anode angle
d. filtration
e. field size

2.21 In abdominal imaging, the scatter to primary ratio of photons leaving the patient is most likely:
a. 0.2
b. 0.5
c. 1
d. 2
e. 5

2.22 The number of scattered photons reaching a radiographic imaging receptor most likely decreases with increasing:
a. field size

b. patient thickness
c. tube voltage
d. beam filtration
e. grid ratio

2.23 The most likely Bucky factor in adult abdominal radiography is:
a. 0.5
b. 1
c. 2
d. 5
e. 10

2.24 Improvement of lesion contrast (%) by the use of a grid in abdominal radiography would most likely be:
a. 10
b. 25
c. 50
d. 100
e. 200

2.25 Which examination would most likely be performed without a scatter removal grid?
a. Extremity
b. Skull
c. Abdomen
d. Mammogram
e. Fluoroscopy

2.26 Air kerma is the kinetic energy released per unit:
a. distance (m)
b. area (m^2)
c. volume (m^3)
d. mass (kg)
e. density (kg/m^3)

2.27 Measuring the charge liberated in a mass of air quantifies:
a. dose
b. exposure
c. equivalent dose
d. HVL
e. LET

2.28 An exposure of 1 R most likely corresponds to an air kerma (Gy) of
a. 0.001
b. 0.01
c. 0.1
d. 1
e. 10

2.29 An air kerma of 1 mGy will most likely to result in an absorbed dose (mGy) to soft tissue (no backscatter) of:
a. 0.5
b. 1.0
c. 1.1
d. 2.0
e. 4.0

2.30 An air kerma of 1 mGy is likely to result in an absorbed dose (mGy) to bone
(no backscatter) of:
a. 1
b. 2

c. 4
d. 8
e. 16

ANSWERS AND EXPLANATIONS

2.1a. The mass number is the total
number of protons and neutrons
(i.e., nucleons) in the atom's nucleus.

2.2d. Barium has 56 protons and a K-shell
binding energy that is slightly
higher than that of Iodine (33 keV).

2.3b. The outer shell binding energy is
∼5 eV (i.e., 0.005 keV).

2.4c. Infrared radiation is nonionizing, as
the photon energy is less than 1 eV.

2.5c. 1,000 ionization events are likely
since it takes 30 eV or so to produce
one ionization and there is 30,000
eV available.

2.6a. Coherent scatter never accounts for
more than 5% of all interactions in
diagnostic radiology.

2.7a. Above the K edge, the photoelectric
effect is proportional to $1/E^3$.

2.8b. There are no scattered photons in
photoelectric absorption; scatter
occurs with Compton interactions.

2.9b. The likelihood of Compton
interactions is approximately
proportional to the electron density.

2.10c. 0.05 cm^{-1}, since Compton
interactions vary as $1/E$, so
doubling the photon energy will
halve the probability of this
interaction.

2.11c. Compton and photoelectric
interactions are equally probable at
40 keV in bone.

2.12b. 10% are lost in 1 cm, so 1% must be
lost in each mm.

2.13c. $e^{-0.5}$ is the fractional transmission of
photons through 1 cm, when the
attenuation of bone is 0.5 cm^{-1}

2.14c. The linear attenuation coefficient is
directly proportional to density; the
mass attenuation coefficient is the
linear attenuation coefficient
divided by the density, which is
therefore independent of density.

2.15d. Each HVL reduces the beam by ½,
so three HVL attenuate the beam by
a factor of 8.

2.16e. Increasing filtration reduces the
x-ray tube intensity; 3 mm or so
would likely halve the x-ray tube
output.

2.17d. A reduction in filtration means that
more x-rays can get out.

2.18d. Increasing (Al) filtration always
increases beam hardening in
radiology.

2.19d. The HVL is a good measure of the
adequacy of filtration and at 80 kV
should be greater than ∼2.5 mm Al.

2.20c. Reducing the anode angle will
increase the heel effect.

2.21e. There are about five scattered
photons exiting the patient for
every one primary photon.

2.22e. A higher grid ratio will reduce the
amount of scatter.

2.23d. Use of a grid will likely increase
patient doses fivefold (i.e., Bucky
factor).

2.24e. Use of grids improves contrast by a
large factor (e.g., 200% or more).

2.25a. In extremity radiography, use of
low kVs means that most
interactions (in bone) will be
photoelectric absorption and not
Compton scatter.

2.26d. Mass (energy transferred to
electrons per unit mass and
measured in Gy).

2.27b. Exposure is the charge liberated per
unit mass, and in the SI system is
measured in C per kg.

2.28b. 1 R equals ∼10 mGy (i.e., 0.01 Gy).

2.29c. An air kerma of 1 mGy will result in
an absorbed dose to tissue of ∼1.1
mGy when there is no
backscatter.

2.30c. An air kerma of 1 mGy will result in
an absorbed dose to bone of ∼4
mGy when there is no
backscatter.

Chapter 3

PROJECTION RADIOGRAPHY I

I. FILM

A. Emulsions
-**Analog radiography** uses **film** to **capture, display,** and **store** radiographic images.
-Film consists of an **~10-μm-thick emulsion** supported by a **150-** to **200-μm**-thick polyester (**Mylar) base.**
-Most radiographic films have an **emulsion layer** on **both sides** of the base.
  -**Laser** and **mammography** films are exceptions and have a **single emulsion.**
-Additional layers on radiographic film can include a **protective coating, antistatic,** or **anti-crossover layer.**
-The emulsion contains **silver halide** (iodobromide) grains, which can be sensitized by radiation or light to hold a **latent image.**
-**Silver halide grains** are typically about **1 μm** in diameter and contain between 10^6 and 10^7 silver atoms.
  -There are about **10^9 grains** per **cubic centimeter.**
-Several **light photons** must be absorbed to **sensitize** each **grain.**
  -A grain may also be sensitized by absorbing a *single x-ray* photon.
-**Absorbed light** photons liberate electrons in the grain, which combine with positively charged silver ions (Ag^+) to produce electrically neutral atoms of **silver.**
-Grains that have been sensitized by absorption of light or x-rays form the **latent image.** Silver halide grains can also be sensitized by thermal and chemical processes without photons (i.e., **fogging**).
-Sensitized grains are relatively stable, but can **fade** over time.
  -**Fading** and **fogging** can be aggravated by **environmental heat** and **humidity.**

B. Film development
-After **exposure,** grains have a **few neutral silver atoms** in the speck along with millions of Ag^+ ions.
-The film development process converts the **invisible latent image** to a **permanent visible** image.
-**Sensitized grains** are **reduced** in the alkaline developer solution by the addition of electrons, which converts the **positive silver ions** to **silver atoms.**
-A **developed grain** results in a **speck** of **silver** that appears black on the film.
  -**Unexposed grains** with no latent image are developed at a **much slower rate.**
-**Film speed, contrast,** and **fog** levels are all affected by **developer chemistry** and **temperature.**
-Increasing the **developer temperature** can **increase film contrast** and **density.**
  -Increasing **development time** has a similar effect to using higher developer temperature.
-Raising the **developer temperature** also increases the level of **fogging** on the processed film.

C. Film processors
-Modern film processors **automatically** run film sequentially through the **developer, fixer,** and **washing** solutions using a series of rollers to transport the film.
-**Developer temperatures** typically range from **31°C** to **35°C.**

-The developer is consumed during the reduction of the sensitized silver halide grains.
-The processor must supply fresh developer as more films are run (**replenishment**).
  -The rate of replenishment depends on the workload of the processor.
-The **fixing solution** contains **acetic acid** to inhibit further development and **remove unexposed silver halide grains.**
-**Fixing** makes the image **stable.**
  -Inadequate fixation can result in a milky appearance to the film.
-After fixing, the film is **washed** again to eliminate all chemicals and is then **dried** by heaters or infrared lamps.
  -Incomplete removal of the fixer causes the film to turn brown.
-The total **processing time** is typically **90 seconds** (e.g., 25 seconds developer time, 21 seconds fixer time, 44 seconds washing and drying time).
-Dirty, uneven, or maladjusted rollers can leave lines or other **artifacts** (e.g., π lines) on the film.
  -Static electricity also causes severe film artifacts.
-Film processor **quality control (QC)** is essential in maintaining film image quality at a high level.
-Processor QC involves measuring **developer temperature** and monitoring the **density** and **contrast** of film exposed to a light source in a sensitometer.

D. Film density
  -After processing, the **blackening** of the **film** represents the **pattern** of **x-rays** reaching the cassette.
  -Film blackening is related to the number of x-ray or light photons that exposed the film.
  -Film blackening is measured using **optical density (OD).**
  -**OD = $\log_{10}(I_0/I_t)$,** where I_0 is the light intensity incident on the film, and I_t is the light transmitted through the film.
  -**OD** can be measured using a **densitometer.**
  -Transmittance is the fraction of incident light passing through the film, where the **transmittance $= I_t/I_0$.**
  -As **OD increases, transmittance decreases.**
  -The **useful** range of **film ODs** is from $\sim$0.3 **(50% transmittance)** to $\sim$2 **(1% transmittance).**
  -Densities greater than about 2 require the use of a **hot (bright) light.**
  -The **OD** of **superimposed films** is **additive,** so two films with an OD of 1.0 (10% transmittance) superimposed would have an OD of 2.0 and transmit 1% of the incident light.
  -Table 3.1 shows the relationship between optical density and transmittance.

E. Characteristic curves
  -The **characteristic curve** represents the relation between radiation intensity (**air kerma**) and resultant film **optical density** as shown in Figure 3.1.
    -Characteristic curves are also known as **H** and **D curves,** named after Hurter and Driffield who first generated such a curve (1890).
  -The **toe** is the low-exposure region, and the **shoulder** is the high-exposure region of the curve.
  -**Fog** is the level of blackening due to a few grains being developed in the *absence* of any radiation exposure.
  -**Base** refers to the density of the film base alone, which will absorb a small faction of any incident light.
  -Base plus fog levels are $\sim$0.2 OD units.
  -An unexposed film that is processed will thus have a film density of $\sim$0.2.

TABLE 3.1   Relationship between Light Transmittance and Film Optical Density

Transmittance (T, %)	Optical Density (OD)	Comments
50	0.3	Base plus fog has a density of $\sim$0.2
10	1.0	Light film density
3	1.5	Average film density
1	2.0	Dark film density[a]
0.1	3.0	Typical *maximum* film density

[a] Darker films require a hot light.

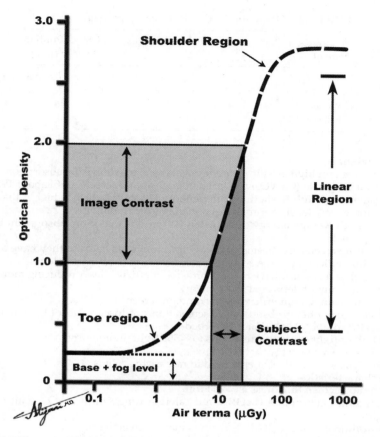

FIGURE 3.1   Characteristic curve showing relation between radiation intensity (air kerma) and optical density for a radiographic film.

  –The **maximum OD** for exposed film is ~3.0 OD units.
  –**Fast films** require **less radiation** to achieve a given film density.
    –**Slow films** require **more radiation.**

II. INTENSIFYING SCREENS

A. Screen rationale
  –A **film alone** (i.e., no screen) **absorbs** only ~1% of the incident x-rays, with the remaining 99% being wasted.
  –**Intensifying screens** contain phosphor crystals that absorb about 50 times more of the incident x-rays than a radiographic film.
  –For each **x-ray absorbed** in a screen, **hundreds** of **visible light photons** are produced that expose the film.
  –The screen therefore converts the **x-ray pattern** to a **light pattern,** which is subsequently recorded on radiographic film.
  –Intensifying screens improve the **efficiency** of radiographic imaging over film alone.
  –The use of **intensifying screens decreases** the **exposure time** required for a given film density.
  –**Shorter exposures** result in a lower patient dose.
    –Shorter exposure times **decrease x-ray tube loading.**
    –Shorter exposures also **decrease blur** caused by patient motion.

TABLE 3.2   Elements Used in Rare Earth Screens

Element	Atomic Number (Z)	K-Shell Binding Energy (keV)
Yttrium (Y)	39	17
Barium (Ba)	56	37
Lanthanum (La)	57	39
Gadolinium (Gd)	64	50

B. Screen materials
–**Screens** contain **high atomic number** materials to maximize the absorption of x-rays.
–**Calcium tungstate ($CaWO_4$)** was used in intensifying screens until about 1970.
–Tungsten has a **high K-shell binding energy (70 keV),** which is higher than the mean photon energy levels normally used in diagnostic radiology.
  –The **high K-edge energy** of **tungsten (W)** means that **x-ray absorption** is **less than optimal.**
–**Rare earth screens** are "faster" than calcium tungstate because they have a higher **absorption efficiency** at the x-ray energies normally used in radiology.
–Rare earth screens also have higher **conversion efficiencies,** producing more light for a given amount of deposited x-ray energy.
–The typical **conversion efficiency** of common screens is ∼**10%.**
–A 10-keV x-ray photon absorbed in a screen thus produces a total of 1 keV of light energy (i.e., 10% of the 10 keV that is absorbed).
  –**1 keV** of **light** energy corresponds to ∼**500 light** photons given that one light photon has ∼2 eV of energy.
–Table 3.2 lists common elements used in **rare earth** screens.
C. Screen characteristics
–A common **screen thickness** is ∼**200 μm.**
–**Lanthanum oxybromide (LaOBr)** and **calcium tungstate ($CaWO_4$)** emit mainly blue light.
–**Gadolinium oxysulfide (Gd_2O_2S)** emits mainly green light.
–The light color from a screen and the light sensitivity of the film must be matched.
–**Matching** the **light** emitted by the **screen** with **film sensitivity** is known as **spectral matching.**
–**Conventional film** is sensitive to **ultraviolet** and **blue** light.
–**Orthochromatic film** is also sensitive to **green** light.
–Screen **absorption efficiency** refers to the percentage of x-ray photons absorbed in the screen.
  –A typical **screen–film** combination used to perform chest radiography absorbs ∼50% of the incident x-ray photons (i.e., **absorption efficiency** is **50%).**
–The **intensification factor** is the ratio of exposures, without and with intensifying screens, required to obtain a given film density.
–Intensification factor depends on the absorption and conversion efficiency of the screen.
–Typical **intensification factors** are 30 to 50.
D. Cassettes
–The film and screens are held in a **light-tight cassette.**
–Figure 3.2 shows a cassette with two screens and a double-emulsion film.
–**Screens** are usually permanently mounted inside the cassette.
–A thin layer of foam backing holds the screen tightly against the film when the cassette is closed.
–The **front** of the **cassette** is made of a minimally attenuating material such as **aluminum** or **carbon** fiber.
–**Dual-screen, dual-emulsion** systems are frequently used to improve x-ray absorption.
–Intensifying screens can be significant sources of **image artifact.**
–**Scratches, stains, hair, dust, cigarette ash,** and **talcum powder** are all potential sources of image **artifacts.**
–As part of a **quality control** (QC) program, all screens should be regularly cleaned.
–Cassettes should also be evaluated for good **screen–film contact.**
–Screen–film contact is evaluated by taking an image of a **wire mesh** and ensuring that the resultant image permits visualization of the mesh.

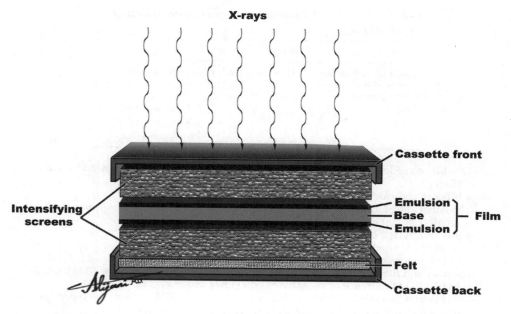

X-rays

Cassette front

Intensifying screens

Emulsion
Base   } **Film**
Emulsion

Felt

Cassette back

FIGURE 3.2   Cross section of a typical screen–film cassette containing double emulsion film and two screens.

–To ensure the correct film density, **automatic exposure control (AEC)** systems are generally used.
  –AEC is also known as **phototiming.**
–An AEC **measures** the actual **amount** of **radiation incident** on the screen–film and **terminates** the **exposure** when the correct amount has been received.
E. **Screen–film speed**
  –An **air kerma** of ~10 μGy produces a satisfactory film density in a **100 speed** screen–film combination.
    –**Both screen** and **film** must be **specified** when assigning speed to any screen–film combination.
  –The **speed** of a screen–film combination is **inversely** related to the **air kerma** required to produce a given density.
    –As the **speed increases,** the **air kerma** required **decreases.**
  –A 200 speed screen–film combination requires an air kerma of 5 μGy, and a 50 speed screen–film combination requires an air kerma of 20 μGy.
  –**Speeds** of screen–film combinations used in radiology **range from 50** to **800.**
  –Screen speed increases with increasing **screen thickness, absorption efficiency,** as well as **conversion efficiency.**
  –**Fast screens** are generally thicker.
    –Whereas slow (detail) screens are thinner.
  –**Fast screen–films** are used for **abdominal** studies whereas **slow screen–films** are used for **extremity** examinations.
  –**Single-emulsion, single-screen** systems are used for **bone detail** and **mammography.**
  –Table 3.3 lists a range of screen types used in radiology.

III. DIGITAL BASICS

A. **Computer basics**
  –Computers use the **binary system** (base two).
  –A **bit** (**bin**ary dig**it**) is the fundamental information element used by computers and can be assigned one of two discrete values.

TABLE 3.3   Screen Characteristics and Common Clinical Applications

	Image Receptor	
Screen Classification	Air Kerma (μGy)	Clinical Uses
Mammography	200	Mammography
Detail	20	Extremity radiography
Medium	5	Chest imaging
Fast	2	Abdominal imaging

–One bit can code for two values, or two shades of gray, which correspond to white and black.
–*n* **bits** can code for **2^n values,** or **gray levels.**
–The American Standard Code for Information Exchange (ASCII) uses 8-bit groups (designated a byte) to represent common letters and symbols.
–**8 bits = 1 byte; 2 bytes = 1 word (16 bits).**
–A total of **256 shades** of **gray** (2^8) can be coded for by **1 byte** (8 bits).
 –4,096 shades of gray (2^{12}) can be coded for by 12 bits.
–Memory and file storage requirements for computers are normally specified using **kilobyte** (kB) (1,024 bytes) or **megabyte** (MB) (1,024 kB).
–One kilobyte is 1,000 bytes in the decimal system and 1,024 bytes in the binary system and which are taken to be equivalent for most practical purposes.
–Large storage requirements are specified using **gigabyte** (GB) (1,024 MB).
–Radiology departments have very large storage requirements, normally measured in **terabyte** (TB) (1,024 GB).

B. Computer hardware
 –Computer **hardware** refers to the physical components of the system including the **central processing unit (CPU), memory,** and **data entry** and **export** devices.
 –Computer memory stores the various bit sequences and is either **random access memory (RAM)** or **read only memory (ROM).**
 –**RAM** is **temporary** (volatile) memory that stores information while the software is used.
  –RAM is the primary memory component in most computers.
 –**ROM** is for **permanent** storage and cannot be overwritten.
  –Important **CPU instructions** for system operation are stored in ROM.
 –**Buffer** memories are normally considered a part of RAM and are used for **video displays.**
 –**Cache** memory provides transitional memory storage and is often built into CPU chips to provide a buffer between RAM and disc memory.
 –**Address** refers to the location of bit sequences in memory.
 –**CPUs** perform calculations and logic operations by manipulating bit sequences under the control of software instructions.
 –**Parallel** processing occurs when several tasks are performed *simultaneously,* and requires multiple CPUs.
 –**Serial** processing refers to performing tasks sequentially.
 –**Array processors** are hard-wired devices dedicated to performing one type of rapid calculation.
 –**Array processors** are used in **CT** and **MR** imaging where large numbers of calculations are needed to convert data into images.
 –A **bus** is a local pathway linking components.

C. Computer software
 –Computers use **operating systems** to perform internal system bookkeeping activities such as storing files.
 –A **file** is a collection of data treated as a unit.
 –Examples of operating systems are **WINDOWS** (IBM), **MAC OS** (Apple), **UNIX** and **LINUX** (SUN), and **VMS** (mainframe computers).
 –**Computer software** instructs the computer where input data are stored, how these data are to be manipulated, and where the results are to be placed.
 –Most computer programs are written using high-level languages such as **C, Pascal, COBOL, dBase, FORTRAN,** or **Basic.**
 –**Object code** or machine language is the machine-specific binary code instructions used by the CPU.

TABLE 3.4   Typical Storage Capacities and Access Times for Computer Storage Media

Media	Storage Capacity	Access Time
Hard disk	20 MB–50 GB	10 ms
Magnetic tape	600 MB–50 GB	10 s to a few minutes
Optical disk	600 MB–10 GB	16 ms
Optical jukebox	500 GB–3 TB	10–60 s

–High-level machine-independent languages are called **source codes.**
–**Java** is a platform-independent programming language designed to run in a network environment.
–A **compiler** is a software program used to convert high-level language (**source code**) to machine language (**object code**).

D. **Computer peripheral devices**
   –Input devices include **keyboards, joysticks, light pens, trackballs,** and **touch screens.**
   –Output devices include **cathode ray tubes (**CRT **), thin film transistors** (TFT) or **liquid crystal displays** (LCD), **laser film** printers, and **paper printers.**
   –Data storage devices include **hard disks, compact disks** (CDs), **optical disks, optical jukeboxes,** and **magnetic tapes.**
   –RAID (**redundant array** of **inexpensive disks**) provides redundant, inexpensive, readily accessible local storage.
   –Table 3.4 summarizes the capabilities of various data storage devices.
   –Computers communicate via **coaxial cables, telephone lines, magnetic tape transfers, microwaves,** and **fiber-optic** links.
   –A **modem** (modulator/demodulator) is used to transmit information over telephone lines.
   –A **cable modem** is used to transmit information over cable television lines.
   –Figure 3.3 shows peripheral devices associated with computers.
   –**Baud rate** describes the rate of information transfer in bits per second.

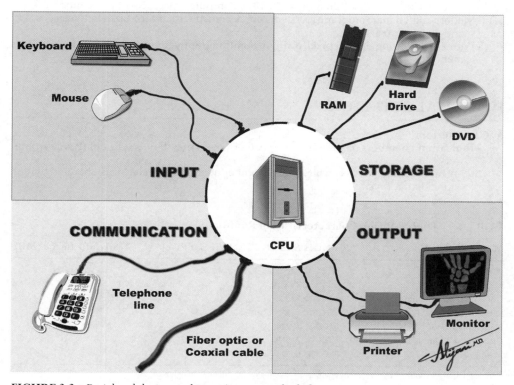

FIGURE 3.3   Peripheral devices and input/output methods for computers.

TABLE 3.5   Local Area Networks and Transfer Times for Chest X-ray (10 MB)

Mode	Nominal Speed (Mbit/s)	Chest X-ray Transfer Time
Modem (telephone)	0.056	~45 min
Ethernet	10	~1 min
Fast Ethernet	100	<10 s
GigabitEthernet	1,000	<1 s

–**A baud rate** of **56,000 corresponds** to **56,000 bits/s or 7,000 bytes/s.**
–Modern computers are linked using networks such as **Ethernet** (10 Mbps), **Fast Ethernet** (100 Mbps), and **Gigabit Ethernet** (1,000 Mbps).
–Table 3.5 lists common network options for transmitting images.

E. Image information
  –**Pixels** are individual *pic*ture *el*ements in a two-dimensional image.
  –In digital images, each pixel intensity is normally coded using either 1 or 2 bytes.
  –The total number of pixels in an image is the product of the number of pixels assigned to the horizontal and vertical dimensions.
  –The number of **pixels** in each dimension is called **matrix size.**
  –If there are 1,024 (1 k) pixels in both the horizontal and vertical dimensions, then the image contains $1 \text{ k} \times 1 \text{ k} = 1 \text{ M, or } 1,024^2$ **pixels.**
  –Table 3.6 lists matrix sizes used in diagnostic radiology.
  –The **information content** of images is the product of the number of pixels and the number of bytes per pixel.
  –An image with a **512 × 512 matrix** and **1-byte** coding of each pixel requires **0.25 MB** of memory (512 × 512 × 1).
    –The same image matrix size, but using 2-byte coding of each pixel, would require **0.5 MB** of memory **(512 × 512 × 2).**
  –A single-view **chest x-ray** digitized to a **2 k × 2.5 k** matrix using **2-byte** coding of each pixel (2,048 × 2,560 × 2) requires **10 MB** of computer space (RAM or memory).
  –Modern digital **mammography** systems are designed with matrix sizes between **4 × 4 k** and **4 × 6 k pixels.**
  –With 2-byte coding of each pixel, a **single mammography** image requires **32** to **48 MB** of memory.

IV. DIGITAL DETECTORS

A. Gas detectors
  –**Ionization chambers,** containing air or other gases, may be used to detect x-ray photons.
    –A **high voltage** across an air or gas chamber measures the electrons liberated by the incident x-rays.

TABLE 3.6   Digital Image Characteristics in Radiology

Modality	Matrix Size	Byte per Pixel	Size of 1 Image (MB)
Nuclear medicine	128 × 128	1	1/64
Magnetic resonance	256 × 256	2	1/8
Computed tomography	512 × 512	2	1/2
Ultrasound	512 × 512	1	1/4
Digital photospot/DSA	1,024 × 1,024	2	2
CR, DR, and film digitizers	2,560 × 2,048	2	10
Mammography	4,096 × 6,144	2	50

DSA, digital subtraction angiography; CR, computed radiography; DR, digital radiography.

–Incident x-rays transfer energy to electrons in **Compton** and **photoelectric** interactions.

–Energetic electrons lose energy by undergoing collisions with atoms and thereby producing many **ionizations.**

–The signal produced by absorption of x-rays is the total **electron charge liberated** in the gas, which is collected by the positive anode.

–Gas detectors (ionization chambers) containing **air** can be used to accurately measure x-ray beam intensities and are calibrated in **air kerma (Gy).**

  –Air-based ionization chambers absorb very little of the incident x-rays.

–For **imaging,** any practical gas detector must have a high x-ray absorption efficiency and would not use air.

  –Imaging detectors use **high atomic number gases** and/or **high pressures.**

–**Xenon** is a high atomic number gas (**Z = 54; K-edge energy 34.6 keV**) and is an efficient x-ray detector at high pressure.

B. Solid state detectors

–In **solid-state crystals** (e.g., NaCl), atoms are arranged in a regular three-dimensional structure.

–Electrons occupy **shells** according to their energy in **atoms,** but in **solid-state crystals, electrons occupy energy bands.**

–In solid-state crystals, only the two outer energy bands of electrons are important.

  –These are called the (inner) **valence** and (outer) **conduction** band.

–When x-rays interact with a solid-state material, energy is transferred to electrons (i.e., **Compton electrons** and **photoelectrons**).

–In **photostimulable phosphors,** some of this energy is stored in "electron traps" and can be released at a later time when the phosphor is stimulated with light.

–In **scintillators,** some of the deposited energy is converted into **light,** or fluorescence.

–In **photoconductors,** this charge is collected and measured directly.

C. Photostimulable phosphors

–**Computed radiography** (CR) uses **photostimulable phosphor** plates made of **barium fluorohalides** (e.g., **BaFBr** and/or **BaFI**).

–X-ray photons interact with the electrons in the phosphor, creating a latent image.

–After exposure, the plates are read out using a **red laser light** to stimulate and empty the **electron traps.**

–**Blue light** is emitted, which can be measured using a light detector (photomultiplier tube).

–The amount of **light detected** is proportional to the incident **x-ray intensity.**

  –The detected signal is digitized and stored in a computer.

–White light is used to erase photostimulable phosphor plates, which can then be reused.

–Photostimulable phosphors have a wide dynamic range.

  –CR plates can tolerate x-ray intensities **100 times lower,** and **100 times higher,** than the **5 μGy** required for **screen–film.**

–Figure 3.4 shows the response of a photostimulable phosphor (PSP) detector.

–The **dynamic range** of CR is **10,000:1** and much higher than a typical value for a **screen–film (40:1)** as shown in Figure 3.4.

–**PSP** can be used with air kerma <**0.1 μGy** up to an air kerma of **1,000 μGy.**

D. Scintillators

–**Scintillators** are materials that emit light when exposed to radiation.

  –Scintillators are also known as phosphors.

–The **conversion efficiency** of a scintillator is the percentage of absorbed energy that is converted into light.

–Between 2% and 20% of the absorbed energy is converted to light (conversion efficiency).

–Radiographic screens are examples of scintillators in which the light output is detected by a film.

–**Gadolinium oxysulfide** (Gd_2O_2S) is a common radiographic screen material.

–Image-intensifier input phosphors are scintillators, typically **cesium iodide** (CsI).

–Scintillators are used in digital x-ray detector systems.

–A typical scintillator has a thickness of up to 0.5 mm.

–**CsI** in flat panel detectors is normally manufactured in **columns** to minimize light diffusion.

E. Photoconductors

–A **photoconductor** is a solid state device that detects x-rays directly.

–**Selenium (Z = 34; K edge energy 12.7 keV)** is the most common photoconductor in use in digital radiography.

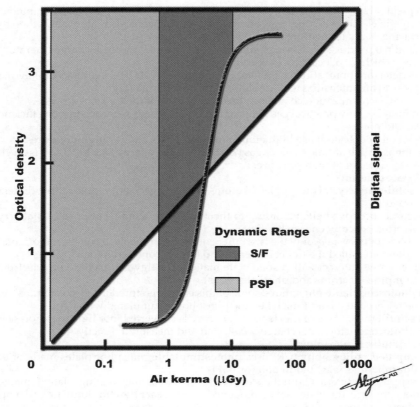

FIGURE 3.4   Dynamic range characteristics of a photostimulable phosphor (PSP) compared to that of screen-film (S/F).

-A typical photoconductor has a thickness of about 0.5 mm.
-A **voltage** across the **photoconductor** detects electrons (charge) produced by the deposition of x-ray energy.
-The electronic signal (i.e., charge collected) in a given region is directly proportional to the amount of **x-ray energy deposited** in the region.
-Photoconductors based on **selenium** have **poor x-ray absorption** properties at higher photon energies because of the relatively low K-shell binding energy.
-Alternatives to selenium include **lead iodide** (PbI) and **mercury iodide** (HgI).
-X-ray absorption characteristics of PbI and HgI are expected to be excellent for x-ray imaging applications.

V. DIGITAL RADIOGRAPHY

A. Film digitizers
-It is necessary to convert a conventional analog **film** print into a **digital image** for electronic transfer **(teleradiology)** or for entering into a PACS (*p*icture *a*rchive and *c*ommunication *s*ystem).
-Commercial film digitizers read the analog image by shining light on the film, and then quantifying (digitizing) the intensity of the **transmitted light.**
-One digitizer uses a **narrow laser light beam** that is scanned across the film.
-The intensity of the *transmitted* light beam is converted to a digital signal.
-Another form of digitizer uses a collimated **light source** and a **charge-coupled device (CCD) linear array.**
  -**Laser digitizers** are more accurate and can digitize to higher film densities.
  -**CCD digitizers** are cheaper and require less maintenance.

–A typical chest x-ray would have **2,000** measurements along 1 line and **2,500** lines to cover the film.

–Output from a film digitizer has about **five million** individual pixel values (i.e., 2,500 × 2,000).

B. Cassette systems

–**Computed radiography** (CR) uses **photostimulable phosphors** to capture x-ray exposure patterns.

–After being exposed, CR plates are read out using a laser, pixel by pixel.

–The **intensity** of the **light** (i.e., signal) released from each pixel is directly **proportional** to the **x-rays absorbed** in this region.

–Acquired CR image data are stored in a computer, and can be **processed** in various ways.

–The processed **CR image** may be printed on a **film** or displayed on a **monitor.**

–CR systems use cassettes and are compatible with analog screen–film imaging systems.

–A **single CR reader** can process CR cassettes from **several radiographic rooms.**

–CR systems are ideal for performing **portable x-ray examinations** where automatic exposure control is not available.

C. Noncassette systems

–**Photostimulable phosphors (CR)** can be **integrated** with the **x-ray generator** including dedicated chest applications and table radiographic systems.

–Most **noncassette** systems consist of **flat panel detectors** that are integrated with the x-ray generator.

–Flat panels have an x-ray absorber that is coupled to a **two-dimensional array** of elements.

–Each element stores charge in proportion to the x-ray intensity, which can be **read** out **electronically.**

–Flat panel x-ray absorbers include **indirect (scintillators)** and **direct (photoconductor)** systems.

–Digital x-ray detectors based on scintillators (e.g., **CsI**) are **indirect** x-ray detectors (Fig. 3.5).

–Absorbed x-rays are first converted to light, which is subsequently stored as charge.

–Digital x-ray detectors based on photoconductors are **direct** x-ray detectors (Fig. 3.5).

–Absorbed x-rays are converted to charge that is directly stored.

–**Noncassette systems** permit the review of an acquired image within seconds of the exposure.

–**Noncassette systems** are **expensive** but can improve **operational efficiency.**

D. Hard copy

–**Hard copy** display refers to printing images onto film using a **laser camera.**

–The film is exposed in a **raster fashion** by a laser that projects a beam of varying intensity light across the film.

–The brightness of the beam at each position depends on the (digital) image intensity value at this location.

–**Lasers** usually **emit red light,** which requires the use of **red-sensitive film.**

–Laser film should not be handled in darkrooms that have a red safe light.

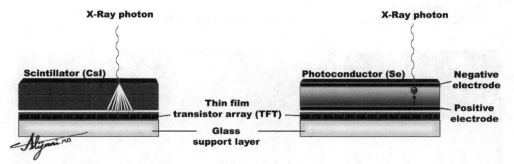

FIGURE 3.5   Indirect (scintillator shown **left**) and direct (photoconductor shown **right**) flat panel detector systems.

–Laser printed images have **excellent resolution** and a **high dynamic range.**
–A matrix of about 4,096 × 4,096 can be written to a 35 × 43 cm film.

E. **Soft copy display**
   –**Soft copy** display refers to presenting images on **cathode ray tubes** (CRT) or **flat panel** monitors.
      –**Flat panel displays** require less frequent checks than CRT monitors.
   –A monitor with a larger horizontal dimension has a **landscape** display, whereas a monitor with a larger vertical dimension has a **portrait** display.
   –**Luminance** of monitors (80–300 cd/m^2) is much lower than that of conventional radiographic viewboxes (1,500–3,500 cd/m^2).
   –**Interpolation** refers to the mapping of an image of one matrix size to a display of another size.
      –**A 2 × 2 k image displayed** on a **1 k** monitor requires that four pixels from the image be mapped to each pixel on the monitor.
   –**Video** displays use **8-bit** images, which register **256 brightness intensity levels** (gray scales).
   –A 2 k × 2.5 k display is known as a **5 megapixel (MP) monitor.**
      –**Five-MP grayscale monitors** are **used** for **mammography.**
   –Grayscale monitors are for **radiography** and **fluoroscopy (3 MP)** and CT/MR **(2 MP).**
   –**Two-MP color monitors** are used in nuclear medicine (**NM**), **ultrasound,** and positron emission tomography **(PET)/CT** fused images.
   –The standard diagnostic workstation uses a **3-MP** monitor.
      –The **matrix size** of a **3-MP monitor** is **2,048 × 1,600.**
   –Test patterns used to evaluate monitor performance have been developed by the Society of Motion Picture and Television Engineers (**SMTPE**).
      –American Association of Physicists in Medicine (**AAPM**) **Task Group 18** has also developed a test pattern for use in radiology.

VI. DIGITAL IMAGE DATA

A. **Image display**
   –Digital radiography separates **image capture, image storage,** and **image display** functions.
      –*All three* functions are performed by *film* in screen–film imaging.
   –In **digital imaging,** each individual picture element (pixel) is assigned a location and gray scale value or intensity by groups of bits.
   –**Look-up tables** are a method of altering the tonal qualities of an image by mapping intensity values to a desired brightness level.
   –Digital images permit the **display window width** and **window level** settings to be adjusted by the operator, which modifies the image brightness and contrast.
   –**Image window width** refers to the range of gray scale values displayed.
   –All pixels with values below the range register as black and all those above as white
   –**Image contrast** within the window range is increased more as the **window** is **narrowed.**
   –**Window level** defines the center value of the window width and therefore overall **image brightness.**

B. **Image processing**
   –**Digital images** can be processed by **manipulating data** (Fig. 3.6).

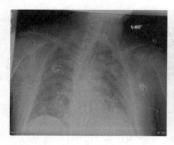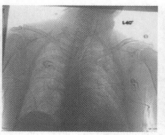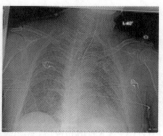

FIGURE 3.6 Conventional portable chest radiograph **(left),** which can be inverted **(middle)** or unsharp mask enhanced **(right).**

–**Histogram equalization** eliminates white and black pixels that contribute little diagnostic information, and expands the remaining data to the full display range.

–**Low-pass spatial filtering** is a method of noise reduction in which a portion of the averaged value of the surrounding pixels is added to each pixel.

–**Unsharp masking** involves subtraction of a smoothed version from the original, which is then added to a replicate original (Fig. 3.6).

  –Visibility of tubes, lines, and catheters is improved, but noise increases and artifacts may be introduced.

–**Background subtraction** can digitally reduce the effect of x-ray scatter to increase image contrast.

–**Energy subtraction** techniques are based on subtracting projection radiographs obtained at two x-ray generator settings (e.g., 60 and 110 kV).

–Chest radiographs obtained at a high and low kV can be subtracted to eliminate bonelike structures, and improve **depiction** of **lung** and **soft tissue.**

  –Conversely, a **bone-only** image can also be produced, which helps distinguish between **calcified** and **noncalcified lung nodules.**

–Digital images also enable the use of **computer-aided detection (CAD)** as well as computer-aided diagnosis methods.

–CAD systems are well established in **mammography** and are being **introduced** into clinical practice in **chest imaging** (planar and CT).

C. Networks

–**Computer networks** allow two or more computers to exchange information.

–Network **protocols** are the codes and conventions under which a network operates.

–**Bandwidth** defines the maximum amount of information that can be transferred over a data channel per unit of time and is measured in Mbit/s or Gbit/s.

–**Topology** refers to the network layout and connection of the various components.

–**Token ring** topology is a closed loop of point-to-point connections.

–**Ethernet** is a standard often used for local area networks.

–**Backbone** refers to a large network that connects smaller networks.

–A **bridge** connects network segments.

–Local area networks **(LANs)** have devices connected by cable or optical fiber.

–Wide area networks **(WANs)** such as the internet use remote telecommunication devices.

–A **hub** allows physical interconnection of multiple devices to a single network.

–A **switch** is a more complicated device for connecting multiple devices to a single network in a point-to-point manner.

–A **router** is a computer system that connects and directs information from one network to another by selecting the best available pathway.

–A **gateway** is a computer system for connecting one network to another.

D. Image transmission

–**Client** refers to a computer requesting information from another computer **(server).**

–**Push technology** refers to an opposite scenario in which a passive client receives information broadcast from a server.

–**Domain** refers to the name identification for a particular machine.

–**E-mail addresses** contain various levels of domain names (local name@domain.top-level domain).

–IP **(internet protocol)** is a low-level protocol for assigning addresses to information packets.

–The internet uses high-level **TCP/IP protocols** (transmission control protocol/internet protocol).

–**Transmission control protocol** (TCP) breaks down information into pieces of manageable size called packets for movement on the internet.

–The **World Wide Web (www)** is the collection of computers that exchange information over the internet using the **hypertext transfer protocol (HTTP).**

–Image data sets are large and benefit from **image compression,** which reduces the size of data files by removing or encoding redundant information.

–**Lossless compression** is completely reversible, and levels of data compression up to **5:1** may be achieved.

–**Lossy compression** achieves higher savings but introduces some degree of irreversible data loss.

–**Joint Photographic Experts Group (JPEG)** and **JPEG 2000** are widely available image standards that accommodate **lossy image compression.**

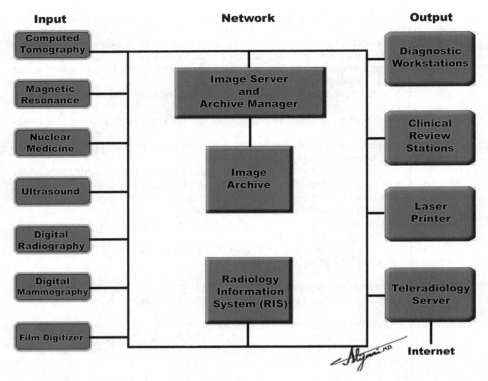

FIGURE 3.7   Components of a PACS.

E. **PACS**
  –**DICOM** (Digital Imaging and Communications in Medicine) is an image-based medical protocol that specifies image formats.
  –DICOM is now an **international standard (ISO).**
  –**ACR-NEMA** is a joint committee of the American College of Radiology and the National Electrical Manufactures Association that developed DICOM.
  –**Picture archive** and **communication systems** (PACS) are digital radiology systems that have the potential to eliminate the use of film.
  –Figure 3.7 shows the components of a PACS.
  –A PACS offers healthcare information integration including radiology records and reports, medical records, and laboratory information.
  –**Health Level Seven (HL7)** is a standard for electronic data interchange in healthcare environments.
  –**HL7** does *not* relate to **medical images.**
  –PACS needs to be integrated to the **radiology information system** (RIS) and **hospital information system** (HIS).
  –**Integrating the Healthcare Enterprise** (IHE) is a joint effort of the **Radiological Society of North America** (RSNA) and **Healthcare Information and Management Systems Society** (HIMSS).
  –The **goal** of **IHE** is to **standardize interoperability among PACS, RIS,** and **HIS.**
  –**Networks** make image data **widely available** to **multiple users** at the same time.
  –**Networks** also permit **instantaneous access** to users in multiple locations.
F. **PACS benefits**
  –**PACS** is expected to **reduce** the **time** and **financial cost** associated with film and paper storage and transfer.
  –**PACS permits rapid image retrieval** and **simultaneous** and **remote viewing.**
  –The use of PACS also **compacts storage, reducing archival space** (file rooms) and requiring **fewer personnel** (file room clerks).
  –Problems of lost, misplaced, and sequestered films are potentially eliminated.

–PACS promises to improve **operational efficiency,** reduce costs, and provide a much **faster service** in terms of **report time** to referring physicians.

–One major limitation to the widespread introduction of PACS is the **high capital costs** involved.

–The amount of image data generated by a radiology department performing **100,000 exams per year** is **very large (i.e., several TB).**

–Technical personnel required to support **PACS** are **expensive.**

–Other difficulties associated with PACS include **security** and **reliability.**

REVIEW TEST

3.1 X-ray film emulsion contains crystals of:
  a. calcium tungstate
  b. silver bromide
  c. lanthanum oxybromide
  d. silver nitrate
  e. cesium iodide

3.2 In film processing, the developer most likely:
  a. modifies developer pH
  b. removes unexposed grains
  c. attaches silver to the base
  d. removes bromine
  e. reduces silver halide

3.3 If I_o is the light incident on a film, and I_t is the light transmitted, optical density is:
  a. $I_o + I_t$
  b. $I_o - I_t$
  c. I_o/I_t
  d. $\log(I_o/I_t)$
  e. $\log(I_o - I_t)$

3.4 The fraction of light transmitted by a film with an optical density of 2 is:
  a. 0.5
  b. 0.1
  c. 0.05
  d. 0.01
  e. 0.005

3.5 The maximum slope of the characteristic curve is called the film:
  a. density
  b. gamma
  c. transmittance
  d. opacity
  e. lambda

3.6 Films used for chest x-ray examinations are likely to have increased:
  a. gradient
  b. gamma
  c. speed
  d. latitude
  e. density

3.7 The percentage of x-ray photons (%) absorbed by a radiographic film alone (no screen) is most likely:
  a. 0.001
  b. 0.01
  c. 0.1
  d. 1
  e. 10

3.8 How many light photons would a screen likely to emit after absorbing a 20-keV photon?
  a. 1
  b. 10

  c. 100
  d. 1,000
  e. 10,000

3.9 Conversion efficiencies (%) of radiography intensifying screens are likely:
  a. 1
  b. 10
  c. 50
  d. 90
  e. 99

3.10 The fraction of 80-kV x-rays absorbed by a standard screen–film cassette is most likely:
  a. 0.1
  b. 0.25
  c. 0.5
  d. 0.75
  e. 0.9

3.11 Which factor is *least* likely to affect the speed of a screen–film imaging system?
  a. Cassette dimensions
  b. Film type
  c. Phosphor material
  d. Screen thickness
  e. Developer temperature

3.12 The air kerma (μGy) required to expose a 200 speed screen–film combination would likely to be:
  a. 1
  b. 2
  c. 5
  d. 10
  e. 20

3.13 How many bits are required to store 512 shades of gray?
  a. 6
  b. 8
  c. 9
  d. 10
  e. 12

3.14 Input devices for a computer do *not* include a:
  a. keyboard
  b. trackball
  c. touch screen
  d. light pen
  e. printer

3.15 A telephone modem with a 56k baud rate likely transmits (bits per second):
  a. 56
  b. 56^2
  c. 56×8
  d. 56,000
  e. $56,000 \times 8$

3.16 How many $1,024^2$ images (2-byte/pixel) can be stored on a 2-gigabyte disk?
   a. 500
   b. 1,000
   c. 4,000
   d. 10,000
   e. 50,000

3.17 What is the most likely pixel size (mm) when a 25 cm × 25 cm region is imaged using a 256^2 matrix?
   a. 0.1
   b. 0.25
   c. 0.5
   d. 1
   e. 2

3.18 Which gas would be most likely used as an x-ray detector for digital medical imaging?
   a. Carbon dioxide
   b. Hydrogen
   c. Nitrogen
   d. Oxygen
   e. Xenon

3.19 Which of the following would most likely be used to acquire digital x-ray images?
   a. BGO
   b. CsI
   c. LiF
   d. LSO
   e. NaI

3.20 Photostimulable phosphors are read out using:
   a. infrared light
   b. microwaves
   c. red light
   d. RF
   e. ultraviolet

3.21 The dynamic range of a photostimulable phosphor is most likely:
   a. 10:1
   b. 10^2:1
   c. 10^3:1
   d. 10^4:1
   e. 10^5:1

3.22 The x-ray absorber material most likely used in indirect flat panel x-ray detectors is:
   a. BaFBr
   b. CsI
   c. NaI
   d. PbI
   e. Se

3.23 Which of the following materials is most likely used as a photoconductor in direct flat panel x-ray detectors?
   a. Xe
   b. Br

   c. Se
   d. Ba
   e. Cs

3.24 A typical pixel size (μm) in a digital diagnostic chest x-ray image is most likely:
   a. 50
   b. 100
   c. 175
   d. 300
   e. 500

3.25 Typical maximum brightness (cd/m^2) of a digital image display is most likely:
   a. 3
   b. 10
   c. 30
   d. 100
   e. 300

3.26 The display capacity (megapixel, MP) of a radiology diagnostic workstation is most likely:
   a. 0.25
   b. 0.5
   c. 1
   d. 2
   e. 3

3.27 Processing a digital x-ray image by unsharp mask enhancement likely increases the:
   a. limiting resolution
   b. visibility of edges
   c. patient dose
   d. matrix size
   e. image magnification

3.28 Reducing image noise by smoothing the acquired data is most likely to reduce:
   a. data content
   b. lesion contrast
   c. matrix size
   d. patient dose
   e. spatial resolution

3.29 The test pattern used to evaluate the display monitor performance is most likely:
   a. SSFP
   b. SONET
   c. SECAM
   d. SMTPE
   e. SCBE

3.30 PACS will most likely result in an increase in:
   a. retrieval time
   b. lost images
   c. viewboxes
   d. capital costs
   e. film clerks

ANSWERS AND EXPLANATIONS

3.1b. Silver bromide grains are the light-sensitive grains found in film emulsions.

3.2e. Film development is the reduction (i.e., addition of electrons) of silver halide grains to "a clump of silver atoms."

3.3d. Film density is $\log(I_o/I_t)$.

3.4d. A film with density of 2 transmits 1% (0.01) of the incident light.

3.5b. Film gamma is the maximum slope.

3.6d. Chest films require wide-latitude films to capture intensities transmitted through the lungs and mediastinum.

3.7d. A film alone absorbs ~1% of the incident x-ray photons.

3.8d. Twenty keV is absorbed, and ~10% (i.e., 2,000 eV) goes into light; since each light photon has ~2 eV, there would be ~1,000 light photons.

3.9b. Most screens convert 10% of the absorbed x-ray energy into light energy.

3.10c. A typical screen absorbs about half the incident x-ray photons (0.5).

3.11a. Cassette *size* is irrelevant for film speed determination.

3.12c. Five μGy is required for a satisfactory film image using a 200 speed screen–film combination.

3.13c. Nine bits are required to generate 512 shades of gray (i.e., 2^9).

3.14e. A printer is an output device, not an input device.

3.15d. Fifty-six thousand since 1 baud means 1 bit per second.

3.16b. Each image has 1 M pixels and 2 bytes per pixel (i.e., is 2 MB), so the disk can store 1,000.

3.17d. Approximately 1 mm because the dimension is 250 mm and the number of pixels is 256.

3.18e. Xenon since it has a high atomic number (54) and has x-ray absorption properties comparable to I and Ba.

3.19b. CsI has excellent x-ray absorption properties and is ubiquitous as an x-ray detector in fluoroscopy and in flat panel radiography.

3.20c. Red light is used to read out photostimulable phosphors (when stimulated, blue light is emitted).

3.21d. The typical dynamic range of a photostimulable phosphor is 10^4:1.

3.22b. Indirect x-ray detectors mainly use CsI as the x-ray absorbing phosphor material.

3.23c. Se is the most common photoconductor in use in medical imaging today (2008).

3.24c. The typical matrix size is 175 microns (i.e., 350-mm width of a chest x-ray film divided by 2,000 pixels, or 430-mm height divided by 2,500).

3.25e. Diagnostic workstations have a maximum image brightness of 300 cd/m^2.

3.26e. Diagnostic workstations typically use 3 MP displays (5 MP are used in mammography).

3.27b. Visibility of edges improves in images processed by unsharp mask enhancement.

3.28e. Average pixel values to reduce random fluctuations (mottle) will blur the image and reduce spatial resolution.

3.29d. SMTPE (Society of Motion and Television Picture Engineers) developed the test pattern.

3.30d. PACS is (very) expensive to install.

Chapter 4

PROJECTION RADIOGRAPHY II

I. MAMMOGRAPHY IMAGING CHAIN

A. X-ray tubes
  - –X-ray tube voltage in **mammography** ranges from **25 kV** to **34 kV.**
  - –**Three-phase** or **high-frequency generators** are used to minimize voltage fluctuations.
  - –For film–screen mammography, **molybdenum (z = 42; K-edge energy 20.0 keV)** is the most common **target** material in the anode because it produces characteristic radiation at optimal energy levels.
    - –**Molybdenum** produces **characteristic x-rays** of **17.9** and **19.5 keV.**
  - –Some commercial x-ray tubes use **rhodium targets (z = 45; K-edge energy 23.2 keV),** which produce characteristic x-rays with a *slightly* higher energy.
  - –**Rhodium** produces characteristic x-rays of **20.2** and **22.7 keV**, which are more penetrating than those of molybdenum.
    - –**Rhodium characteristic x-rays** have an energy ∼3 keV **higher** than **molybdenum** characteristic x-rays.
  - –**Tungsten targets** are also available on some machines, which do not produce characteristic x-rays in the mammography range.
    - –**Filters** for **tungsten targets** may be **molybdenum, rhodium,** or **sliver (Z = 47; K-edge energy 25.5 keV).**
  - –The **normal focal spot** is **0.3 mm,** which is much smaller than conventional radiography (1.2 mm).
    - –The **0.3 mm focal spot** uses tube currents of **100 mA.**
  - –The **small focal spot (0.1 mm)** is used for **magnification** mammography.
    - –The **small focal spot** can tolerate only low currents of ∼**25 mA.**
  - –A **beryllium (Z = 4)** x-ray tube window is used to minimize x-ray beam attenuation.
  - –The **heel effect** (higher x-ray intensity on the cathode side) is used to **increase** the **intensity** of **radiation near** the **chest wall** where greater penetration is needed.
  - –Table 4.1 shows the physical characteristics of the key components of mammography x-ray tubes.

B. Filtration
  - –For screen–film **mammography,** the x-ray energy level that **optimizes contrast** for an average-sized breast is ∼**19 keV.**
  - –**Lower-energy** x-ray photons have **inadequate breast penetration** and increase dose.
  - –**Higher-energy x-rays** photons **decrease contrast.**
  - –The **optimum mammographic photon energy increases** with increasing breast **thickness** and breast **density.**
  - –**Filters** are used to achieve the **optimal photon energies** that minimize *both* high- and low-energy x-ray photons.
  - –**Filters** in **mammography** may be made of **molybdenum, rhodium,** or **silver.**
    - –Filters in mammography are ∼**30 μm thick.**
  - –Filters **remove** most **bremsstrahlung radiation above** the **filter K-edge.**
  - –Removal of this higher-energy bremsstrahlung radiation improves contrast.
  - –All **filters** remove **very low-energy x-rays** that contribute *only* to patient dose.
  - –Figure 4.1 shows the x-ray spectra from a molybdenum target.

TABLE 4.1   Specifications for a Screen–Film Mammography Unit

Parameter	Specification
Target material	Molybdenum, rhodium, or tungsten
Window material	Beryllium
Added filtration	Molybdenum, rhodium, or silver
Half-value layer	~0.3 mm Aluminum

–Compared to a Mo filter, a Rh **filter transmits** more photons between **20 keV** and **23 keV.**

–Compared to a Rh filter, **silver (K-edge 25.5 keV)** transmits more photons between **23 and 25.5 keV.**

C. Grids

–**Scatter** to **primary ratios** in mammography ranges from **0.6** to **1.0.**

–Reduced scatter is due to the use of low-energy photons that interact primarily by **photoelectric absorption.**

   –For **soft tissue,** x-ray photon **energies >25 keV would produce more Compton** scatter than photoelectric absorption.

–Scatter to primary ratios in mammography are lower than for general radiology.

   –Scatter in mammography nonetheless reduces image contrast.

–The importance of **scatter increases** with increasing **breast thickness** and increasing **x-ray tube voltage.**

–**Contact mammography** is performed using a **moving grid.**

–**Carbon fiber** is the most common interspace material for linear grids as aluminum would attenuate too many of the low-energy x-rays used in mammography.

–One manufacturer produces a **high transmission cellular** (HTC) grid with a honeycomb pattern and an **air-interspace material.**

–Values for **linear grid line densities** are ~**50 lines per centimeter.**

–Mammography imaging systems use **grid ratios** of ~**5:1.**

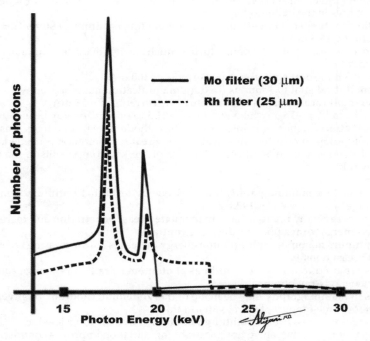

FIGURE 4.1   X-ray spectra from a molybdenum target at 30 kV showing the effect of adding a molybdenum (or rhodium) filter.

–Mammography grids have a **Bucky factor** (ratio of radiation intensity incident on the grid to that transmitted) of ∼**2.**

–Use of a **grid doubles** the **patient dose** relative to nongrid examination.

D. Screen–films

   –**Rare earth** intensifying screens made of **gadolinium oxysulfide (Gd_2O_2S)** are used in screen–film mammography.

   –**Single screens** are used, which may incorporate light absorbers to limit screen diffusion and improve resolution.

   –**Single-emulsion films** are used to reduce receptor blur.

      –**Crossover** and **parallax** effects are **eliminated** by using a single emulsion.

   –X-rays are mainly absorbed at the front of the screen which should be located as close as possible to the film to minimize blur.

      –This is achieved by having the **film between** the **x-ray source** and **screen.**

   –Mammography films generally have **high gradients (>3.0)** and, accordingly, **low film latitude.**

      –Limited latitude is acceptable when there is **adequate breast compression** and the film is **properly exposed.**

   –Mammography films have relatively **thick *single* emulsions,** which make them sensitive to **processor artifacts.**

   –**Optimal film densities** in mammography are between **1.6** and **2.0,** higher than in radiography.

   –**Higher film densities** are needed in mammography because this results in the **best film contrast.**

E. Digital detectors

   –Full field of view **digital systems** are **replacing screen–film mammography.**

      –In **2008,** about **one third** of all mammography facilities were using **digital mammography.**

   –**Higher-energy x-ray spectra** are used in digital mammography.

   –A typical matrix size in digital mammography is **3k × 4k.**

   –**Pixel sizes** are ∼**80** μm, whereas the smallest visible **microcalcifications** are ∼**150** μm.

   –**Photostimulable phosphors** with a 50-μm pixel size have also been used to perform digital mammography.

   –Digital mammograms may be processed using **computer aided diagnosis (CAD)** software, which attempts to identify malignant lesions, and microcalcification clusters.

   –CAD systems can assign a **probability** of **malignancy** for each identified lesion.

   –**Mammography CAD** software has been shown to have **sensitivities** as high as **90%** and can identify lesions missed by radiologists.

   –CAD systems can have a **high false-positive** rate of up to one or two false positives per image.

   –**CAD** has a **high accuracy** for detection of **clusters** of **microcalcifications.**

F. Compression

   –**Optimal mammography** requires the use of breast **compression.**

   –Compression is achieved using **radio translucent paddles.**

   –**Compression reduces** the **thickness** of the **breast,** and as a result reduces breast dose.

      –Compression also **immobilizes** the **breast** and **spreads** the **breast tissue.**

   –**Lower x-ray tube voltages** can be used with **compression,** which will **increase contrast.**

   –Compression brings the breast closer to the image plane, minimizing image magnification and **reducing focal spot blur.**

   –Compression **reduces exposure times,** and thus **minimizes patient motion blur** associated with long exposure times.

   –Compression force is normally between **111** and **200 newtons (25** and **45 lb).**

   –The principal drawback of compression is patient discomfort.

II. CLINICAL MAMMOGRAPHY

A. Cancer Detection Task

   –Mammography is a **low-cost** and **low-dose** procedure that can **detect early-stage breast cancer.**

   –Recognition of breast cancer depends on detection of subtle **architectural distortion, masses** near normal breast tissue density, **skin thickening,** and **microcalcifications.**

TABLE 4.2   Properties of Breast Tissue

Tissue Type	Density (g/cm³)	Linear Attenuation Coefficient at 20 keV (cm⁻¹)
Adipose	0.93	0.45
Fibroglandular	1.035	0.80
Carcinoma	1.045	0.85
Calcification	2.2	12.5

–Microcalcifications are specks of **calcium hydroxyapatite** [$Ca_5(PO_4)_3OH$], which may have diameters as small as **0.1 mm** (100 μm).

–Detection of microcalcifications is difficult because of their small dimensions.

–Table 4.2 summarizes the key physical properties of the major breast tissues and pathologic conditions.

–*X-ray attenuation properties of breast cancer are similar to those of normal fibroglandular tissue.*

–The small differences in attenuation between normal and malignant tissue result in **low contrast** and make **cancer detection difficult.**

–Mammography imaging systems are designed to **maximize image contrast.**

–Image contrast in screen–film mammography is improved by use of **low photon energies, high film gradients, breast compression,** and scatter-removal **grids.**

B. Contact mammography

–Screening mammography normally includes a **craniocaudal** and a **mediolateral oblique** view of each breast.

–Compressed breasts are normally 3 to 8 cm thick, with an **average** of $\sim$**4.5 cm.**

–Typical x-ray **tube currents** are $\sim$**100 mA.**

–**Exposure times** are **generally longer than** $\sim$**1 second.**

–Exposure times may be up to 4 seconds for dense and/or thick breasts.

   –Exposures in excess of about 2 to 3 seconds may introduce motion artifacts.

–X-ray beam **half-value layers** in mammography are $\sim$**0.3 mm Al.**

–For a normal compressed breast (4.5 cm), a typical x-ray tube voltage in screen-film mammography is **25 kV.**

   –Higher tube voltages are used in digital mammography.

–The tube current exposure time product is $\sim$**150 mAs.**

–**Compression** results in **greater sharpness, less scatter,** and **reduced patient dose.**

–A mammogram requires an air kerma of $\sim$**0.2 mGy** at the image receptor.

–Table 4.3 summarizes techniques used in **contact mammography.**

C. Magnification mammography

–**Magnification mammography** improves visualization of **mass margins** and **fine calcifications.**

–Magnification is achieved by moving the breast away from the film using a **15-** to **30-cm standoff** and keeping the **source** to **image** receptor distance **constant.**

–The geometric principles of magnification are illustrated in Figure 4.2.

–The magnification is the ratio of the source to image receptor distance (SID) to the source to object distance (SOD); magnification is given as **SID/SOD.**

–A typical **SID** is **65 cm,** and **SOD** in magnification is **35 cm,** so that **magnification** is **normally 1.86.**

–**Small focal spots (0.1 mm)** are essential to minimize geometric unsharpness with tube currents of $\sim$25 mA.

–The breast area that can be imaged in a single magnification radiograph is reduced.

TABLE 4.3   Technique Summary for Mammography

Parameter	Typical Value
Generator power	$\sim$3 kW
X-ray tube voltage	25–34 kV
Tube current (0.3 mm focal spot)	100 mA
Exposure time (0.3 mm focal spot)	1–2 seconds

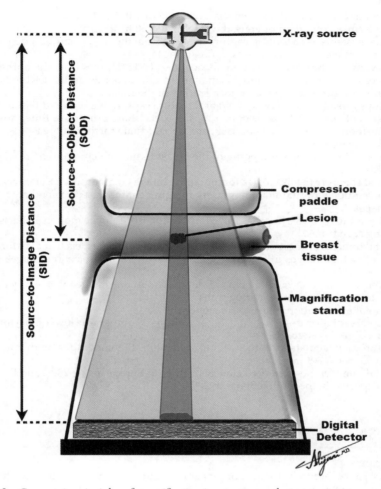

FIGURE 4.2 Geometric principles of magnification in mammography.

- –The presence of an **air gap reduces** the **amount** of **scatter** reaching the film and **eliminates** the **need** for a **grid.**
- –The **absence** of a **grid reduces** the required **mAs** by ~**30%,** since there is no loss of primary photons by any grid.
- –Compared with contact mammography, **reduced** x-ray tube currents **(i.e., 25 mA) increase exposure times** by a factor of about three.
- –Longer exposure times markedly increase the chance of **patient motion (blur).**

D. Viewing mammograms
- –**High luminance viewboxes** and complete film masking are required.
- –Viewboxes with luminance values of ~**3,000 candelas per square meter (cd/m^2)** are used.
  - –Conventional viewboxes are ~1,500 cd/m^2.
- –**Extraneous light decreases contrast perception.**
- –A **magnifying glass** should be used to view microcalcifications.
- –**Viewing rooms** should be **darkened** (<50 lux), and hot lights should be available.
- –A digital screening examination and prior examination contain **400 MB** of data.
- –Viewing digital mammograms requires high quality and high performance monitors.
- –**Five-MP monitors** are essential for viewing digital mammograms.

E. Stereotaxic localization
- –**Stereotaxic localization** has been developed to perform **core needle biopsies.**
- –**Digital imaging systems** are used for stereotaxic localizations, eliminating time-consuming film processing.

–The matrix size of digital systems is **512 × 512** or **1,024 × 1,024.**
–For a **5 cm × 5 cm field** of **view,** the pixel size is 50 to 100 μm.
–Digital systems use a CCD to capture the light from the screen and a 2:1 demagnification of the image via optical lenses or fiberoptic tapers.
–Two views of the breast are normally acquired (**±15 degrees** from the **normal**).
–Images of the lesion will shift by an amount that depends on the lesion depth, which permits a **three-dimensional localization** of the lesion.
–A **biopsy needle gun** is positioned and fired to capture the required tissue sample.
–Benefits of core needle over open biopsies are a **short procedure time, minimal local anesthetic, reduced cost** and **risk,** and **no residual scarring** of breast tissue.

F. **Digital Tomosynthesis**
–Compression causes overlapping of the breast tissue, which reduces breast cancer visibility.
–**Digital tomosynthesis** creates **tomographic images** that improve lesion visibility.
–A conventional **digital mammography imaging chain** is used to generate tomographic images.
–Digital tomosynthesis requires **full compression** to minimize motion artifacts during the **long scan times.**
–Digital tomosynthesis takes a **number** of **projection images,** each at a **different angle.**
–The x-ray tube moves in an arc around the breast, with projection **images** obtained at selected angles.
  –The total angular movement is 15 degrees, with one image taken every degree, for a total of 15 projection radiographs.
–The total examination time is ∼**5 seconds.**
–The total **radiation dose** in digital tomosynthesis is **comparable** to a **contact mammogram** on a digital system.
–Acquired image data are processed to generate ∼45 tomographs, with a nominal **slice thickness** of ∼**1 mm.**
–Digital tomosynthesis entered clinical practice in Europe in late 2008, and FDA approval is expected in the United States in 2009.

III. MQSA

A. **Breast cancer**
–Breast cancer accounts for **32%** of **cancer incidence** and **18%** of **cancer deaths** in women in the United States.
–The National Cancer Institute estimated that there were ∼**180,000 new cases** of breast cancer in the United States in 2007, including 2,000 males.
  –The number of breast **cancer deaths** was **40,000.**
–*One in eight women in the United States ultimately develops breast cancer.*
–Figure 4.3 shows breast cancer incidence and mortality rates.
–Early detection with screening mammography **reduces breast cancer mortality** rates by between **15%** and **35%.**
–The **American Medical Association, American Cancer Society,** and **American College of Radiology (ACR)** all recommend **screening** of *asymptomatic* women.
–The ACR recommends a **baseline mammogram** by age **40,** biannual examinations between ages 40 and 50, and **yearly examinations** after age **50.**

B. **MQSA**
–The **Food and Drug Administration** (FDA) developed the **Mammography Quality Standards Act** (MQSA) requiring all of the more than **10,000 mammography facilities** in the United States to be **certified.**
  –MQSA was passed in 1992, and the final rules became effective April 1999.
–It is **against federal law** to practice **mammography without certification** by the FDA.
–To obtain **certification,** the facility must receive **accreditation** by an approved body such as the **American College of Radiology** (ACR).
–The ACR initially developed a voluntary mammography accreditation program in 1987 to improve the quality of screen–film mammography.
–Accreditation is currently based on the five steps listed in Table 4.4.
–Some states (e.g., **Arkansas, California, Iowa,** and **Texas**) have mammography accreditation programs that are similar to the ACR program.

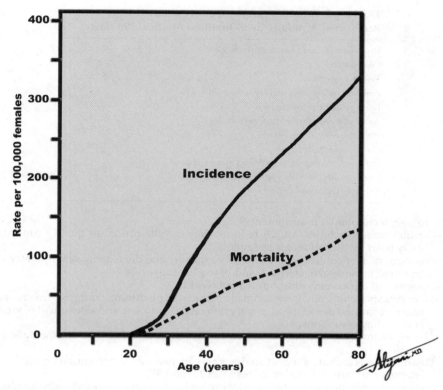

FIGURE 4.3   Breast cancer incidence and mortality.

–Mammography facilities meeting the ACR standards receive a **certificate** of **accreditation** in mammography.
–Optimal mammography performance requires the combined efforts of **physicians, technologists,** and **medical physicists.**
C. **Physician requirements**
    –MQSA specifies requirements for **interpreting physicians** and does not specifically use the term *radiologist.*
    –The **lead interpreting physician** is responsible for ensuring that quality assurance requirements are met.
    –All interpreting physicians participate in the facility **medical outcomes audit.**
    –Interpreting physicians are required to have documented that they have interpreted at least **200 mammograms** in the previous **24 months.**
    –The lead interpreting physician is responsible for ensuring technologists have **adequate training,** and identifying a single technologist to oversee the **QC program.**
    –The lead interpreting physician is also responsible for selecting a **medical physicist** to perform the annual testing.
    –A **qualified individual** must be designated to oversee the **radiation protection program.**

TABLE 4.4   American College of Radiology Accreditation Requirements

Site survey questionnaire completed
Assessment of image quality using a phantom
Dosimeter assessment of mean glandular dose
Assessment of clinical images by independent radiologists
Assessment of quality control program

TABLE 4.5   Mammography Quality Control Tests to Be Performed Annually by a Qualified Medical Physicist

Unit assembly and cassette performance
Collimation
System resolution
Peak voltage accuracy and reproducibility
Beam quality (half-value layer)
Automatic exposure control performance
Uniformity of screen speeds
Radiation output
Entrance skin exposure and mean glandular dose
Image quality (mammography phantom)
Artifact evaluation

D. Radiologic technologist requirements
  –For film–screen facilities, MQSA requirements include **processor quality control** on a **daily** basis by the radiologic technologist.
  –Processor quality control is performed by exposing and developing **sensitometry strips** and measuring **speed, contrast,** and **base plus fog** levels.
  –**Screens** and **darkrooms** must be **cleaned weekly.**
  –**Weekly tests** include obtaining an image of the ACR **phantom;** scoring the image quality, film background density, and density difference (contrast); and assessment of **viewbox** and reading conditions.
  –The x-ray imaging equipment should be visually inspected by a technologist every month.
  –**Quarterly tests** include a **repeat analysis** and analysis of **fixer retention** on film.
    –Repeat rates are expected to be between **2% and 5%.**
    –Repeats may be caused by positioning, patient motion, and overexposure/underexposure.
  –**Darkroom fog, screen–film contact,** and **compression** are performed on a **semiannual basis.**
  –The technologists; **QC program** is **reviewed** annually by a qualified **medical physicist.**
E. Physicist requirements
  –The responsibilities of the **medical physicist** include assessing **image quality** and **equipment performance** as well as evaluating patient **dose.**
  –Medical physicists must be adequately trained in mammography, perform at least six annual medical physics surveys every 2 years, and receive the required CME credits.
  –Imaging tests performed annually by medical physicists are shown in Table 4.5.
  –Phantom images are used to assess film optical **density, contrast, uniformity,** and **image quality** produced by the imaging system and film processing.
  –Phantoms are equivalent to a compressed breast (4.2 cm) with equal glandular and adipose components.
  –The **ACR phantom** contains various-sized **fibers (6), speck groups (5),** and **masses (5).**
  –To pass, the phantom image must show a **minimum** of **four fibers, three speck groups,** and **three masses.**
    –**Image artifacts** must also be **minimal.**
  –The **automatic exposure control (AEC)** needs to maintain film optical density within 0.15 of the mean density.
  –The **ACR** requires that the **average glandular dose (AGD)** for a 4.2-cm-thick breast should be **<3 mGy** per image with a grid.
  –If **no grid** is used, the AGD should be **<1 mGy** per image.

IV. IMAGE INTENSIFIERS

A. Image intensifier tubes
  –**Image intensifiers** (II) convert x-rays exiting the patients into a **bright light image.**
    –The II image can be viewed on a monitor or recorded.
  –An II consists of an **evacuated envelope** made of glass or nonferromagnetic material such as aluminum.

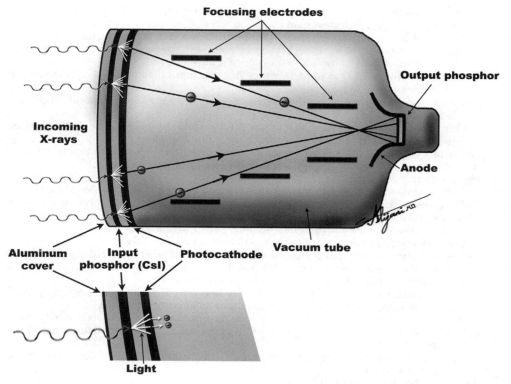

FIGURE 4.4   Schematic view of an image intensifier, which converts an incident pattern of x-ray photons into a bright light image at the output phosphor.

–Important II components include an **input phosphor, photocathode, electrostatic focusing lenses, accelerating anodes,** and **output phosphor** (Fig. 4.4).
  –IIs have diameters that range up to 57 cm.
–**Large IIs** cover larger organs such as the **chest** and **abdomen.**
–**Small IIs** are used for smaller anatomic regions such as the **heart.**
–The **input phosphor absorbs x-ray photons** and re-emits part of the absorbed energy as a large number of light photons.
  –Approximately **10%** of the **absorbed x-ray energy** is emitted in the form of **light** photons.
–The input phosphor is a ~300-μm-thick **cesium iodide** (CsI) screen.
–X-rays are efficiently absorbed by this screen because the **K-shell binding energies** of **Cs** and **I** are ~**35 keV.**
–Light photons emitted by the input phosphor are absorbed by a **photocathode,** which emits **photoelectrons.**
–The photoelectrons are accelerated across the II tube and focused onto the **output phosphor** by an **electrostatic lens.**
–The **accelerating voltage** across the II is ~**30 kV,** and the accelerated electrons gain a kinetic energy of **30 keV.**
–These energetic electrons are absorbed by the **output phosphor** and emit a large number of light photons.
–The output phosphor is **ZnCdS,** which emits green light.
–**Electronic magnification** can be accomplished by focusing photoelectrons from a smaller II area onto the output phosphor.
  –*Electronic magnification* irradiates a *smaller area* of the II.
B. Image intensification
–The II converts the pattern of **incident x-ray intensities** at the input phosphor into an intense pattern of visible **light** at the **output phosphor.**
–The light image on the output of an II is **several thousand** times **brighter** than that on the input phosphor.

–The increase in brightness at the output phosphor relative to the brightness at the input phosphor is the **brightness gain (BG).**

–The **BG** of an II equals the product of the **minification gain** and **flux gain.**

–**Minification gain** is the increase in image brightness that results from reduction in image size from the input phosphor to the output phosphor.

   –**Minification gain** $D = (d_i/d_0)^2$, where d_i is the input diameter and d_0 is the output diameter.

–The output phosphor is typically 2.5 cm in diameter so for a 25-cm II, minification gain is **100** (i.e., $[25/2.5]^2$).

–**Flux gain** is the number of light photons emitted from the output phosphor compared to number of light photons produced in the input phosphor.

–The **flux gain** is typically **50**, which means that for each light photon emitted at the input phosphor, there are 50 light photons emitted at the output phosphor.

C. Light output

–The **conversion factor** is a modern method of measuring the **light output** of the II.

–The conversion factor is the ratio of the **luminance** of the output phosphor measured in candelas per square meter **(cd/m²)** to the input **air-kerma rate** measured in **mGy/s.**

   –A candela is a measure of luminance intensity or light brightness.

–The **conversion factor** of modern IIs is ~**10 to 30 cd/m² per μGy/s.**

–The **air kerma** at the input phosphor must be **increased** when the **field size** is **reduced** to maintain a constant brightness level at the II output phosphor.

–Table 4.6 gives light conversion factors for different sizes of IIs.

–The II **contrast ratio** is the ratio of periphery to central light intensities (output) when imaging a lead disc one tenth the diameter of the II input phosphor.

–A typical II contrast ratio is **20:1,** and several factors contribute to the loss of contrast.

–Some x-ray photons pass through the input phosphor and photocathode and strike the output phosphor.

–Contrast is reduced by **veiling glare,** which is the result of light scattered within the output phosphor.

D. Automatic brightness control

–A variable **optical diaphragm (aperture)** is used to control the amount of light that is transmitted to the television camera.

   –As image intensifiers age, the **optical diaphragm size** is **adjusted** to compensate for the **loss** of **light** produced in the input phosphor.

–The **automatic brightness control** (ABC) regulates the radiation required to maintain a constant TV display.

–The amount of radiation is changed by **adjusting** the **technique factors** to maintain a constant light level at the II output phosphor.

–Modern systems adjust both **tube current** (mA) and **tube voltage** (kV) to control image brightness.

–The **light output** of an II is proportional to the **input area** of the II and the radiation exposure.

–Reducing the **II size** by a **factor** of **two** reduces the **exposed region** by a **factor** of **four.**

–A fourfold increase in radiation exposure would be required to **maintain** a **constant brightness** at the output of the II.

   –This assumes that technical factors (**kV, optical diaphragm,** etc.) are kept constant when the **field of view** is **changed.**

–**Electronic magnification** by decreasing the exposed area of the II results in **increased skin doses.**

   –An unnecessarily high dose can be delivered to the patient if magnification is overused.

TABLE 4.6   **Representative Values of Conversion Gain for Image Intensifiers**

Image Intensifier Diameter (cm)	Conversion Gain (cd/m² per μGy/s)
57	60
33	20
23	10

E. Artifacts

  –**Lag** is the continued luminescence at the output phosphor after x-ray stimulation has stopped.
  –Modern **CsI tubes** have a **low lag** time of about 1 ms, which is of little concern.
  –The **II input** is **curved,** and projecting this surface onto a flat output phosphor results in **geometrical distortions.**
    –A curved input permits the **window** to be **thin,** which minimizes the absorption of incident x-rays.
  –**Pincushion** distortion is produced by all IIs, where straight lines appear curved.
  –For 23-cm IIs, pincushion distortion is ∼**3%,** which increases with II diameter.
  –**Vignetting** is a falloff in brightness at the periphery of the II field; it is typically <∼**25%.**
  –The **curvature** of the II faceplate gives rise to both **pincushion** distortion and **vignetting.**
    –**Imperfections** in **electron focusing** also contribute to pincushion distortion and vignetting.
  –**Pincushion** distortion and **vignetting** are of **less** concern with **smaller field sizes** (i.e., less minification).
  –There is also **S distortion** due to local magnetic fields, which can be a major problem.
    –S distortions can vary as an II rotates due to changes in orientation with respect to the **earth's magnetic field.**

V. TELEVISION

A. TV cameras operation

  –Fluoroscopy systems use a **television** (TV) camera to view the image output of the II.
  –An **aperture** between the lenses controls the light intensity incident on the TV camera.
  –The aperture is adjusted to control the (different) doses that are required in fluoroscopy and radiography.
    –The **aperture** is normally **open** for **fluoroscopy** and **closed** down for **radiographic imaging.**
  –Output images from IIs are focused onto the **photoconductive target** in the TV camera using optical lenses.
  –TV cameras **convert light** images into **electric (video) signals** that can be recorded or viewed on a monitor.
  –The TV target is scanned with an electron beam in horizontal lines (**raster scanning**) to read the image light intensity.
    –Raster scanning may be progressive or interlaced.
  –The **display monitor** converts video signals back into a visible image for direct viewing.

B. Scan modes

  –North American TV displays images at **30 frames per second,** with each frame taking 1/30 of a second.
  –**In field no. 1, 262.5 odd lines** are first scanned in 1/60 second, followed by **262.5 even lines (field no. 2)** in another 1/60 second.
  –**One frame** is the **sum** of **two fields (odd plus even) totaling 525 lines** that are *interlaced.*
  –**Interlacing prevents flickering** when only 30 full frames are updated every second.
    –Cinemas display film at 48 frames per second to prevent flicker.
  –**European** TV systems generally use **625** lines and **25** frames per second (50 fields per second).
    –European TV is therefore *not* compatible with North American TV.
  –When a TV camera is operated in a **progressive** scan mode, **each line** is **read sequentially** (i.e., line 1 followed by line 2 and so on).
  –**Progressive** scan modes are used in digital systems and **reduce motion artifacts.**

C. Camera types

  –Conventional TV systems were classified as **vidicon** or **Plumbicon** camera systems.
  –**Vidicon** systems had **high image lag,** improving image quality by averaging sequential image frames.
  –**Plumbicon** cameras had **less lag** than vidicon cameras.
    –Low lag permits motion to be followed with minimal blur, but quantum mottle is increased.

–Most current fluoroscopy systems make use of **CCD cameras.**
  –**CCD** cameras have **minimal lag.**
–CCD systems usually incorporate **digital recursive filtering** to provide noise averaging. This may be an operator-selectable parameter.
–**CCD** and **TV cameras** produce **similar fluoroscopy image quality.**
–TV cameras are available with **1,000 lines.**
–One thousand line TV cameras require special **1,000 line monitors** to satisfactorily display images at full resolution.
–TV cameras in high-quality imaging (e.g., angiography) require **low noise** levels and **high stability.**

D. Digitizing TV frames
–The **analog voltage** signal from a TV camera must be **converted** to a **digital** bit sequence (analog to digital) before it can be processed.
  –An **analog-to-digital converter (ADC)** changes varying voltage levels to the closest binary equivalent.
–The TV output video signal of a fluoroscopy unit may be digitized and stored in a computer for further processing or subsequent display.
–If the TV is a nominal **525-line** system, **one frame** generally consists of 525^2 **pixels.**
  –A standard TV frame has ~250,000 individual pixels.
–Each **pixel** requires **10 bits** (two bytes) to record the signal level.
  –**Ten bits** per pixel corresponds to **1,024 shades of gray.**
–In **1,000-line mode,** a single **frame** has $1,000^2$ **(1 million)** pixels.
–The information content of a **1,000-line TV frame** is **2 MB.**

E. Digital TV
–**Digital TV** was first introduced in the 1990s and involves the transmission and reception of moving images (plus sound) by means of discrete (digital) signals.
  –Conventional TV uses analog signals.
–In the **United States,** use of analog TV signals will cease in **February 2009.**
–Digital TV makes use of two formats, **standard definition TV** (SDTV) and **high definition TV** (HDTV).
–In the United States, **SDTV** uses a **640 × 480** format for a **4:3 aspect ratio.**
  –For a **16:9** aspect ratio, a **704 × 480** format is used.
–**HDTV** uses **1,280 × 720** in **progressive** scan mode **(720p)** or **1,920 × 1,080** in **interlaced** mode **(1,080i).**
  –Both of these HDTV modes use a **16:9 aspect ratio.**
–Digital TV channels have a maximum bandwidth of **19 Mbit** per second (2.4 MB/s).

VI. II/TV IMAGING

A. Fluoroscopic imaging
–**Fluoroscopy** allows **real-time observation** and imaging of dynamic activities such as barium moving through the gastrointestinal (GI) tract or the flow of iodinated contrast material through blood vessels.
–Figure 4.5 is an overview of a digital fluoroscopic imaging system based on image intensifiers.
–**Fluoroscopy** is performed using low **tube currents** between **1** and **5 mA.**
–X-ray **tube voltages** range between **70** and **110 kV** (Table 4.7).
–Fluoroscopy systems use **grids** to remove scatter radiation, with a typical grid ratio of **10:1.**
–Imaging a smaller patient area using electronic magnification results in a magnified image **(electronic zoom).**
–In **electronic zoom** mode, the **x-ray field** is reduced to **match** the displayed **field of view** (FOV).
  –*At a given FOV,* additional *collimation reduces patient doses* with *no loss of image quality.*
–**Portable fluoroscopy** systems are C-arm devices, with 18- and 23-cm-diameter IIs being most common.
–**Flat panel detectors,** similar to those used in digital radiography, are now **replacing image intensifiers.**
–Flat panel detectors offer good image quality at radiation doses comparable to image intensifiers but are **expensive.**

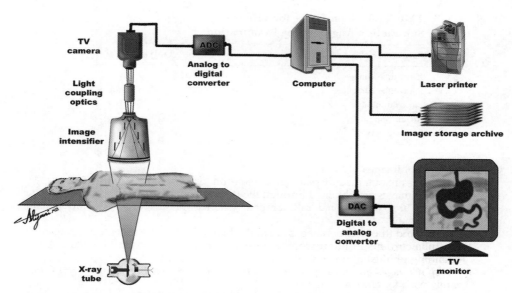

FIGURE 4.5   Digital fluoroscopy imaging system based on an image intensifier.

B. Digital fluoroscopy

–**Digital fluoroscopy** is a fluoroscopy system whose **TV camera** output is **digitized.**

–The image data can be passed through a computer to **process** the **images** before being displayed on a monitor.

–Because the images are acquired by a computer, **last image hold** (LIH) software permits the visualization of the last image when the x-ray beam is switched off.

  –**Last image hold** is a **regulatory requirement** for all fluoroscopes sold in the United States after **June 2006.**

–**Image processing** in digital fluoroscopy occurs in **real time.**

–**Road mapping** permits an image to be captured and displayed on a monitor while a second monitor shows live images.

–Road mapping may also be used to capture images with contrast material, which can be overlaid onto a live fluoroscopy image.

–**Digital temporal filtering** (i.e., frame averaging) is a technique of adding together and then averaging the pixel values in successive images.

–Temporal filtering reduces the effect of random **noise.**

–Appreciable temporal filtering causes **noticeable lag** but much lower noise levels.

  –Temporal **filtering** could **reduce patient doses.**

–**Pulsed fluoroscopy** can reduce dose by **acquiring** frames that are **less than real time** (i.e., **<30 frames per second).**

  –Frame rates in **pulsed fluoroscopy** are **7.5** or **15 frames per second.**

–**Pulsed fluoroscopy** generally **increases** the **dose per frame** to reduce the perceived level of random noise.

TABLE 4.7   Typical Values of X-ray Tube Voltage Used in Common Fluoroscopic Examinations

Clinical Examination	X-ray Tube Voltage for Average Patient (kV)
Gall bladder	~70
Myelogram	~75
Upper GI	~100
Barium enema	~110

TABLE 4.8   Techniques for a Neurologic Digital Subtraction Angiography Examination

Parameter	Typical Value
X-ray tube voltage	75 kV
X-ray tube current	300 mA
Pulse duration	50 ms
Acquisition rate	4 frames/s
Image matrix size	$1,024^2$

C. Spot/photospot images

- **Spot** images are obtained by placing a screen-film or a CR *in front* of the II.
- **Photospot** images are obtained through the II imaging chain.
- Spot films are conventional radiographs, whereas photospot images are obtained through the II.
- Photospot and fluoroscopy images are both obtained using the same II imaging chain.
- X-ray tube currents in **fluoroscopy** are ~3 mA, but are increased to ~300 mA when obtaining **photospot images.**
- *Photospot images* are of *diagnostic quality,* whereas a *last image hold (LIH) frame* is rarely used for *clinical diagnosis.*
- Current photospot images are digital with a matrix size of $1,024^2$.
- Photospot images can be processed, transmitted, and stored.
  - Hard copy images may be obtained using a **laser printer** (Fig. 4.5).

D. Cardiac imaging

- A **cine film** is a series of photospot images obtained in rapid sequence.
- **Cine** historically used **35-mm film** and images were 18 × 24 mm.
- Film has now been replaced by digital images that are stored electronically and displayed on a monitor.
- In digital cardiac imaging of adults, **15 frames per second** acquisitions are used for fluoroscopy and cine.
- With exact framing, the II circle fits exactly within the rectangular frame.
- With total overframing, the rectangular frame fits within the II circle, and the outer part of the II image is lost.
  - Rectangular collimators prevent irradiation of nonvisualized portions of the II.

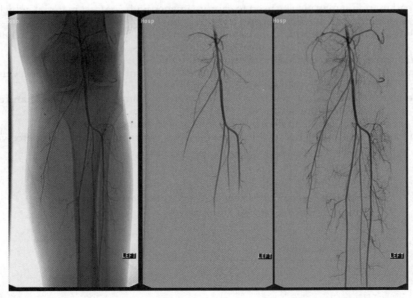

FIGURE 4.6   Digital subtraction angiography of the femoral artery with the left image showing all the patient anatomy and the two right images showing the vasculature alone.

E. **Digital subtraction angiography**
    –In **digital subtraction angiography** (DSA), a digital **mask** image (no vascular contrast) is subtracted from subsequent frames following **contrast administration.**
    –**DSA** images show only the **contrast-filled vessels.**
    –Table 4.8 shows the typical exposure factors used in DSA imaging.
    –**DSA** can detect **low-contrast objects,** so less contrast material is needed.
    –DSA can be used to visualize contrast differences of <**1%** in **x-ray transmission.**
        –Differences of 2% to 3% may often be missed with film–screen or nonsubtracted digital acquisitions.
    –Studies of the venous system use direct venous contrast injections, and studies of the arterial system use direct arterial contrast injections.
    –The **mean rate** of **flow** of **iodine** contrast through a vessel can be determined.
        –The degree of **vessel stenosis** may also be estimated.
    –DSA and temporal subtraction techniques in general are quite susceptible to **patient motion** including breathing, cardiac motion, and vascular pulsation.
    –**Corrections** for **patient motion** may be made by computer manipulation of the digital images stored in memory.
        –Methods of motion correction may incorporate **spatial displacement** of the mask frame or selection of a later frame for use as the mask **(remasking).**
    –Figure 4.6 shows a clinical example of DSA.

REVIEW TEST

4.1 The ideal photon energy (keV) for performing mammography is most likely:
a. 10
b. 15
c. 19
d. 25
e. 33

4.2 The standard focal spot size (mm) in mammography is:
a. 0.1
b. 0.2
c. 0.3
d. 0.6
e. 1.2

4.3 Molybdenum filters in mammography most likely have a thickness (μm) of:
a. 1
b. 3
c. 10
d. 30
e. 100

4.4 The most likely grid ratio in contact mammography is:
a. no grid used
b. 2:1
c. 5:1
d. 8:1
e. 12:1

4.5 The average gradient of a mammography film is most likely:
a. 1
b. 2
c. 3
d. 5
e. 10

4.6 The optimum film density in mammography is:
a. 0.8
b. 1.4
c. 1.8
d. 2.2
e. 2.6

4.7 Calcifications in mammograms are visible because of their:
a. atomic number
b. physical density
c. electron density
d. cross-sectional area
e. linear thickness

4.8 Compression in mammography increases:
a. tube loading
b. breast thickness

c. x-ray penetration
d. average glandular dose
e. image magnification

4.9 Power (kW) supplied to a mammography x-ray tube is most likely:
a. 1
b. 3
c. 10
d. 30
e. 100

4.10 The most likely x-ray tube voltage (kV) in a screening film mammogram is:
a. 17
b. 20
c. 25
d. 30
e. 35

4.11 The exposure time (s) for magnification film mammogram is likely:
a. 0.1
b. 0.3
c. 1
d. 3
e. 10

4.12 Viewing mammography films would likely use viewboxes with a luminance (cd/m^2) of:
a. 500
b. 1,000
c. 1,500
d. 3,000
e. 5,000

4.13 The number of breast cancer deaths in the United States (2007) was:
a. 10,000
b. 20,000
c. 40,000
d. 80,000
e. 160,000

4.14 To pass ACR accreditation, a phantom image must show all the following *except*:
a. four fibers
b. three groups of microcalcifications
c. three masses
d. minimal artifacts
e. film density <1.2

4.15 Which repeat rate (%) is most likely to occur in screen–film mammography?
a. 0.1
b. 0.3
c. 1
d. 3
e. 10

4.16 The II input phosphor is most likely made of:
a. NaI
b. PbI
c. LiF
d. CsI
e. Se

4.17 The II flux gain is most likely:
a. 2
b. 5
c. 10
d. 25
e. 50

4.18 The brightness gain of a 250-mm-diameter II is most likely:
a. 3
b. 10
c. 30
d. 100
e. >100

4.19 Image intensifier output brightness during fluoroscopy is *least* influenced by:
a. tube voltage
b. tube current
c. exposure time
d. II diameter
e. phosphor thickness

4.20 Falloff in brightness at the periphery of a fluoroscopic image is called:
a. vignetting
b. pincushion distortion
c. barrel distortion
d. S-wave distortion
e. edge packing

4.21 The aspect ratio of high-definition TV is:
a. 4:3
b. 5:4
c. 7:5
d. 12:7
e. 16:9

4.22 Replacing a TV camera with a CCD would likely improve (%) fluoroscopy signal to noise ratio by:
a. 0
b. 25
c. 50
d. 100
e. >100

4.23 The most likely tube current (mA) in fluoroscopy is:
a. 3
b. 10
c. 30

d. 100
e. 300

4.24 Pulsed fluoroscopy would likely *acquire* images at a rate (frames per second) of:
a. 15
b. 30
c. 45
d. 60
e. >60

4.25 Automatic brightness control (ABC) in fluoroscopy attempts to maintain a constant:
a. tube voltage
b. tube current
c. exposure time
d. patient dose
e. II brightness

4.26 For constant techniques (kV/mA), switching an II from 250 mm to 125 mm input diameter likely increases skin doses (%) by:
a. 25
b. 50
c. 100
d. 200
e. 400

4.27 Tube currents (mA) in photospot imaging are most likely:
a. 0.3
b. 3
c. 30
d. 300
e. 3,000

4.28 What is the most likely matrix size of digital photospot image?
a. 256^2
b. 512^2
c. $1,024^2$
d. $2,048^2$
e. $4,096^2$

4.29 Use of temporal filtering in digital fluoroscopy would likely increase:
a. noise
b. scatter
c. dose
d. lag
e. contrast

4.30 Increasing the DSA matrix size would likely *decrease*:
a. pixel size
b. digitization rate
c. image contrast
d. data storage
e. processing time

ANSWERS AND EXPLANATIONS

4.1c. Photons of 19 keV have sufficient energy to penetrate the breast but are low enough to offer high image contrast.

4.2c. The standard focal spot size in mammography is 0.3 mm.

4.3d. A typical molybdenum filter thickness is 30 μm.

4.4c. Mammography imaging systems usually use grids of ~5:1 because there is less scatter at the low energies that are used (e.g., 25 kV).

4.5c. Mammography films have gradients of ~3.

4.6c. The optimum for mammography is ~1.8, as this maximizes image contrast.

4.7a. The high atomic number of calcium (Z = 20) strongly absorbs the low-energy x-rays used in mammography.

4.8c. X-ray penetration will increase with compression.

4.9b. Mammography x-ray tubes require about 3 kW of electrical power.

4.10c. Mammography techniques typically use 25 kV and 100 mAs; note that the average energy in mammography is likely to be ~19 keV, and it is primarily influenced by the Mo characteristic x-rays.

4.11d. Exposure times in mammography are long (>1 s), and 3 s for a magnification view is typical.

4.12d. The ACR accreditation program requires a viewbox luminance of at least 3,000 cd/m^2.

4.13c. It is estimated that in the United States, ~180,000 women are diagnosed with breast cancer each year and that ~40,000 die from this disease (2007).

4.14e. Film density would be >1.2 and typically ~1.6.

4.15d. A repeat rate of 3% is typical for a screen–film mammography facility.

4.16d. The input to an image intensifier is normally made of CsI, which has excellent x-ray absorption properties.

4.17e. A typical II flux gain is ~50.

4.18e. II brightness gains are ~5,000 (flux gain of ~50 and minification gain of ~100).

4.19c. Exposure time does not affect image brightness during fluoroscopy.

4.20a. Fall off in brightness at the periphery of a fluoroscopic image is called vignetting.

4.21e. HTDV uses a 16:9 aspect ratio, whereas traditional (analog) TV uses a 4:3 aspect ratio.

4.22a. Fluoroscopy is quantum noise limited imaging, which means that the TV/CCD will not be an additional source of significant noise.

4.23a. Low tube currents (~3 mA) are the norm in fluoroscopy.

4.24a. Since pulsed fluoroscopy uses <30 frames per second, it would *acquire* 15 frames per second.

4.25e. Automatic brightness control (ABC) is used to maintain a constant brightness at the output of an II.

4.26e. Halving the II input diameter will reduce the exposed CsI phosphor area to a quarter and require a fourfold increase (400%) in the radiation intensity if the II output brightness intensity is to be kept constant.

4.27d. A typical tube current used to generate a digital photospot image is 300 mA.

4.28c. The most common matrix size in digital photospot imaging is 1,024^2.

4.29d. Filtering requires frame averaging, which must increase image lag.

4.30a. Pixel size always decreases with increasing matrix size.

Chapter 5

COMPUTED TOMOGRAPHY

I. HARDWARE

A. X-ray tubes
- **High-frequency power** supplies are used in computed tomography (CT), capable of providing **stable tube currents** and **voltages.**
- Modern CT scanners make use of **slip ring** technology in which high voltage is supplied to the tube through contact rings in the gantry.
- Tube **voltages** range from **80** to **140 kV.**
- Tube currents can range up to **1,000 mA.**
- **Tube currents** are frequently **modulated** as the x-ray tube rotates around the patient.
    - **Tube currents** increase when the **path length increases,** as in a lateral abdominal projection compared to an anteroposterior (AP) projection.
- Time for a **360-degree rotation** of the x-ray tube currently ranges between **0.3** and **2 seconds.**
- Table 5.1 shows how x-ray tube rotation times have been reduced since the introduction of CT scanners into clinical practice in the early 1970s.
- Tube current of **800 mA** and rotation time of **0.3 s** corresponds to **240 mAs.**
- **Power** loading on CT x-ray tubes can be as high as ~**100 kW.**
    - A tube voltage of **120 kV** and tube current of **830 mA** corresponds to **100 kW.**
- Table 5.1 shows how x-ray tube power capabilities have increased since the early 1970s.
- CT x-ray tubes have a **large focal spot** with a size of ~**1 mm,** which can tolerate a power loading of **100 kW.**
- **Small** x-ray tube focal spots are about **half** the **size** of the large focal spot and can tolerate no more than ~**25 kW.**
- **Heat loading** on CT x-ray tubes is generally **high,** requiring high anode heat capacities.
- X-ray tube **anode heat capacities** are high, and can **exceed 4 MJ.**
    - **Anode heat dissipation** rates are ~**10 kW.**
- Recent innovations in x-ray tube design include a **rotating envelope vacuum vessel (Straton tube).**
    - The Straton tube is relatively light and has very **high heat dissipation** rate that is >**60 kW.**
- **CT x-ray tubes** are very **expensive,** with the price of some tubes exceeding $200,000.

B. Filtration
- The x-ray tube **anode–cathode axis** is positioned **perpendicular** to the **imaging plane** to reduce the heel effect.
- **Copper** or **aluminum filters** are used to filter the x-ray beam.
- The typical filtration on a CT x-ray tube is ~**6 mm Al.**
- The heavy filtration used with CT scanners typically produces a beam with an aluminum **half-value layer (HVL)** of up to **10 mm Al.**
    - **Heavy x-ray beam filtering reduces** x-ray **beam hardening** effects.
- A **bow tie filter** is used to **minimize** the **dynamic range** of exposures at the **detector.**
- Bow tie filters attenuate little in the center, but attenuation increases with increasing distance from the central ray.

TABLE 5.1   Representative Values of X-ray Tube Power and Minimum Scan Times in CT Scanning

Year (Approximate)	X-ray Tube Power (kW)	Minimum 360-degree Tube Rotation Time (s)
1975	2	300
1985	25	3
1995	50	1
2005	100	0.33

–**Bow tie filters** are made of a low Z material such as **Teflon** to minimize **beam hardening** differences.

–Bow tie filters also **reduce scatter** and **patient dose.**

C. Collimation

–**Collimators** are located at the **x-ray tube** as well as at the x-ray **detectors.**

–Collimation defines the **section thickness** on a single-slice scanner.

    –Collimation defines the total **beam width** in **multidetector CT (MDCT)** systems.

    –The **beam width** on a **64**-slice CT scanner is ∼**40 mm.**

    –The beam width on a **320-slice** scanner is ∼**160 mm.**

–Collimators also help reduce the amount of scatter radiation reaching the CT detectors.

–Some scanners have (optional) **antiscatter collimation** in the form of thin lamellae (e.g., 100-μm tantalum sheets).

    –Antiscatter collimation is located between the detector elements oriented along the long patient axis and aligned with the x-ray focus.

–Some CT scanners use a **high-resolution comb** whose teeth serve to reduce the detector aperture width.

–Use of a **high-resolution comb improves resolution** but will also **reduce dose efficiencies.**

D. Radiation detectors

–**Each detector** measures the intensity of radiation transmitted through the patient along **one ray.**

–Detectors are separated from each other by a **dead space** of ∼0.1 mm, which **reduces** the **geometric efficiency.**

    –**Geometric efficiencies** are ∼**90%** for detectors that are 1 mm wide.

–Modern CT scanners use **scintillators** that produce light when x-ray photons are absorbed.

–Scintillation detectors are coupled to a **light detector.**

    –Common light detectors are **photomultiplier tubes** and **photodiodes.**

–CT detectors should have a good **temporal response** and **rapid signal decay.**

    –CT detectors should also have **low afterglow characteristics.**

–Detectors have **high quantum efficiency,** which is the percentage of incident x-ray photons that are absorbed.

    –CT detectors have a **quantum efficiency** of >**90%.**

–**Scintillators convert** ∼**10%** of the **absorbed x-ray energy** into **light energy** (conversion efficiency).

–In CT detectors, an **electric signal** is produced that is **proportional** to the **incident radiation intensity.**

    –The signal acquired by each detector is digitized and stored in a computer.

–The most common material used in solid-state detectors is **cadmium tungstate (CdWO$_4$),** which is an efficient x-ray detector.

–**Cesium iodide, calcium fluoride,** and **bismuth germanate** may also be used.

E. Detector arrays

–**Single-slice CT scanners** had a **single detector array.**

    –A **detector array** contains ∼**800 individual detectors** in axial plane for each slice that is acquired.

–A single-slice CT scanner generates **one tomographic image (slice)** for each 360-degree rotation of the x-ray tube.

–Single-slice CT scanners are rapidly being replaced by **multidetector CT (MDCT)** scanners.

–MDCT scanners have a number of detector arrays that allow multiple tomographic images to be acquired per 360-degree rotation of the x-ray tube.

–**Four-slice MDCT** were introduced into clinical practice in 1998, which produce **four images (slices) per 360-degree x-ray tube rotation.**

–By 2004, 64-slice MDCT were in clinical operation.

–A **64-slice MDCT** has **64 detector arrays,** each with a dimension of ~0.6 along the long patient axis, which can generate **64 × 0.6 thick slices** for **each x-ray tube rotation.**

   –The beam width for this 64 slice CT scanner is ~40 mm (i.e., 64 × 0.6 mm).

   –Figure 5.1 shows a schematic depiction of a 64-slice CT scanner.

–MDCT scanners have been developed to acquire **320 slices** in one 360-degree rotation of the x-ray tube, with each slice having a thickness of 0.5 mm.

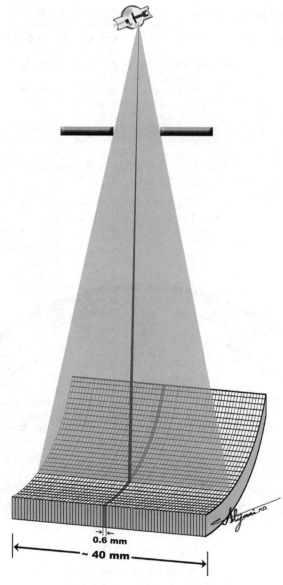

FIGURE 5.1   Schematic depiction of a MDCT with 64 rows of detector aligned along the long patient axis.

–A 320-slice CT scanner has a beam width of 160 mm (i.e., 320 × 0.5 mm) and covers the **brain** or **left ventricle** in **one x-ray tube rotation.**
–MDCT scanners with thin patient axis slices now have **isotropic resolution.**
  –Isotropic resolution permits **nonaxial reconstructions** *without* stretching pixels.

II. IMAGES

A. Image acquisition
  –For each position of the x-ray tube, a **fan beam** is passed through the patient.
  –In body imaging, the **fan beam angle** is ∼**50 degrees.**
    –A fan beam of 50 degrees corresponds to a **field** of **view** with a **50-cm diameter.**
  –Measurements of the **transmitted x-ray beam intensities** are made by an array of detectors.
  –The total **x-ray transmission** measured by **each detector** is the result of the **sum** of the **attenuation** by **all** the **tissues** the **beam** has **passed through** (i.e., **ray sum**).
  –The **collection** of **ray sums** for all the detectors at a **given tube position** is called a **projection.**
  –Each **projection** has ∼**800 individual data points** corresponding to the ∼800 individual detectors in a single array (single-slice scanner).
  –Figure 5.2 shows the acquisition of a single projection at one position of the x-ray tube.
  –**Projection data** sets are acquired at **different angles** around the patient.
  –A **CT image** generally requires ∼**1,000 projections** for a single rotation of the x-ray tube.
  –A graphic plot of **projections** as a **function** of **x-ray tube angle** is called a **sinogram.**
  –Figure 5.3 shows a typical sinogram that consists of projections acquired through all the angular positions of the x-ray tube as it rotates 360 degrees around the patient.
  –**CT images** are derived by mathematical **analysis** of **projection data sets (sinograms)** at each location along the long patient axis.
B. Image reconstruction
  –Generating an **image** from the acquired data involves determining the **linear attenuation coefficients** of the **individual pixels** in the image matrix.
  –A mathematical **algorithm** takes the multiple **projection data** (raw data) and reconstructs the **cross-sectional CT image** (image data).

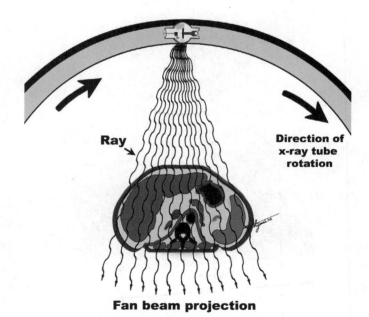

Ray

Direction of x-ray tube rotation

Fan beam projection

FIGURE 5.2 Schematic depiction of a single projection transmitted through the patient, consisting of ∼700 individual rays.

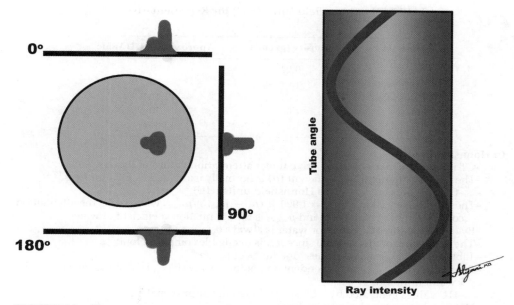

FIGURE 5.3 Three projections as acquired at x-ray tube angles of 0 degrees, 90 degrees, and 180 degrees **(left),** and the resultant sinogram **(right)** showing all projections stacked on top of each other.

–**Back projection** allocates the measured total attenuation **(ray sum)** *equally to each pixel along the x-ray path* through the patient.
–Modern scanners use **filtered back projection** image reconstruction algorithms.
–**Projection data** are **convolved** with a **(mathematical) filter** before being back projected.
  –Convolution is a type of mathematical multiplication.
 –Image reconstruction involving millions of data points may be performed in less than a second using **array processors** (number crunchers).
–Different **filters may** be used in **filtered back projection reconstruction.**
  –Commercial CT scanners typically offer six or seven filters for clinical use.
–The **choice** of **filter** in the reconstruction algorithm offers **tradeoffs** between spatial **resolution** and **random noise.**
–Some filters (e.g., **bone**) permit **reconstruction** of **fine detail** but with **increased noise.** Other filters (e.g., **soft tissue**) **decrease noise** but also **decrease resolution.**
–Table 5.2 shows how the amount of noise in reconstructed CT images varies with the type of reconstruction filter.
–The choice of the **best filter** to use with the reconstruction algorithm **depends** on the **clinical task.**
–**Iterative (trial** and **error)** methods such as **algebraic reconstruction techniques (ART)** have been used for image reconstruction.
–There is a **resurgence** of **interest** in **iterative reconstruction techniques** in CT.
  –**Iterative reconstruction** algorithms may offer an effective means for **minimizing CT artifacts** (e.g., streak).

TABLE 5.2   Relative Image Noise Values as a Function of the Choice of CT Image Reconstruction Filter

Reconstruction Filter	Relative Noise (Approximate)
Smooth	1
Standard or soft tissue	1.5
Bone	3
Bone plus or edge	5

TABLE 5.3   Hounsfield Units (HU) for Representative Materials

Material	Density (g/cm^3)	Approximate HU Value
Fat	0.92	−90
White matter	1.03	30
Gray matter	1.04	40
Muscle	1.06	50
Cortical bone	1.8	1,000+

C. Hounsfield units
   –CT **images** are maps of the **relative linear attenuation values** of **tissues.**
   –The *relative* **attenuation coefficient (μ)** is normally expressed as **CT numbers.**
      –**CT numbers** are known as **Hounsfield units (HU).**
   –The HU of material x is **HU$_x$ = 1,000 × (μ_x − μ_{water})/μ_{water}** where μ_x is the attenuation coefficient of the material x and μ_{water} is the attenuation coefficient of water.
   –By definition, the **HU value** for **water** is **always 0.**
   –**The HU** value for **air** is **–1,000** since μ_{air} is negligible compared to μ_{water}.
   –Table 5.3 lists typical HU values for a range of tissues.
   –Because μ_x and μ_{water} are dependent on photon energy (keV), HU values depend on the kV and filtration.
      –**HU values** generated by a CT scanner are only **approximate.**
   –**HU** may be used to **characterize tissue.**
      –For example, a HU of –100 suggests that the tissue being examined is fat and a HU of +50 suggests the tissue being examined is muscle.
D. Field of view
   –The **field of view (FOV)** is the diameter of the body region being imaged.
      –A **head** CT normally has a **FOV** of ~**25 cm.**
      –A **body** CT normally has a **FOV** of ~**40 cm.**
   –The **matrix size** in CT is normally **512 × 512.**
   –CT **pixel size** is determined by dividing the FOV by the matrix size.
   –Pixel sizes are **0.5 mm** for a **25-cm diameter FOV head** scan (25 cm divided by 512).
      –Pixel sizes are **0.8 mm** for a **40-cm FOV body** scan (40 cm divided by 512).
   –**Voxel** is a volume element in the patient.
      –**Voxel volume** is the product of the **pixel area** and **slice thickness.**
   –In the early days of CT, the acquired slice thickness ranged from 1 to 10 mm.
   –For **MDCT,** the acquired slice thickness is generally ~**0.5** to ~**0.6 mm.**
   –Figure 5.4 shows voxel and pixel sizes encountered in CT.
   –The field of view may be reduced by reducing the **fan beam angle.**
   –Unlike diagnostic x-rays, **regions outside** of a **reduced FOV** will receive a **direct dose.**
E. Image display
   –A **35-cm-long chest CT scan,** acquired with a **0.5-mm slice thickness,** would result in **700 images.**
      –**CT images** are normally **viewed** with a **3-** or **5-mm slice thickness,** which combines six to 10 thin slices.
   –CT images viewed on **monitors** have a **pixel brightness** related to the **average attenuation coefficient.**
   –Each pixel is normally represented by **12 bits,** or **4,096 gray levels.**
   –**Window width** and **level** optimize the **appearance** of **CT images** by determining the contrast and brightness levels assigned to the CT image data.
   –Figure 5.5 shows how the choice of window and level value affects the appearance of a given CT number (HU value).
   –CT images with a window width of 100 HU and a window level (center) of 50 HU have HU <0 black, HU >100 white, and HU ~50 mid-gray.
   –Window **(width** and **level)** settings **affect** only the **displayed image,** *not* the reconstructed **image data** stored in the computer.
   –Table 5.4 shows typical window and level settings used in clinical CT.
   –**Multiplanar reformatting** (MPR) generates **coronal, sagittal,** or **oblique** images from the original axial image data.
   –**Maximum intensity projection** (MIP) is useful to visualize tortuous vessels with contrast agent.

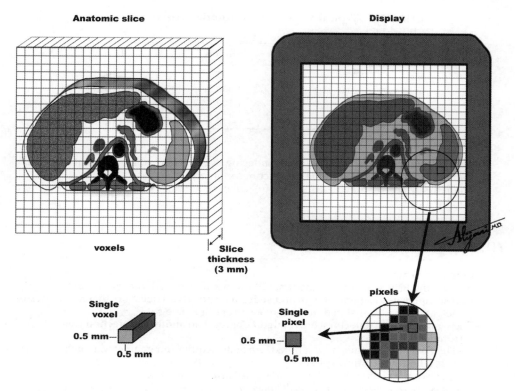

FIGURE 5.4   Schematic representation of an anatomic slice **(left)** and the corresponding image display **(right)** showing typical pixels and voxels in CT imaging.

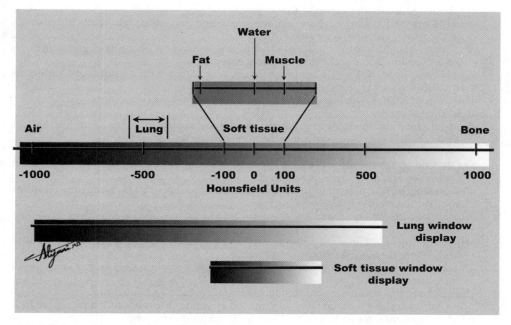

FIGURE 5.5   The CT number scale (Hounsfield unit) ranges from −1,000 to ∼+1,000. Its appearance depends on the choice of window level and window width.

TABLE 5.4   Typical Window/Level Settings Used in
Clinical CT

Type of Examination	Window	Level
Head	80	40
Chest (mediastinum)	450	40
Chest (lung)	1,500	−500
Abdomen (liver)	150	60

- **Three-dimensional (3-D)** or **volume rendering** of CT data requires segmentation of the image data to select the tissue or structures of interest.
- **Shaded surface display** is a method for creating surface renderings that simulate a lighted object.

III. SCANNER OPERATION

A. Acquisition geometry
  - In 1972, the **EMI** scanner was the first CT scanner introduced into clinical practice.
  - EMI scanners used a **pencil beam** and **sodium iodide** (NaI) detectors that moved across the patient (i.e., **translated**) to obtain one projection data set.
  - The **x-ray tube** and **detector** were **rotated 1 degree,** and **another projection** was obtained (rotation).
    - The EMI scanner thus used a **translate/rotate acquisition geometry,** which is known as a **first-generation system.**
  - The **CT scanner generation** defines the **acquisition geometry.**
    - *An old generation is not (necessarily) inferior.*
  - **Second-generation** scanners also use translate-rotate technology but have multiple detectors and a fan-shaped beam.
  - **Third-generation** scanners use a wide rotating fan beam coupled with a large array of detectors (**rotate-rotate** system).
    - The geometric relationship between the tube and detectors does not change as it rotates 360 degrees around the patient.
  - **Fourth-generation** scanners have a rotating tube and fixed ring of detectors (up to 4,800) in the gantry (rotate-fixed system).
  - For single-slice CT scanners, **third-** and **fourth**-generation acquisition geometries resulted in **similar patient doses** and **image quality.**
  - The advent of **MDCT** made the manufacture of scanners with a **fourth-generation acquisition geometry cost prohibitive.**
  - **All current MDCT** systems use **third-generation acquisition geometry.**
B. Single-slice scanners
  - In **axial** scanning, the **table** and **patient** remain **stationary** while the x-ray tube rotates through 360 degrees and acquires the necessary projection data.
    - A single-slice CT scanner generates one slice per 360-degree x-ray tube rotation.
  - At the completion of the x-ray tube rotation, the **table** is **moved** a distance (e.g., beam width W), and the process is repeated.
  - A **scan length** of L will normally require a total of approximately **L/W x-ray tube rotations** to cover the anatomic region of interest.
  - For some examinations, the table increment distance can be much greater than the section thickness.
  - **High-resolution CT** in chest imaging may be performed using a **1-mm detector width** and a **table increment distance** of **10 mm.**
  - A table increment distance greater than the x-ray beam width results in a sampling of the anatomic region.
  - Sampling in this manner risks missing lesions but greatly reduces doses.
    - A table **increment distance** of **10 mm,** and a section **thickness** of **1 mm,** will **reduce** the **patient dose** to **10%** of the dose for contiguous imaging.
  - In **helical CT** acquisitions, the patient is moved along the horizontal axis as the x-ray tube rotates around the patient.

–The **x-ray beam** central ray follows a **helical path** during the CT scan.

–The relation between patient and tube motion is called **pitch,** defined as the **table movement** during each x-ray tube rotation divided by the total **x-ray beam width.**

–For a 5-mm beam width, if the patient moves 10 mm during the time it takes for the x-ray tube to rotate through 360 degrees, the pitch is 2.

–**Increasing pitch reduces** the **scan time** and **patient dose.**

–Image reconstruction is obtained by **interpolating projection data** obtained at selected locations along the patient axis.

–**Images** can be **reconstructed** at **any level** and in **any increment** but have a thickness equal to the collimation used.

    –**Reconstructed images** can have a greater thickness than the collimation, but *cannot* be **less** than the **collimation.**

C. Electron beam CT

–**Electron beam CT** (EBCT) uses an electron gun that deflects and focuses a fast-moving electron beam along a 210-degree arc of a large-diameter tungsten target ring in the gantry.

    –**EBCT** is also known as **fifth-generation CT** or **ultrafast CT.**

–The x-ray beam produced is collimated to traverse the patient and strike a detector ring.

–Two detector rings permit the simultaneous acquisition of two image sections.

–There is **no motion** by the **x-ray tube** or **detector array,** which allows images to be obtained in as little as **50 ms** with **minimum motion artifacts.**

–The major advantage of electron beam CT is the **speed** of **data acquisition,** which can **freeze cardiac motion.**

–Images of the **whole heart** can be acquired in ∼**0.2 s (eight images).**

–Serial images of a given section can be acquired **every 50 ms (cine mode).**

–The advent of MDCT, as well as (fast) dual-source CT scanners, is now rendering **EBCT obsolete.**

D. Multidetector

–Table 5.5 shows the historical evolution of multislice CT scanning.

–An **N-slice MDCT** scanner generates **N projections** at **each position** of the x-ray tube.

–In **axial mode, one complete rotation** of the x-ray tube will **generate N slices.**

–*Acquisition* **slice thickness** is determined by the **detector width.**

–Detector widths are normally **0.5 to 0.6 mm,** which offers a **slice thickness** that is *comparable* to the (in plane) **pixel dimension.**

–The **beam width** in MDCT equals the **number** of **slices multiplied** by **acquisition slice thickness (detector width).**

–In helical mode, different classes of **interpolation algorithms** are used by different vendors.

    –Common modes of interpolation are **linear** and **z-filtering.**

–Use of **linear interpolation** algorithms **restricts** the **choice** of pitch to a few fixed values.

–Use of **z-filtering** offers **much greater flexibility** in the choice of **pitch.**

–Scanners with N detector rows can simulate scanners that have N/2 detector rows by adding data from adjacent slices.

–The **number** of x-ray tube rotations is given by the **scan length** (L) divided by the **beam width.**

    –A 64-slice CT (∼40-mm beam width) scanner performing an abdominal scan with a length of 32 cm requires only eight x-ray tube rotations.

–**A 360-degree x-ray tube rotation** takes between **0.3** and **2 seconds.**

–**Longer rotation** times are **used** to **increase mAs.**

TABLE 5.5   Historical Evolution of MSCT Technology

Year	Number of Slices per X-ray Tube Rotation
1994	2^a
1998	4
2001	16
2004	64
2008	320

[a] Original EMI (1973) also used two NaI detectors generating two slices per x-ray tube rotation

–Slow rotation times are common in head CT where motion is minimal.

–Fast rotation times are used in body imaging to reduce motion artifacts.

–With a **0.3-second rotation time,** an **abdominal CT scan** (eight rotations) can be completed in **2.4 seconds.**

E. Dual-source CT

–A **dual-source CT** has recently been developed that offers improved **temporal resolution** for **cardiac imaging.**

–The scanner has **two x-ray tubes** and **two detector arrays.**

–Both acquisition systems are mounted on a rotating gantry with **angular offset** of **90 degrees.**

–One detector array covers a **field of view** of **50 cm** (fan angle 52 degrees).

–The second detector array has a **smaller FOV** of **26 cm** (fan angle 27 degrees).

–Gantry space limitations restrict the size of the second detector array.

–Gantry rotation time is 0.33 second.

–**Two 80-kW** generators power each x-ray tube.

–**Partial scans** (half scans) are used for electrocardiographically gated CT image reconstruction.

–**Temporal resolution** is approximately **half** of the **gantry rotation time** for a **single-source** CT scanner.

–The dual-source CT scanner has **temporal resolution** of a quarter of the gantry rotation time

–Dual-source CT permits a temporal resolution as short as **83 ms.**

–**Data from** only **one cardiac cycle** are used, and **temporal resolution** is **independent** of **heart rate.**

–Dual-source CT can perform **multisegment reconstruction,** further improving temporal resolution.

IV. DOSIMETRY

A. Dose distributions

–A **single rotation** of the x-ray tube will deposit approximately **one half** of the absorbed energy in the **directly irradiated volume.**

–The remaining half of the absorbed energy is deposited in **scattered tails** adjacent to the directly irradiated slab.

–A scanned volume may have **absorbed doses** that **vary** between the **center** and **peripheral** (surface) regions.

–In **head** scans, **central** and **surface** doses are very **similar.**

–In **body** scans, **surface** doses are generally **higher** than the **central** dose.

–In a **32-cm-diameter acrylic phantom,** the **surface** dose is **twice** that obtained at the **center** of the phantom.

–Tissues beyond the directly irradiated region are always exposed to **scatter radiation.**

–Scattered radiation intensities fall rapidly as one moves away from the directly irradiated region.

–**Scatter radiation intensities** are **reduced** because of the loss of intensity from the **inverse square law,** as well as from **attenuation** by the intervening tissues.

–Absorbed **doses** in body regions that **receive only scattered** radiation are *much lower* than organ doses in the directly irradiated volume.

B. CT dose index (theory)

–Manufacturers specify CT doses by the **CT dose index (CTDI).**

–CTDI is obtained from the **dose distribution** that occurs when the x-ray tube performs **one single 360-degree rotation** with no table motion.

–An acrylic cylinder with a **16-cm diameter** is normally taken to represent an adult patient **head.**

–The head CT dosimetry phantom can also represent a pediatric abdomen.

–An acrylic cylinder with a **32-cm diameter** is normally taken to represent an adult **body.**

–Most patients are smaller than a 32-cm acrylic phantom, and dose measurements made in this phantom will *underestimate* patient doses.

–The **CTDI** is obtained by **integrating** the **axial dose profile** for a single CT slice and then dividing this integral by the beam width (i.e., slice thickness).

–**CTDI** values are measured in terms of **air kerma** and are specified in **mGy.**

–Integration of the axial dose profile is normally achieved using a pencil-shaped ionization chamber that is **100 mm** long.
   –Measurements made with 100-mm-long pencil-shaped ionization chambers are expressed as **CTDI$_{100}$**.
–CTDI measurements *include* the energy deposited in the **scatter tails.**
–Values of **CTDI predict** the **dose** that results from a series of **contiguous scans.**
–CTDI measurements can also be made at the **scanner isocenter** in the **absence** of **any patient** or **phantom.**
   –Air measurements are expressed as **CTDI$_{air}$.**
–At 120 kV, typical **CTDI$_{air}$** values for commercial CT scanners are ~**0.25 mGy/mAs.**

C. **CT dose index (practice)**
   –CTDI measurements may be made at the surface **(periphery)** of the phantom and specified as **CTDI$_p$.**
   –Measurements made at the **center** of the phantom are specified as **CTDI$_c$.**
   –A weighted CTDI (i.e., **CTDI$_w$**) is defined as **2/3 CTDI$_p$ + 1/3 CTDI$_c$.**
   –CTDI$_w$ is taken to approximate the average dose in the dosimetry phantom when the phantom is scanned contiguously.
   –For a **head** phantom (16-cm diameter acrylic), CTDI$_w$ is ~**0.2 mGy/mAs** (120 kV).
      –Head phantom CTDI doses are about 75% of those measured free in air (CTDI$_{air}$).
   –For a **body** phantom (32-cm-diameter acrylic), CTDI$_w$ is ~**0.1 mGy/mAs** (120 kV).
   –At the same techniques, body phantom doses are generally about half those of head phantoms.
   –Doses in **helical scanning** modes with a **pitch** of **1.0** are **similar** to those resulting from **contiguous axial scanning.**
   –If the **pitch** is <**1.0, doses increase** because of overlapping scans.
   –When **pitch increases** to **more than 1.0, doses decrease** because the energy is spread out over a larger volume.
   –To account for different pitch values in helical scanning, the **volume CTDI$_{vol}$** has been introduced as **CTDI$_w$/pitch.**
      –For a **pitch** of 1.0, CTDI$_w$ and CTDI$_{vol}$ are **equal.**
   –CTDI$_{vol}$ is **independent** of the total **scan length,** whereas the amount of radiation received by the patient is directly proportional to the scan length.
   –The **dose length product** (DLP) is the **product** of **CTDI$_{vol}$** and **scan length.**
      –The **DLP** is **proportional** to the **total dose (energy) imparted** to the **patient.**
   –**DLP** is a good indicator of the total amount of **radiation incident** on a **patient.**

D. **CT techniques**
   –CT **doses** are directly **proportional** to the **mA** and the **scan rotation time.**
   –Figure 5.6 shows how CTDI doses vary with x-ray tube voltage.
   –Increasing the x-ray tube voltage from **80 kV** to **140 kV increases doses fivefold.**
      –Body doses in Figure 5.6 are lower because the larger phantom attenuates the x-ray beam much more than the head phantom.
   –**CT doses** are **inversely proportional** to **pitch.**
      –A pitch of 2 halves the dose, and a pitch of 0.5 doubles the dose.
   –**Tube current modulation** can reduce patient doses without adversely affecting image quality.
   –The tube current may be modulated as the x-ray tube rotates around the patient (**angular**).
      –In scanning the abdomen, the tube current would be **reduced** for **anteroposterior (AP)** and **posteroanterior (PA) projections relative** to those used for **lateral projections.**
   –The tube current may be modulated as the patient passes through the CT scanner.
      –Tube currents are **reduced** in the **chest (lung) region relative** to the **shoulders** and **abdomen.**
   –In cardiac CT, **temporal modulation** is used to reduce the tube current in the **systolic** part of the cardiac cycle.
      –Images acquired during **systole have increased mottle** because of the reduced mA but are **adequate** for **functional analysis** (cardiac ejection fraction, etc.).

E. **Patient doses**
   –Patient dose is directly proportional to the product of the **acquired slice thickness** and the total **number** of **slices** in the CT examination.
   –Performing **multiphase studies** can substantially increase patient doses.
      –For constant techniques, performing four-phase examinations (precontrast, arterial, venous, and equilibrium) would **quadruple** the **patient dose.**

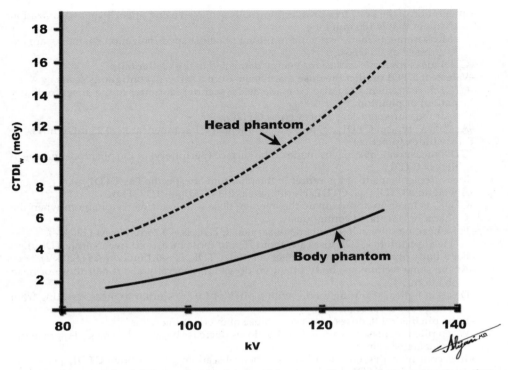

FIGURE 5.6 Weighted CTDI$_w$ values (mGy) per 100 mAs as a function of x-ray tube voltage (kV) in head and body phantoms.

- –**Multidetector CT** has radiation **doses similar** to those of **axial CT** for *similar image quality.*
- –The **American College of Radiology** runs a CT Accreditation Program, including CT dosimetry data.
- –Data are acquired pertaining to **adult head** scans, **adult abdomen** scans, and **pediatric body** scans.
- –The mean value of **CTDI$_{vol}$** for an **adult head** is **58 mGy** (16-cm phantom), and for an **adult abdomen** is **18 mGy** (32-cm phantom).
- –**Reference doses** are set by considering the **75th percentile value** of the doses reported to the ACR CT Accreditation Program.
- –Values that exceed the 75th percentile should be investigated, and reduced if this is possible without adversely affecting diagnostic performance.
- –Doses that are higher than published **reference values** need to be justified by a corresponding improvement in diagnostic performance.
- –Table 5.6 shows the current (2008) values of reference doses for CTDI$_{vol}$ in CT in the United States.

F. **Pediatric doses**
- –For a **5-year-old pediatric abdomen** examination, the mean **CTDI$_{vol}$** is **16 mGy** as measured in a 16-cm-diameter phantom.
- –When scanning **children,** it is essential that **reduced techniques (mAs)** are used.

TABLE 5.6   ACR CT Accreditation Program Reference Doses for CTDI$_{vol}$ in 2008

Examination Type	Reference CTDI$_{vol}$ (mGy)	Diameter of Phantom Used for Dose Measurement (cm)
Adult head	75	16
Adult abdomen	25	32
Pediatric abdomen (5-year-old)	20	16

TABLE 5.7   Percentage (%) Transmission through the Abdomen of Patients of Varying Weight (120 kV).

Weight (kg)	% Transmission through Abdomen
20	3.1
30	2.0
50	0.90
70	0.41
100	0.13

–Table 5.7 shows the relationship between patient size and x-ray beam penetration.
  –**Increasing** the **patient** size from **20** to **100 kg reduces x-ray beam penetration** by a **factor** of **30.**
–Reduced techniques are possible because x-ray penetration is much greater in children than in adults.
–**Large dose reductions** may be possible when performing **body CT examinations** in **very young children.**
–Table 5.8 shows typical dose reductions that should be achievable when performing body CT examinations in pediatric patients.
–**Dose reductions** when performing **pediatric head CT** examinations are much more **modest.**
–Technique factors (mAs) for a 5-year-old head examination would be only ~5% lower than for an adult.
–**Technique reductions** would be ~**15%** for a **1-year-old** and ~**25%** in a **newborn** undergoing a standard head CT examination.

V. MISCELLANEOUS

A. Clinical techniques
–Most CT scans are performed using **120 kV.**
–Higher kV values **(140 kV)** may be used in head CT scanning (posterior fossa) to help minimize beam hardening artifacts.
  –A **higher kV** may also be used to **improve penetration** of **larger patients.**
–Reduced x-ray tube voltages **(80 kV)** are used when imaging **iodinated contrast** material.
–Lower x-ray tube voltages **(80 kV** or **100 kV)** may be used in **pediatric CT** to help **reduce patient doses.**
–In **head CT** scanning, x-ray tube **rotation times** are **longer (~1 s)** where motion is minimal, and higher radiation intensities are required to minimize quantum mottle.
–In body CT scanning, the faster rotation speeds are used to minimize the scan time.
  –**Short scan times reduce motion artifacts** and help **minimize** the amount of **iodinated contrast** material administered to the patient.
–**Tube currents** are selected based on the **total mAs required** for a given CT examination.
–Routine adult **head CT** scans use ~**300 mAs** (i.e., CTDI$_{vol}$ ~**60 mGy**).
  –Adult **chest CT** scans use ~**150 mAs** (i.e., CTDI$_{vol}$ ~**15 mGy**).
  –Adult **abdominal CT** scans use ~**200 mAs** (i.e., CTDI$_{vol}$ ~**20 mGy**).

TABLE 5.8   Approximate Techniques (mAs) for Routine Body CT Examinations (Adult mAs Is 100%)

Pediatric Patient Age (Years)	Thorax CT Examination (%)	Abdomen CT Examination (%)
Newborn	40	45
1	50	55
5	60	65
10	65	70
15	75	80

–**Clinical protocols** should specify **CTDI$_{vol}$,** and not just the mAs.
    –There are **large dose differences** between **scanners** at the **same mAs** resulting from variations in x-ray tube design and filtration.

B. CT and planar imaging
–All CT examinations begin with acquisition of a **projection radiograph.**
    –Projection radiographs are also known as **topographic** or **scout images.**
–Projection radiographs have markedly different properties from CT tomographic images in terms of detection performance, spatial resolution, and radiation dose.
–CT images are superior to projection radiographs because they **eliminate overlapping tissues.**
–CT images also permit the visualization of planes in any orientation (volume imaging).
–**CT** can **detect lesions** that differ about **0.3%** from the surrounding tissues.
    –**Screen–film radiography** requires the lesion to differ by ~3% for **detection.**
–Fine detail visibility in CT is less than in projection radiography.
–**Pixels** in **CT** (~0.6 mm) are **three times larger** than in a **chest radiograph** (~0.2 mm).
–**Radiation doses** in **CT** are much **higher** than those for conventional **radiographs.**
–A single **chest CT** scan is normally taken to have a radiation dose (risk) that is comparable to **100 conventional chest x-rays.**

C. Cardiac imaging
–**Cardiac imaging** is best performed in the **diastolic phase** of the cardiac cycle.
–During diastole, cardiac motion can be minimal for periods of 250 ms at moderate heart rates.
–**Calcium scoring** makes use of prospective cardiac triggering and sequential (**step** and **shoot**) scanning.
–To cover the complete heart with prospective triggering can take a long time (up to 30 seconds).
–**Long scan times** in cardiac imaging result in **registration problems** from slice to slice because of respiration-related motion.
–Most **cardiac imaging** using **64-slice MDCT** is currently performed using helical scanning and **retrospective electrocardiogram (ECG)-correlated image reconstruction.**
–**Retrospective** cardiac imaging requires the use of **low pitch** values that are typically between 0.2 and 0.3 and depend on the patient's heart rate.
–Use of **low pitch** in cardiac imaging **markedly increases** the **patient dose.**
    –**Patient doses** with **retrospective** imaging are **three** or more times **higher** than those associated with **prospective imaging.**
–**Temporal resolution** in single-source scanners is **generally half,** or slightly greater than, the x-ray tube **rotation time.**
    –With a **300-ms** rotation time, **temporal resolution** can be as low as **150 ms.**
–**Image reconstruction windows** during the cardiac cycle are selected by the operator and chosen where cardiac motion is minimal.
–**Multisegment reconstruction** makes use of image data from multiple heart beats.
    –Multisegment reconstructions offer **improved temporal resolution** but require use of **lower pitch** values and **increase patient dose.**

D. CT fluoroscopy
–CT images can be reconstructed in near real time during continuous rotation of the tube.
–In **CT fluoroscopy,** the CT image is **constantly updated** to include the latest projection data (e.g., 60-degree increments).
–Images are typically updated at the rate of **six per second,** which provides **excellent temporal resolution.**
–Any **motion** at the image level can then be **followed** in **nearly real time** by observing the updated reconstruction.
–This facilitates advancement of a needle for **biopsies** or **drainage** procedures.
–**Low tube currents (20–50 mA)** are used to **minimize radiation** doses.
–Radiation dose are often reduced even further for some diagnostic tasks (e.g., tracking a biopsy needle).

E. Dual energy
–**Dual-energy** CT requires the acquisition of projection data using **two x-ray tube voltages** that produce spectra that differ in their average energies.
    –Dual-energy CT would likely use **80 kV** and **140 kV** for data acquisition.
–In dual-energy CT, the **HU value** of **each pixel** is obtained at **two different average energies.**

–One way of performing dual-energy CT is to **rapidly switch** the **x-ray tube voltage** and acquire similar projections at two energies.

–Use of two x-ray tubes **(dual-source CT)** also **permits** the acquisition of two sets of similar projection data at two **different energies.**

–Dual-energy CT **improves** the **delineation** of **different materials** that have **similar linear attenuation coefficients.**

  –Dual-energy CT improves the differentiation of **iodine** and **bone.**

–**Clinical applications** of dual-energy CT are under **active investigation.**

F. **Artifacts**

–CT images may have **artifacts** that degrade diagnostic quality.

–**Partial-volume** artifact is the result of averaging the linear attenuation coefficient in a voxel that is heterogenous in composition.

–**Motion** artifacts result from involuntary (e.g., cardiac) and voluntary patient motion.

  –Random or unpredictable motion (e.g., if the patient sneezes) produces **streak artifacts** in the direction of motion.

–In high-density structures, such as metal implants, the detector may record no transmission, complicating the filtered back projection and resulting in **star artifacts.**

  –In these cases, the reconstruction algorithm generates streaks adjacent to the high-density structures.

–**Beam hardening** artifacts are caused by the polychromatic nature of the x-ray beam (beam hardening).

–As the lower-energy photons are preferentially absorbed, the beam becomes more penetrating, causing underestimation of the attenuation coefficient (HU).

  –Software algorithms have been developed to reduce beam hardening artifacts that incorporate prior knowledge of the patient (e.g., skull in head CT).

–**Ring artifacts** may arise in third-generation systems if a single detector is faulty or the CT scanner is not properly calibrated.

REVIEW TEST

5.1 The heat capacity of a CT x-ray tube anode (kJ) is most likely:
a. 0.4
b. 4
c. 40
d. 400
e. 4,000

5.2 The power (kW) applied to a modern CT x-ray tube is most likely:
a. 1
b. 3
c. 10
d. 30
e. 100

5.3 A CT beam shaping filter (bow tie) is most likely made out of:
a. aluminum
b. copper
c. molybdenum
d. Teflon
e. tin

5.4 CT collimation is most likely used to change the x-ray beam:
a. width
b. intensity
c. HVL
d. FOV
e. isocenter

5.5 The most likely x-ray beam width (mm) on a 64-row CT scanner is:
a. 0.5
b. 5
c. 10
d. 20
e. 40

5.6 The total number of individual detector elements on a 64-row CT scanner is most likely:
a. 64×100
b. 64×200
c. 64×400
d. 64×800
e. $64 \times 1,600$

5.7 The percentage (%) of incident radiation likely captured by a CT x-ray detector is:
a. 30
b. 45
c. 60
d. 75
e. >75

5.8 The number of projections obtained per 360-degree rotation of the x-ray tube in a single-slice CT scanner is most likely:
a. 500
b. 1,000

c. 2,000
d. 4,000
e. 8,000

5.9 Use of a bone filter, as opposed to a soft tissue filter, to reconstruct CT images would likely improve:
a. subject contrast
b. image contrast
c. scatter rejection
d. spatial resolution
e. data storage

5.10 The CT number (HU) is directly proportional to the pixel:
a. mass attenuation
b. linear attenuation
c. physical density
d. electron density
e. atomic number

5.11 Which of the following most likely has a Hounsfield unit of −90?
a. Fat
b. Gray matter
c. Water
d. Bone
e. Lung

5.12 The CT number is *least* likely to be affected by x-ray tube:
a. voltage
b. filtration
c. ripple
d. current
e. collimation

5.13 Increasing the width of the CT image display window will most likely reduce the:
a. display contrast
b. average brightness
c. image magnification
d. field of view
e. average HU

5.14 Increasing the CT image matrix from 256^2 to 512^2 will likely improve:
a. patient throughput
b. anode cooling
c. patient dose
d. spatial resolution
e. reconstruction time

5.15 The pixel size (μm) in a head CT image is most likely:
a. 50
b. 100
c. 250
d. 500
e. 1,000

5.16 What is the pitch when the x-ray beam width is 40 mm and the table moves 60 mm per x-ray tube rotation?
   a. 0.67
   b. $(0.67)^2$
   c. 1.5
   d. 1.5^2
   e. 1.5/0.67

5.17 The fastest x-ray tube rotation speed (second per x-ray tube rotation) is likely:
   a. 0.1
   b. 0.2
   c. 0.3
   d. 0.5
   e. 0.75

5.18 Replacing a single-slice CT with multislice CT most likely improves x-ray beam:
   a. production
   b. quality
   c. utilization
   d. intensity
   e. detection

5.19 The best temporal resolution (ms) in cardiac imaging on a dual-source CT is most likely:
   a. 20
   b. 40
   c. 80
   d. 160
   e. 320

5.20 The number of x-ray tube rotations required to measure the $CTDI_c$ in a head phantom is:
   a. 1
   b. 2
   c. 3
   d. 7
   e. 10

5.21 The ratio of the peripheral CTDI to the central CTDI in a body phantom is most likely:
   a. 0.25
   b. 0.5
   c. 1
   d. 2
   e. 4

5.22 If the peripheral CTDI is 12 mGy and the central CTDI is 6 mGy, the weighted $CTDI_w$ (mGy) is:
   a. 7
   b. 8
   c. 9
   d. 10
   e. 11

5.23 What is the dose length product (mGy-cm) for a $CTDI_w$ of 20 mGy, pitch of 2, and scan length of 100 cm?
   a. 200
   b. 400
   c. 500
   d. 800
   e. 1,000

5.24 The reference dose ($CTDI_{vol}$ mGy) recommended by the ACR (2008) for an adult head CT is:
   a. 25
   b. 50
   c. 75
   d. 100
   e. 125

5.25 If an adult head CT scan uses 100%, the most likely technique (%) for a 1-year-old is:
   a. 15
   b. 30
   c. 45
   d. 60
   e. 85

5.26 CT fluoroscopy best minimizes radiation doses by reducing:
   a. beam filtration
   b. focus size
   c. tube current
   d. slice thickness
   e. matrix size

5.27 The optimal x-ray tube voltage (kV) for performing CT angiography is most likely:
   a. 80
   b. 100
   c. 120
   d. 140
   e. >140

5.28 The most likely voltages (kV) used in dual-energy CT are:
   a. 80 and 100
   b. 80 and 120
   c. 80 and 140
   d. 100 and 140
   e. 120 and 140

5.29 Ring artifacts in CT are most likely caused by:
   a. beam hardening
   b. metallic implants
   c. faulty detectors
   d. patient motion
   e. scattered x-rays

5.30 CT beam hardening artifacts are minimized by increasing the:
   a. tube voltage
   b. tube current
   c. scan time
   d. matrix size
   e. helical pitch

ANSWERS AND EXPLANATIONS

5.1e. The typical anode heat capacity of a modern CT x-ray tube anode is 4,000 kJ (4 MJ).

5.2e. The most common power level in CT today (2008) is 100 kW.

5.3d. Teflon (i.e., tissue like) is used as the CT beam shaping filter material to minimize beam hardening artifacts.

5.4a. CT collimation changes the x-ray beam width.

5.5e. The most likely x-ray beam width is 40 mm because the detector thickness is comparable to the in-plane pixel size of ~0.6 mm.

5.6d. 64 × 800 Since each slice would make use of ~800 individual detectors.

5.7e. CT x-ray detectors are very efficient and capture well over 75% of the incident radiation (e.g., 90%).

5.8b. In CT, ~1,000 projections are obtained for a single rotation of the x-ray tube.

5.9d. Bone filters improve spatial resolution but also result in higher mottle (noise).

5.10b. CT numbers are directly proportional to the pixel linear attenuation.

5.11a. Fat has a Hounsfield Unit of about −90.

5.12d. The tube current should not affect CT number value.

5.13a. Display contrast will be reduced when the width of the CT image display window increases.

5.14d. Spatial resolution increases when the matrix goes from 256^2 to 512^2.

5.15d. A typical pixel size in head CT is 500 μm (i.e., 0.5 mm).

5.16c. The pitch is 1.5 for a beam width of 40 mm and a table movement of 60 mm per x-ray tube rotation (i.e., 60/40).

5.17c. Modern CT scanners rotate their x-ray tubes in about 0.3 seconds.

5.18c. Utilization of the x-ray beam improves (for single slice scanners, >95% of the x-ray beam is wasted).

5.19c. Temporal resolution of ~80 ms can be achieved in cardiac imaging using a dual-source CT scanner.

5.20a. One, as each individual computed tomography dose index (CTDI) measurement is obtained for a single x-ray tube rotation.

5.21d. Two, since the peripheral dose in a 32-cm acrylic cylinder is generally double that of the central dose.

5.22d. Ten mGy ($CTDI_w$ is one-third the central CTDI plus two thirds the peripheral CTDI).

5.23e. One thousand mGy obtained by multiplying the scan length by $CTDI_{vol}$, which is the $CTDI_w$ divided by the pitch (i.e., 100 cm × 20 mGy/2).

5.24c. The $CTDI_{vol}$ reference dose (mGy) currently recommended by the ACR for an adult head CT (2008) is 75 mGy.

5.25e. Head techniques in a 1-year-old are reduced by 15%, so 85% would be used.

5.26c. Tube currents are generally reduced in CT fluoroscopy.

5.27a. A voltage of 80 kV maximizes iodine contrast by bringing the average x-ray energy closer to the iodine K-shell energy (33 keV).

5.28c. Voltages of 80 kV and 140 kV would likely be used.

5.29c. Faulty detectors can result in ring artifacts.

5.30a. Increasing tube voltage in CT minimizes beam hardening.

Chapter 6

IMAGE QUALITY

I. CONTRAST

A. Subject contrast
  –**Depiction** of **lesions** results from **differential attenuation** of the **x-ray beam** between the lesion and background tissues.
  –**Subject contrast** is the **difference** in **x-ray intensity** that is **transmitted** through a **lesion** in comparison to the **adjacent tissues.**
  –Important **lesion characteristics** include the **size, density,** and **atomic number.**
  –**Subject contrast** can be **positive** if the **lesion absorbs fewer x-rays** compared to the surrounding tissues.
    –**Positive contrast** will result in **darker lesions** in conventional radiographs.
  –Contrast can be **negative** if the **lesion absorbs more x-rays** compared to the surrounding tissues.
    –**Negative contrast** will result in **lighter lesions** in conventional radiographs.
  –**Contrast** is **reduced** by **scattered radiation** captured by the image receptor.
  –Use of scatter removal **grids** to **improve** ∼**contrast** is **substantial** (i.e., hundreds of percent).
  –**Subject contrast** is an **essential** prerequisite for producing **image contrast.**
  –The presence of **subject contrast,** however, does **not guarantee image contrast.**
    –**Underexposed films** look all **white** and thus display no image contrast, even when **subject contrast** is **present.**
B. Image contrast (screen–film)
  –In **screen–film** radiography, **image contrast** is the **difference** in the **film density** of a lesion in comparison to the film density of the **adjacent tissues.**
  –**Image contrast** in screen–film radiography is *primarily* dependent on **film density.**
  –**Underexposed films** with low densities (e.g., <0.5 OD) have **little image contrast.**
  –**Overexposed films** with high densities (e.g., >2.0 OD) show **little image contrast** under normal viewing conditions.
  –**Correct density** in screen-film imaging (e.g., **1.5 OD**) is achieved by having the correct image receptor air kerma (e.g., **5 μGy air kerma** for a **200 speed** system).
  –Correct image receptor air kerma can be achieved by an **automatic exposure control** (AEC), with the x-ray duration terminated by a radiation sensor at the detector.
  –**Film contrast** is determined by the **slope** (gradient) of the **characteristic curve** (Fig. 3.1).
  –The **film gradient** is the **mean slope** between two specified film densities (normally 0.25 and 2.0 OD units).
  –**High film gradients** are, by definition, high contrast films.
  –Gradients >1.0 result in subject contrast being amplified.
  –**Radiographic films** have **gradients** of ∼**2,** but in **mammography,** characteristic curves have gradients >**3.**
C. Contrast and latitude
  –**Film latitude** is the **range** of **air kerma** values that results in a satisfactory **image contrast.**
    –Latitude is known as **dynamic range** in engineering.
  –The **latitude (dynamic range)** of film is ∼**40:1.**
  –**Film latitude** and film gradient (contrast) are **inversely related.**
  –The **higher** the **film gradient,** the **narrower** the range of air kerma values that result in a good image contrast.

–A **wide-latitude** film has a **low film gradient,** which results in a **low contrast.**

–**Wide-latitude** films are used for **chest** radiographs because of large differences in **air kerma** between **lungs** and **mediastinum.**

–**High-contrast films** are used in **mammography.**

–**Breast compression** *reduces* variation of air kerma in **mammography,** and permits the use of **high-contrast film.**

D. Contrast and digital imaging

–**Image contrast** in **digital imaging** is the **difference** in the **monitor brightness** of a **lesion** in comparison to the monitor brightness of the **adjacent tissues.**

–Displayed image contrast is the result of **subject contrast,** together with the effect of the **recording device** and **digital image processing.**

  –**Monitor display characteristics** and **window control** settings also affect **display contrast.**

–**Displayed contrast** in digital imaging can be controlled by the operator by adjusting the **display level** and **display window** width.

–**Increasing** the **window width** will generally **reduce display contrast** and vice versa.

–It is possible to **record** images with a **wide dynamic range** receptor and then **display** them with a **narrow window** to **enhance contrast** in the displayed image.

–In chest CT, a **narrow window** offers **excellent soft tissue contrast,** but the lungs become invisible (all black).

  –Use of a **wider window** in chest CT **permits visualization** of **most tissues,** but the contrast between soft tissues is markedly reduced.

–**Digital imaging** modalities permit **good contrast** over **all** the **image data** by viewing **multiple images.**

E. Contrast and photon energy

–For a given lesion, **subject contrast** is primarily affected by the **photon energy.**

–The average **photon x-ray energy** is **increased** by increasing the x-ray **tube voltage** (kV) or by adding **filters.**

  –*Reducing* the **ripple** on the x-ray tube voltage (e.g., using a constant potential) also **increases** the average **photon energy.**

–**Low photon energies** result in **high subject contrast** and vice versa.

–Figure 6.1 shows how subject contrast depends on the kV.

–At low kV, intensity differences between adjacent tissues are relatively high, but these differences are markedly reduced at higher photon energies.

  –As **photon energy increases, contrast decreases** because of increased x-ray photon penetration.

–For correctly exposed (and displayed) imaging systems, **changes** in **subject contrast** will generally result in **corresponding changes** in **image contrast.**

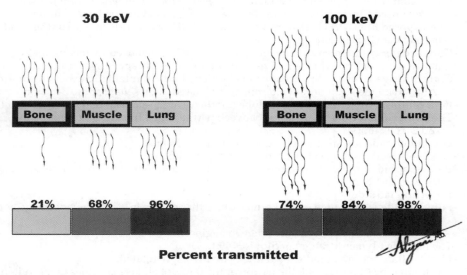

FIGURE 6.1   X-ray penetration increases with increasing photon energy, which reduces x-ray intensity *differences* (i.e., contrast) between bone, muscles, and lung.

TABLE 6.1   CT Image Contrast of a Lesion in a Water Background as a Function of X-ray Photon Energy (Normalized to 100% at 50 keV)

X-ray Energy (keV)	Soft Tissue Lesion (Z = 7.6)	Iodinated Vessel (Z = 53)
50	100	100
60	93	68
70	88	48
80	84	37

–Reduced subject contrast generally results in a reduction of image contrast, and vice versa.

–Photon energy also affects contrast in CT imaging (Table 6.1).

   –Increasing the photon energy from 50 to 80 keV reduces soft tissue contrast (i.e., soft-tissue HU) by 16% and reduces iodine contrast by 63%.

–**Reducing CT tube voltage improves visibility** of iodinated **contrast agents.**

   –For large patients, reducing kV may not be practical because of insufficient patient penetration.

F. **Contrast agents**

–**Contrast agents** including **air, barium,** and **iodine** are used to improve subject contrast.

–**Barium** is administered as a contrast agent for visualization of the **GI tract** on radiographic examinations.

–Barium attenuation is high because of its high density and high **atomic number (Z = 56)** that places the **K-edge** at **37 keV.**

–The barium K-edge energy matches the mean photon energies used in fluoroscopy.

–**Iodine (Z = 53)** is also an **excellent contrast agent** for similar reasons to those for barium **(i.e., K-edge = 33 keV).**

–Iodinated contrast agents can be injected intravenously or arterially.

   –Dilution and the osmolar limitations of intravascular fluids limit the achievable iodine concentration.

–**Air** is a **negative contrast agent** and increases subject contrast because it is less attenuating than tissue.

–**Carbon dioxide** is also sometimes used as a contrast agent in **angiography.**

II. RESOLUTION

A. **What is resolution?**

–**Resolution** is the ability of an imaging system to display **two** adjacent objects as **discrete entities.**

   –Resolution is also known as **spatial resolution, high-contrast resolution, sharpness,** or **blur.**

–Two small adjacent objects such as microcalcifications will appear sharp and distinct in an image obtained with a system that has good resolution.

   –Adjacent microcalcifications might appear as one blurred entity in images obtained with a system that has poor resolution.

–Resolution may be *quantified* using a **parallel line bar phantom.**

   –Bar phantoms possess very high intrinsic contrast.

–**One line pair per millimeter (1 lp/mm)** is a bar phantom that has **0.5 mm lead (Pb)** bars **separated** by **0.5 mm** of **radiolucent material.**

   –A 2 lp/mm bar phantom has 0.25 mm Pb bars separated by 0.25 mm of radiolucent material, and so on.

–**Large objects** correspond to **low** values of **line pairs/mm**

   –**Smaller structures** correspond to **higher** values of **line pairs/mm.**

–The **limiting spatial resolution** is the maximum number of line pairs per millimeter that can be recorded by the imaging system.

   –Table 6.2 shows the limiting resolution of x-ray based imaging modalities.

–The **human eye** resolves ~**5 lp/mm** at a viewing distance of ~**25 cm.**

   –Humans can resolve up to ~30 lp/mm on close inspection.

–**Focal spot** size, **detector blur,** and patient **motion** affect **resolution** in radiography.

TABLE 6.2   Approximate Values of Limiting Resolution in Radiologic Imaging

Imaging Modality	Limiting Spatial Resolution (lp/mm)
Screen–film mammography	15
Screen–film (200 speed)	5
Digital chest imaging	3
Digital photospot/DSA	2
Fluoroscopy (525-line TV)	1
CT	0.7

B. Focal spot blur
   –The finite **size** of a **focal spot** results in **blurred images.**
   –The **blurred margin** at the edge of objects produced by a finite focal spot is called a **penumbra.**
   –The penumbra is the result of x-rays arriving from slightly different locations in the focal spot.
   –The resultant loss of sharpness is called **focal spot blur** or **geometric unsharpness.**
   –**Focal spot blur increases** with increasing **focal spot size** as shown in Figure 6.2.
      –A **point focal spot,** or one that is negligibly small, produces **no focal spot blur.**
   –There is **no focal spot blur** in **contact radiography** (i.e., no magnification) as shown in Figure 6.2.
      –**Focal spot blur** is **minimal** in extremity radiography (i.e., negligible magnification).
   –In **magnification radiography,** it is always very important to use **small focal spot** sizes.
      –Reducing the focal spot size in magnification imaging increases the sharpness of edges by minimizing the penumbra.
   –**Magnification** in **mammography** improves visibility of microcalcifications but needs a **0.1-mm focal spot** to minimize geometric unsharpness.
   –**Magnification** is sometimes used in **angiograms** to improve the visibility of very small blood vessels and makes use of a **0.3-mm focal spot.**
C. Detector blur
   –The **physical size** of any radiation detector will **limit** the **ability** to **resolve small objects.**
   –**Screen thickness** introduces a limit on the achievable spatial resolution performance in radiography.
   –**Light** produced by absorbed x-rays in a screen produces a **blurred image** because the **light diffuses** before being absorbed by a film.

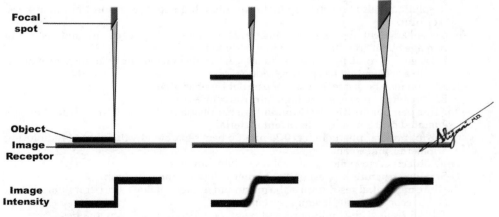

FIGURE 6.2   Focal spot blur in radiography showing that in contact radiography **(left),** the edge is very sharp with negligible blur but becomes less sharp (blurrier) with magnification **(middle),** and the blur further increases with a larger focal spot size **(right).**

–A screen that is **0.4-mm thick** will introduce a **blur** in the resultant image that is comparable to the **screen thickness.**

–Capturing an image with **x-ray film alone** without any screen can a produce **sharp image.**

–Film (i.e., no screen) images are only sharp with minimal motion and focal spot blur.

–In **fluoroscopy,** the **width** of a **TV line** places a lower limit on the visibility of small details.

–In **digital radiography,** the **pixel size** limits the size of small objects that may be visualized.

–In **CT,** each **detector element** produces an average intensity of the x-ray pattern that is incident on the detector, with (any) **finer details** being lost.

–In general, the key **image receptor dimensions** (thickness or detector area) should be **smaller** than the smallest **objects** that are to be resolved.

D. Motion blur

–**Patient motion** introduces **blur** into a radiograph by smearing out the object in the image.

–**Movement** of organs such as the **heart** contribute to patient motion.

–Gross movement of the patient is another source of motion blur.

–Increasing the mA to **reduce** the **exposure time** will minimize motion blur.

–Increasing the mA may not be possible, however, because of limits on the focal spot loading of the x-ray tube.

–**Motion blur** is **independent** of image **magnification.**

–Patient motion can be reduced by the use of **immobilization devices** such as the **compression paddle** in **mammography.**

E. Point spread function (PSF) and line spread function (LSF)

–An image of point (e.g., hole) is called a **point spread function (PSF).**

–The point appears blurred because of the combined effects of the focal spot, motion, and the dimensions of the imaging receptor.

–The image of a narrow line source is called a **line spread function (LSF),** and its width may be taken as a measure of the blur or resolution.

–Normally, width is measured at half the maximum value, termed **full width half maximum (FWHM).**

–A **wide LSF implies poor spatial resolution** and vice versa.

–**Narrow LSFs** (<1 mm or so) are difficult to measure, and **bar phantoms (i.e., lp/mm)** are used to measure spatial resolution performance.

–**Wide LSFs** (>3 mm or so) are easy to measure and are routinely obtained as FWHM in **nuclear medicine.**

–The limiting spatial resolution in lp/mm can be converted to FWHM and vice versa.

–**FWHM ~1/(2 × LSF)**

–A **line spread function** with a **FWHM** of 0.1 mm can thus be taken to have a limiting resolution of **~5 line pairs per mm.**

–A resolution of **1 lp/mm** corresponds to a **FWHM of 0.5 mm.**

F. Modulation transfer function

–The **modulation transfer function (MTF)** is a curve that describes the resolution capability of an imaging system.

–The **MTF** is the ratio of **output** to **input modulation** (signal amplitude) in an imaging system at each **spatial frequency.**

–**Output modulation** of all imaging systems is **less** than the **100%** input because of **blur** introduced by the **focal spot, motion,** and **receptor size.**

–The importance of **blur increases** as the **spatial frequency increases** (i.e., as the objects of interest get smaller).

–At **low spatial frequencies,** the **MTF** is close to **1.0** and corresponds to excellent visibility of large features.

–At **high spatial frequencies,** the **MTF** always falls to **zero,** which corresponds to the poor visibility of small features.

–The **MTF** of the **imaging *system*** is the **product** of the **MTFs** of the **respective *subcomponents.***

–If for a given spatial frequency, the MTF due to the focal spot is 0.9, due to motion is 0.8, and due to the screen is 0.7, the imaging system MTF is the product of the individual components (i.e., $0.9 \times 0.8 \times 0.7$, or 0.5).

–Imaging scientists use **MTF analysis** which permits each component to be analyzed separately (focal spot, motion, detector blur) and weak links to be identified.

–**MTF** analysis also helps scientists to **predict imaging performance** for any specified diagnostic **imaging task.**

III. IMAGING SYSTEM RESOLUTION

A. Screen–film
–Film *alone* (i.e., no screen) has a **limiting spatial resolution** of ∼**100 lp/mm.**
  –Film resolution is limited by the size of the individual grains of silver.
–With **screen–film** combinations, the **film** is **exposed** to **light** photons produced within the **screen.**
–**Light** produced in the screen *spreads out* as it **moves toward** the **film** (Fig. 6.3) producing a blurred image.
–**Screen blur** is determined by the **thickness** of the **intensifying screen.**
  –Screen thickness ranges between 50 and 400 μm.
–**Thicker screens** have greater light diffusion in the screen and, therefore **more blur.**
  –Thicker screens (fast screens) also have improved x-ray absorption efficiencies and reduced exposures.
–**Reduced exposures** may also result in **shorter exposure times.**
  –**Short exposure times minimize motion blur.**
–A screen–film system (**200 speed**) has limiting spatial resolution of ∼**5 lp/mm.**
–The limiting spatial resolution of a **mammography screen—film** is ∼15 lp/mm.
–The **ACR accreditation** program requires the resolution in screen–film mammography to be **11** to **13 lp/mm.**
  –The minimal specifications correspond to 11 lp/mm when measurements are perpendicular to the anode–cathode axis and 13 lp/mm parallel to this axis.
–**Magnification** imaging in **mammography** is performed with a **small focal spot (0.1 mm)** to ensure that the resolution remains within the limits set by accreditation bodies.

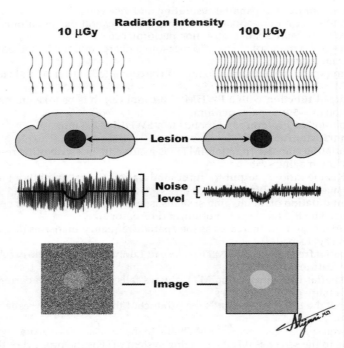

FIGURE 6.3   Increasing x-ray air kerma from 10 μGy **(left)** to 100 μGy **(right)** reduces random fluctuations by $\sqrt{[10]}$ whereas lesion contrast is unchanged; as a result, the lesion becomes visible because lesion contrast is larger than the level of image noise.

B. TV

–**Vertical resolution** of a TV system is determined by the number of **TV lines.**
–A TV system with **N lines** can (theoretically) produce **N/2 line pairs** (i.e., one line pair has one black line and one white line).
–If a TV system views an object that has size L mm, the theoretical limiting spatial resolution is the number of line pairs divided by the object size (i.e., **[N/2]/L) lp/mm**).
–The theoretical vertical resolution for a **525-line TV** system when displaying a **250-mm object** is thus $\sim$**1 lp/mm.**
–**Only $\sim$70%** of this **theoretical TV vertical resolution** is **actually achieved.**
–The ratio of actual (i.e., measured) to theoretical vertical resolution is called the **Kell factor.**
–A typical **TV Kell factor** is $\sim$**0.7,** which means that best achievable TV vertical resolution is 70% of the theoretical resolution of (N/2)/L lp/mm.
–TV **vertical resolution** is **improved** by using TVs with **more TV lines.**
    –A 1,000-line TV system has **twice** the **limiting vertical spatial resolution** of a conventional **525 TV.**
–**Horizontal resolution** is determined by the **bandwidth** of the TV system.
    –TV bandwidth reflects the ability of the electronics to fluctuate between a white signal and a black signal along a single TV line.
–The bandwidth of a 525-line TV system is $\sim$5 MHz.
    –The **bandwidth** of a **1,000-line TV** system is $\sim$20 MHz (i.e., **four times higher**).
–**Horizontal TV resolution** is normally designed to be the same as **vertical TV resolution.**

C. Analog fluoroscopy

–In **fluoroscopy, focal spot blur** is **negligible,** because fluoroscopy uses a small focal spot.
    –Small focal spots are possible in fluoroscopy because of the **very low power** loadings used (e.g., **100 kV** and **3 mA** is **only 300 W**).
–The **limiting resolution** of an **image intensifier** is determined by the characteristics of the **input phosphor (CsI).**
–The CsI II input phosphor is $\sim$400-μm thick, but is made of thin columns to limit the spread of light photons.
–The **limiting resolution** of an **image intensifier** is $\sim$**5 lp/mm.**
    –**Viewing** the **output** phosphor directly yields the **full II resolution.**
–When the II is viewed through a **TV camera**, the limiting **resolution** is **markedly reduced** because TV has much worse resolution performance than an II tube.
–The **limiting resolution** in **fluoroscopy** with a standard **525-line TV** is $\sim$**1 lp/mm.**
–Fluoroscopy resolution can be **improved** to $\sim$**2 lp/mm** by use of a **1,000-line TV system,** including a high-resolution display monitor.
–**Fluoroscopy resolution** can also be **improved** by the **use** of an **electronic zoom** or magnification mode, where the field of view is reduced.
    –**Halving** the **II field** of view *electronically* **doubles resolution.**
    –Reducing the II field of view by **physical collimators** has **no effect** on **resolution.**

D. Nyquist frequency

–The **matrix size** in all digital images determines the **sampling frequency** of digital images.
–A 1 k matrix along a line 100 mm long corresponds to a sampling frequency of $\sim$10 per mm (i.e., 1,000 samples per 100 mm).
–**Each sample** produces a **single pixel value.**
    –The **pitch** is **1/(sampling frequency).**
–**Doubling** the **matrix size** for a constant image size **doubles** the **sampling frequency.**
    –**Doubling** the **matrix size reduces** the **pixel size** by one **half.**
–The **sampling frequency** determines the **limiting spatial resolution** that is achievable by the digital imaging modality.
–The **limiting spatial resolution** is **half** the **sampling frequency.**
    –The limiting spatial resolution in digital imaging is the **Nyquist frequency.**
–A sampling frequency of **10 per mm** has a **limiting resolution** of **5 lp/mm.**
    –That is, 1 mm containing 10 pixels can display five pairs of black and white pixels (i.e., 5 lp/mm).
–**Doubling** the **sampling frequency** will **double** the limiting spatial **resolution** (Nyquist frequency).
–**Nyquist frequency** defines the **highest spatial frequency** in an object that can be *faithfully* reproduced in **digital images.**

–**High spatial frequencies** correspond to **small** features and/or **sharp edges** in the **object.**
–The presence of **higher spatial frequencies** in an imaged object results in **aliasing artifacts.**
–**Aliasing artifacts** are always **caused** by **insufficient sampling** and are **ubiquitous** in digital imaging.
  –**Aliasing** is seen in MR (**wraparound**) and **Doppler ultrasound.**

E. **Digital imaging**
–A **chest x-ray** (35 cm × 43 cm) typically has a matrix size of **2k × 2.5k.**
–The **sampling frequency** along the image length is 2k per 350 mm, or ∼**5.7 per mm.**
  –Limiting **resolution** is half the sampling frequency, or **2.9 lp/mm.**
–The sampling frequency along the height is 2.5k pixels per 430 mm, or ∼5.8 per mm.
  –The limiting resolution is half the sampling frequency, or 2.9 lp/mm.
–The **limiting resolution** for **chest radiography** is ∼**2.9 lp/mm.**
–The **matrix size** in **digital fluoroscopy** with a 1,000-line TV system is **1k × 1k.**
–Digital fluoroscopy for a 250-mm field of view corresponds (1,000 line TV) to a sampling frequency of four samples (i.e., TV lines) per mm.
  –**Digital fluoroscopy resolution** using a 1k line TV is ∼**2 lp/mm.**
–Digital photospot and **digital subtraction angiography** (DSA) images use a **1k × 1k** matrix size.
–**The limiting resolution** in photospot and DSA imaging is ∼**2 lp/mm** (∼25 cm FOV).
–**Improved resolution** can be achieved by maintaining matrix size and **reducing FOV.**
–II-based imaging systems **improve spatial resolution** with magnification zoom (i.e., reducing the field of view *electronically*).
–The **sampling frequency** of a **flat panel detector** is **fixed** (i.e., each pixel is always ∼0.17 mm), and resolution is *independent of the field of view.*
–**Digital mammography** with a **50-μm pixel** size has a limiting resolution of ∼**10 lp/mm.**
  –A 70-μm pixel size would have a resolution of ∼7 lp/mm.

F. **Computed tomography (CT)**
–A **head CT** image has a dimension of **250 mm** and a **matrix size** of **512 × 512**
–The **sampling frequency** in head CT is **2 pixels per mm.**
  –Head CT has a limiting **resolution** of ∼1 lp/mm.
–A **body CT** image has a dimension of ∼350 mm and a matrix size of 512 × 512
–The **sampling frequency** in body CT is thus ∼**1.4 pixels per mm.**
  –Body CT has a liming **resolution** of ∼**0.7 lp/mm.**
–**CT resolution** is *much lower* **than** achieved with a **200 speed screen film** (i.e., **5 lp/mm**) or a **digital chest** x-ray unit (∼**2.9 lp/mm**).
–Larger matrix sizes would not improve CT resolution because of focal spot blur and detector blur.
–Axial **resolution within** the **scan plane** may be improved by operating in a **high-resolution mode** using a **smaller FOV.**
–CT spatial resolution could be improved by using a smaller focal spot as well as designing systems with smaller detectors.
–**Detail (bone) reconstruction filters** are used to achieve the best possible **resolution.**
–Detector width affects resolution in the longitudinal plane (acquired slice thickness).
–Modern **MDCTs (64** slices or more) for body imaging have **isotropic resolution** (∼**0.8 lp/mm**).

IV. NOISE

A. **What is noise?**
–**Noise** describes the content of an image that **limits** the ability to **visualize lesions** or **pathology.**
–**Anatomic structures** can inhibit the visibility of lesions.
  –**Nodules** may be **masked** by the **rib cage** in **chest radiographs.**
–At a **constant air kerma,** x-ray images exhibit **random variations** in image intensity.
–**Random variations** in intensity are known as **mottle,** because the resultant image has a mottled appearance (i.e., **grainy**).
–**Random variations** of **photons** incident on a radiation detector are known as **quantum mottle.**

–**Quantum mottle** generally depends on the **number** or **concentration** of x-ray **photons used** to **produce** an **image.**

–The photon concentration is directly related to the **air kerma** at the image receptor.

–**Increasing** the number of **photons reduces quantum mottle** and vice versa, as depicted in Figure 6.3.

–Figure 6.3 shows that at low air kerma (10 μGy), the level of mottle is high, which will prevent the detection of the low-contrast lesion (noise > contrast).

–Increasing the air kerma to 100 μGy reduces the level of mottle, making the lesion visible (noise < contrast).

–Lesion contrast (i.e., height of the dip beneath the lesion) is *not* affected by the radiation intensity.

–Quantum mottle can be quantitatively described by the use of Poisson statistics.

B. Poisson statistics

–For a *uniform* **x-ray exposure,** adjacent areas of the x-ray image have photons in each mm^2 that **differ** from the **mean value N** in a *random manner.*

–Each mm^2 will have a slightly different number of photons, and the resultant image will have a grainy appearance.

–In other words, a perfectly uniform exposure results in a grainy image.

–The distribution of the number of photons in each mm^2 is described by **Poisson statistics.**

–For a Poisson distribution, the **mean** is equal to the **variance (σ^2).**

–In Poisson statistics, the **standard deviation (σ)** is given by the square root of the mean number of counts **($\sigma = N^{0.5}$).**

–**Sixty-eight percent** of the regions contain counts within one standard deviation of N($N \pm \sigma$).

–**Ninety-five percent** have counts within two standard deviations of N($N \pm 2\,\sigma$).

–**Ninety-nine percent** have counts within three standard deviations of N($N \pm 3\,\sigma$).

–For a uniform object imaged with an average of 100 photons per square millimeter [mean (N) = 100; $\sigma = 100^{0.5} = 10$], 68% of sampled areas are in the 90 to 110 range.

–In this example, 95% are in the 80 to 120 range, and 99% are in the 70 to 130 range.

–A **Gaussian distribution** is a good approximation to the **Poisson** distribution if the **mean** number of events is <**10.**

–When the number of **photons increases,** the **relative standard deviation** is **reduced.**

–When **N** is **100,** the standard deviation is $100^{0.5}$ or 10, and the relative standard deviation is **10%.**

–When **N** is increased to **10,000,** the standard deviation is $10,000^{0.5}$ or 100, and the relative standard deviation is **1%.**

–The **relative standard deviation** is important because it **quantifies** the magnitude of **fluctuations** about the **mean level.**

–The absolute standard deviation (i.e., $N^{0.5}$) is of little practical importance.

C. Screen–film mottle

–**Radiographic mottle** describes the **random fluctuations** in **screen–film images.**

–Sources of radiographic mottle include **screen mottle, film mottle,** and **quantum mottle.**

–**Screen mottle** (structure mottle) is caused by **nonuniformities** in screen construction and is negligible with modern screens.

–**Film mottle** (graininess) is caused by the **grain structure** of **emulsions** and is of little importance.

–**Quantum mottle** is the **major source** of random noise in screen–film.

–For **screen–film,** the air kerma incident on the image receptor determines the amount of quantum mottle.

–If screens are made thicker (faster), quantum mottle remains the same because the same number of x-ray photons is absorbed.

–Thicker screens are faster because they require fewer *incident* photons, while the number actually absorbed remains exactly the same as shown in Figure 6.4

–In diagnostic **radiography,** the number of x-**ray photons** used to create a radiographic image is $\sim$**10^5/mm^2.**

–In **photography,** the corresponding number of light photons required to expose a film is $\sim$10^9/mm^2.

–**Photographs** have **10,000** times **more** photons than **radiographs,** so **photographic mottle** is **negligible.**

–Table 6.3 shows the number of photons used to make one image or frame in projection x-ray imaging.

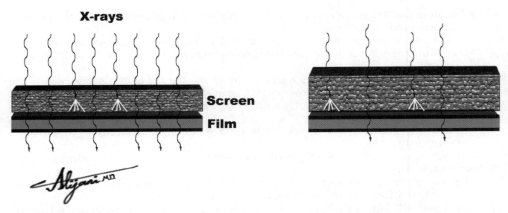

FIGURE 6.4   The speed of a screen–film combination can be increased by increasing the screen thickness, which will require fewer incident x-rays to make the radiographic image. However, since the thick screen still absorbs *exactly the same number of x-rays,* image mottle will be the same.

–There is a **20,000-fold difference** in receptor air kerma between **mammography** and a **single fluoroscopy frame.**

D. Digital radiography
   –In **screen–film** radiography, the amount of **radiation** required to generate a **satisfactory radiograph** is **fixed.**
   –A **200-speed screen–film** requires an image receptor air kerma of **5 μGy.**
   –Table 6.4 shows the receptor air kerma values in digital radiography.
   –Flat panel detectors that use **CsI detectors** are **more efficient** x-ray absorbers than radiographic screens because of their high K-shell binding energies (∼35 keV).
      –CsI indirect flat panel detectors require less radiation than screen–film.
   –Direct flat panel detectors that use **Se** are **efficient only** at **low photon energies** because of the low K-shell binding energy (13 keV).
   –Direct **Se** flat panel detectors are **moderate x-ray absorbers** at typical x-ray tube voltages in radiography (i.e., **60–80 kV)**
   –**Se** detectors have a **poor x-ray absorption** at high voltages (**120 kV**) used in **chest radiography.**
   –**CR** image receptor plates are relatively **thin** to minimize light scattering in the readout process.
      –**CR** requires **more radiation** than CsI detectors to achieve the same amount of quantum mottle.

E. II-based imaging
   –In fluoroscopy, the amount of **radiation used** to **produce** a *single* frame is **more than** a **hundred times lower than in radiography.**
   –Fluoroscopic **quantum mottle** is **much larger** than radiographic mottle.
      –**One hundred-fold more photons** in radiography means **ten times less quantum mottle.**
   –**Fluoroscopy** image intensifier input air kerma is ∼**0.01 μGy** per frame.

TABLE 6.3   Image Receptor Air Kerma Required to Produce a *Single* Radiographic Image or Frame

Imaging Modality	Typical Receptor Air Kerma (μGy)
Fluoroscopy	0.01
Cardiac imaging	0.2
Digital photospot	1
DSA	5
Mammogram (screen–film)	200

TABLE 6.4   Digital Image Receptor Air Kerma That Would Result in the Same Quantum Mottle as a 200 Speed Screen–Film (i.e., S/F Air Kerma ~5 μGy)

Imaging Modality	Receptor Air Kerma (μGy)
Photostimulable phosphor (BaFBr)	10
Indirect flat panel (CsI)	3
Direct flat panel detector (Se) with low kV x-rays	5
Direct flat panel detector (Se) with high kV x-rays	10

- **Digital fluoroscopy** uses image receptor air kermas **comparable** to those of **analog fluoroscopy.**
- **Digital fluoroscopy** permits reduced noise by **averaging frames.**
    - **Frame averaging** in digital fluoroscopy introduces **image lag.**
- A **single photospot** image requires an air kerma of ~1 μGy.
    - Air kermas for **photospot** images are about **five times less** than for conventional **radiographs.**
- **Digital subtracted angiography (DSA) images** use **two acquired images,** which include **noise from each image.**
- **Subtracted images** contain **no anatomic structures,** making DSA image mottle much more visible.
- To minimize DSA noise, **image receptor air kerma** is higher than photospot images and generally ~5 μGy.
    - DSA improves vasculature visibility by the removal of anatomic background, which is of greater importance than quantum mottle.

F. **Computed tomography (CT)**
- **Mottle** in CT is ~3 HU, which represents random fluctuations in attenuation coefficient of only **0.3%.**
- An image of a uniform water phantom has **68%** of the **pixels** with **HU values** between 0 ± 3 HU.
- The primary determinant of **CT mottle** is the **number** of **x-ray photons** used to make the image.
- The number of photons in a CT image is directly **proportional** to the **mA** and to the x-ray **tube rotation time (s).**
- CT mottle is thus inversely proportional to $mAs^{0.5}$, where **quadrupling** the **mAs** would **halve** the **mottle.**
- **Doubling** the **slice thickness** will **double** the number of **x-ray photons** and **reduce CT mottle.**
- When CT images are **acquired** at a slice thickness of **1.25 mm,** displaying these as **5-mm slices** will **halve CT mottle.**
- CT mottle will also be reduced by increasing the kV because more photons are produced and the patient penetration is increased.
- Increasing the x-ray tube voltage from **80** to **140 kV** substantially **reduces CT mottle.**
    - At 140 kV, CT detector air kerma increase approximately eightfold compared to 80kV, and the resultant image mottle is reduced almost threefold (i.e., $8^{0.5}$).
- **Mottle** in **reconstructed images** is also affected by choice of **reconstruction filter.**
- Use of filters with good resolution performance (i.e., **detail, lung, bone, edge,** etc.) will also **increase CT mottle.**
- **Soft tissue (standard) filters reduce CT mottle,** but at the price of inferior spatial resolution performance.

V. MEASURING PERFORMANCE

A. Data Analysis
- **Mean** is the arithmetic average of a group of data.
- **Median** is a measure of the central tendency and is the value that separates the data in half and defines the 50th percentile.
- **Mode** is the most common data point.
- **Range** is the difference between the highest and lowest values and is a measure of dispersion of the data distribution.

–**Standard deviation** (defined for a population) is used to describe the spread or distribution of a data set and is the square root of the average of the square of all the sample deviations.

–**Bias** is the presence of systematic error.

–**Precision** is the reproducibility of a result but does not imply accuracy.

–**Accuracy** refers to how close a measured value is to the true value.

B. Diagnostic Tests

–Excellent diagnostic performance is the primary objective of any radiologic imaging system.

–One measure of good diagnostic performance is to **maximize true positives** and **true negatives.**

–**True positives** (TPs) are positive test results in patients who have the disease.

–**True negatives** (TNs) are negative test results in patients who do not have the disease.

–Another goal of good diagnostic performance is to minimize false positives and false negatives.

–**False positives** (FPs) are positive test results in patients who do not have the disease.

–**False negatives** (FNs) are negative test results in patients who have the disease.

C. Test Results

–Table 6.5 is a truth table that may be applied to any diagnostic test.

–**Sensitivity** is the ability to detect disease and is **TP/(TP + FN),** also known as the true-positive fraction.

–A **sensitive test** has a **low false-negative rate.**

–**Specificity** is the ability to identify the absence of disease and is **TN/(TN + FP),** also known as the true-negative fraction.

–A **specific test** has a **low false-positive rate.**

–**Accuracy** is the fraction of correct diagnosis and is **(TP + TN)/(TP + FP + TN + FN).**

–**Positive predictive value** is the probability of having the disease given a positive test and is **TP/(TP + FP).**

–**Negative predictive value** is the probability of not having the disease given a negative test and is **TN/(TN + FN).**

–Diagnostic performance will generally depend on the disease prevalence.

–**Prevalence** of the disease is **(TP + FN)/(TP + FP + TN + FN).**

D. Receiver operator characteristic curve

–A **receiver operator characteristic (ROC)** curve is used to compare the performance (sensitivity and specificity) of diagnostic tests at various thresholds of interpreter confidence.

–Figure 6.5 shows a typical ROC curve.

–An **ROC curve** is a plot of the **true-positive fraction (sensitivity)** against the **false-positive fraction (1-specificity)** as the threshold criterion is relaxed.

–**Threshold criteria** for accepting a positive diagnosis range from the most **strict** to the most **lax.**

–**Strict thresholds mean underreading** whereas **lax thresholds mean overreading.**

–At the most restrictive threshold criterion, both sensitivity and the false-positive fraction are 0.

–At the most lax threshold criterion, both sensitivity and the false-positive fraction are 1.

–**Threshold criteria** represent different compromises between the need to **increase sensitivity** while **minimizing** the number of **false positives.**

E. Area under the ROC curve

–As the **threshold criterion** is **relaxed,** both the **sensitivity** and the **false-positive fraction** increase from **0** to **1.**

–The **area under** an **ROC curve (AUC)** is a measure of overall **imaging performance** and is commonly called A_Z.

TABLE 6.5   Truth Table for Any Diagnostic Test

Patient Status	Diagnostic Test Result	
	Positive	Negative
Disease present	True positive (TP)	False negative (FN)
Disease absent	False positive (FP)	True negative (TN)

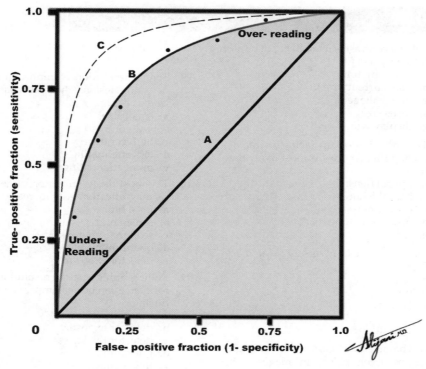

FIGURE 6.5   Three ROC curves where curve A ($A_z = 0.5$) corresponds to random guessing, and curve C ($A_z \sim 0.95$) corresponds to a performance level that is markedly better than curve B ($A_z \sim 0.85$). Also depicted are regions of underreading (i.e., number of true positives is too low) and overreading (i.e., number of false positives is too high).

–The maximum area under the curve is 1.0 (i.e., 100%).
–For **random guessing,** the ROC curve is a straight line through the points (0,0) and (1,1), and the **area** under the curve is **0.5 (i.e., 50%).**
–As the imaging performance improves, the ROC curve moves toward the upper left-hand corner, and the area under the ROC curve increases.
–**ROC** analysis is generally considered a good scientific way of **comparing two imaging modalities.**
–For any imaging modality, as **diagnostic performance improves** the **ROC curve** moves to the **upper left-hand corner.**
–One logistic **difficulty** of **ROC** analysis is **determination** of the **clinical truth** that is needed to compute sensitivity and specificity.

REVIEW TEST

6.1 Subject contrast is most likely to be affected by the:
  a. exposure time
  b. tube current (mA)
  c. tube voltage (kV)
  d. focus size
  e. display window

6.2 The most important factor for maximizing film contrast is most likely the film:
  a. optical density
  b. base thickness
  c. exposure time
  d. processing time
  e. fog level

6.3 Film contrast is inversely related to film:
  a. fog
  b. noise
  c. latitude
  d. speed
  e. resolution

6.4 A characteristic curve with a high gamma likely results in images with a high:
  a. patient dose
  b. film density
  c. quantum mottle
  d. image contrast
  e. fog level

6.5 Screen–film mammography contrast is likely improved by increasing:
  a. tube voltage
  b. target atomic number
  c. screen thickness
  d. film latitude
  e. film gradient

6.6 Increasing the kV alone in CT scanning would most likely reduce:
  a. anode loading
  b. image mottle
  c. patient dose
  d. reconstruction time
  e. scan time

6.7 Increasing the amount of scatter in a radiograph reduces:
  a. image contrast
  b. focal blur
  c. screen blur
  d. image mottle
  e. patient dose

6.8 Which of the following is *least* likely a measure of spatial resolution?
  a. ROC
  b. PSF
  c. LSF
  d. FWHM
  e. MTF

6.9 Spatial resolution is important when detecting lesions that are characterized as being:
  a. small size
  b. low contrast
  c. high contrast
  d. less attenuating
  e. more attenuating

6.10 The most likely limitation of geometric magnification is an increase in:
  a. focal blur
  b. screen blur
  c. scattered photons
  d. quantum mottle
  e. detector exposure

6.11 Radiographic spatial resolution performance can be best improved by reducing:
  a. beam filtration
  b. detector exposure
  c. detector thickness
  d. grid ratio
  e. tube voltage

6.12 Increasing the detector thickness to absorb more x-rays will most likely increase image:
  a. contrast
  b. magnification
  c. blur
  d. mottle
  e. brightness

6.13 When the full width half maximum of an imaged slit is 0.1 mm, the limiting resolution (line pairs per mm) is most likely:
  a. 1
  b. 2
  c. 3
  d. 5
  e. 10

6.14 The MTF value (%) at the lowest spatial frequencies is most likely:
  a. 100
  b. 75
  c. 50
  d. 25
  e. 0

6.15 The limiting spatial resolution (lp/mm) of a (dedicated) chest screen–film unit is likely:
  a. 0.5
  b. 1
  c. 2.5
  d. 5
  e. 10

6.16 Actual vertical resolution (line pairs) achieved with a 525-line TV monitor is:
- **a.** 180
- **b.** 262
- **c.** 370
- **d.** 425
- **e.** 525

6.17 The horizontal resolution of a TV system is primarily determined by the:
- **a.** image lag
- **b.** bandwidth
- **c.** TV lines
- **d.** frame rate
- **e.** camera size

6.18 Digital fluoroscopy spatial resolution would most likely be improved by increasing the:
- **a.** grid ratio
- **b.** II input diameter
- **c.** air kerma
- **d.** tube voltage
- **e.** image matrix

6.19 The maximum number of line pairs that can be observed using a 1k matrix size is:
- **a.** 50
- **b.** 100
- **c.** 250
- **d.** 500
- **e.** 1,000

6.20 The best achievable head CT limiting resolution (line pairs/mm) using a 512^2 matrix and 25 cm field-of-view is most likely:
- **a.** 0.25
- **b.** 0.5
- **c.** 1.0
- **d.** 2.0
- **e.** 4.0

6.21 If an average of 10,000 photons are detected per mm^2, the chance (%) of detecting between 9,700 and 10,300 counts in any exposed mm^2 is:
- **a.** 67
- **b.** 90
- **c.** 95
- **d.** 99
- **e.** 99.9

6.22 X-ray quantum mottle is best characterized by quantifying:
- **a.** x-ray beam filtration
- **b.** detector air kerma
- **c.** average photon energy
- **d.** scintillator conversion efficiency
- **e.** image receptor thickness

6.23 For comparable image mottle in an abdominal radiograph, which image receptor would likely result in the highest patient dose?
- **a.** Screen-film
- **b.** Photostimulable phosphor
- **c.** Direct flat panel detector
- **d.** Indirect flat panel detector
- **e.** Digital photospot

6.24 The dominant source of image mottle in a radiographic flat panel detector is most likely:
- **a.** detector granularity
- **b.** electronic noise
- **c.** digitization noise
- **d.** quantum mottle
- **e.** monitor structure

6.25 The detector air kerma (μGy) producing a digital photospot image in a Ba enema examination is most likely:
- **a.** 1
- **b.** 5
- **c.** 25
- **d.** 100
- **e.** 500

6.26 The II air kerma (μGy) needed to produce a single digital fluoroscopy image (frame) is most likely:
- **a.** 0.01
- **b.** 0.03
- **c.** 0.1
- **d.** 0.3
- **e.** 1

6.27 CT image mottle is *least* likely to be affected by changing the:
- **a.** section thickness
- **b.** reconstruction algorithm
- **c.** patient size
- **d.** x-ray intensity
- **e.** window width

6.28 Sensitivity is given by the:
- **a.** true-negative fraction
- **b.** true-positive fraction
- **c.** (1 − true-positive fraction)
- **d.** (1 + true-negative fraction)
- **e.** true positives + true negatives

6.29 Specificity is given by the:
- **a.** true-negative fraction
- **b.** true-positive fraction
- **c.** (1 − true-positive fraction)
- **d.** (1 + true-negative fraction)
- **e.** true positives + true negatives

6.30 Relaxing the threshold criterion in a ROC study increases false-positive fraction as well as the test:
- **a.** performance
- **b.** specificity
- **c.** ROC area
- **d.** sensitivity
- **e.** accuracy

ANSWERS AND EXPLANATIONS

6.1 c. The x-ray tube voltage (average photon energy) is the most important factor that affects subject contrast.

6.2 a. Film optical density is critical (light and dark films have very little image contrast).

6.3 c. Film contrast (i.e., gradient) is inversely related to film latitude.

6.4 d. Gamma is the maximum film gradient; high gamma produces a high image contrast.

6.5 e. A high film gradient in mammography (~3 or more) results in high image contrast.

6.6 b. Mottle will be reduced at higher kV because more x-rays are produced, and the x-ray beam is more penetrating, which will increase the number of detected photons.

6.7 a. Image contrast is reduced when scatter increases.

6.8 a. ROC is receiver operating characteristic, which measures diagnostic performance (PSF is the point spread function; LSF is the line spread function; FWHM is the full width half maximum; and MTF is the modulation transfer function).

6.9 a. Spatial resolution is important for detecting, differentiating, and characterizing lesions that have a small size.

6.10 a. Focal blur is extremely important in magnification imaging.

6.11 c. Detector thickness (e.g., screen thickness) is important for determining the spatial resolution performance.

6.12 c. Image blur will increase with a thicker x-ray detector.

6.13 d. Five line pairs per mm, since the achievable number of lp/mm is normally taken to be $\sim 1/(2 \times \text{FWHM})$.

6.14 a. The MTF value is 100% for all imaging systems; this effectively means that huge objects can very easily be seen.

6.15 d. Screen–film (200 speed) should achieve 5 lp/mm.

6.16 a. A TV with 525 lines can display 262.5 line pairs, but TV achieves only 70% of this value, so actual vertical TV resolution is 180 line pairs.

6.17 b. The TV bandwidth determines the horizontal TV resolution (usually the same as the vertical resolution).

6.18 e. Increasing the image matrix size will normally improve spatial resolution.

6.19 d. A 1k matrix can display 500 line pairs (1 line pair needs two pixels, one that is white and one that is black).

6.20 c. One line pair per mm, since the pixel size is 0.5 mm.

6.21 d. Ninety-nine percent, since the standard deviation is 100, and the limits correspond to three standard deviations.

6.22 b. The detector air kerma determines the number of x-ray photons used to make an image.

6.23 b. Photostimulable phosphor requires more radiation as it must be *thin* to minimize light scatter during the readout process.

6.24 d. Quantum mottle, as virtually all radiographic and CT imaging is quantum noise limited.

6.25 a. The detector air kerma in digital photospot imaging is 1 μGy.

6.26 a. The air kerma that produces a single digital fluoroscopy frame is 0.01 μGy.

6.27 e. The display window width will not affect the image data, only the way it appears on the monitor.

6.28 b. The true-positive fraction is the sensitivity.

6.29 a. The true-negative fraction is the specificity.

6.30 d. Sensitivity will increase as the threshold criterion increases and one moves up the ROC curve from lower left to upper right.

Chapter 7

RADIOBIOLOGY/ PATIENT DOSIMETRY

I. BASICS

A. Energy transfer
  –**Ionizing radiation transfers energy** to **electrons** in the absorbing medium.
  –Interacting x-rays produce *energetic* **recoil Compton electrons** and **photon electrons.**
    –Figure 7.1 illustrates the fate of an energetic photoelectron, which results in a large number of additional **ionization events.**
  –**Ionizing radiations** have **sufficient energy** to **break** apart **chemical bonds.**
  –**Direct action** occurs when Compton/photoelectrons **directly ionize** a target molecule.
  –**Indirect action** occurs when Compton/photoelectrons interact with water to produce a (free) **hydroxyl radical.**
    –**Free radicals** are **chemically reactive** molecules with unpaired electrons produced by ionizing radiation.
  –Hydroxyl radicals exist long enough to **diffuse** to, and **damage,** target molecules.
  –About **two thirds** of the **biologic damage** by x-rays is caused by **indirect action** and the remaining one third by direct action.
  –The **physics** and **chemistry** are very rapid, and occur in **less** than a **millisecond.**
  –Energy deposited in a cell can damage biologically important molecules (e.g., DNA).
    –The **DNA** molecule carries the code needed for cell metabolism and is duplicated when cells divide.
  –Radiation may damage a DNA molecule, possibly causing **cell death, somatic damage,** or a **mutation** that results in **hereditary effects.**
B. Cells
  –**Radiobiology** is the study of the effects of ionizing radiation in cells and animal models.
  –Cell cycles for mammalian cells include **mitosis (M), G1, DNA synthesis (S),** and **G2.**
  –Cells are generally most **sensitive** in **M** and **G1** and most **resistant** during **S.**
  –Energy from x-rays is deposited unevenly and produces **double-strand DNA breaks.**
    –**Chromosome breaks** and **aberrations** are examples of biologic damage caused by radiation.
  –**Double-strand** breaks are **important factors** for **cell death, carcinogenesis,** and **mutations.**
    –By contrast, **single-strand breaks** are much more **likely** to be **repaired.**
  –Health consequences of cell death occur on a time scale measured in hours and weeks.
  –A small amount of **energy deposited** in a cell may cause **cell function** to be **modified.**
  –**Damaged somatic cells** can result in the induction of **cancer** (fatal and nonfatal).
    –Induction of cancer by radiation takes years and decades to develop.
  –**Damaged sperm** and **eggs** (i.e., germ cells) can result in **hereditary effects** (mutations).
    –Hereditary effects are sometimes called genetic effects.
  –**Changes** in the **genetic code** of a **germ cell** can **affect future generations.**
C. Cell sensitivity
  –The amount of **biologic damage** produced depends on the total amount of **energy deposited** in a cell or tissue (i.e., absorbed dose).

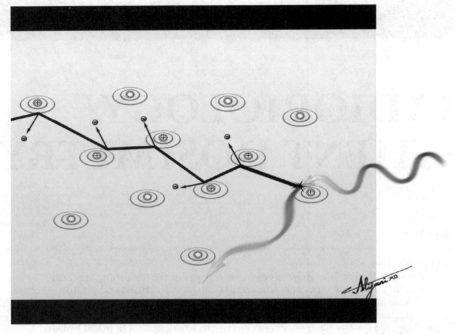

FIGURE 7.1   Fate of an energetic Compton electron showing some of the hundreds of ionization events this electron will produce.

- –A plot of the **surviving fraction** of cells versus **radiation dose** is called a **cell survival curve.**
- –Cell survival curves for x-ray exposures are not straight lines, but are curved.
- –Cells may die attempting to divide (**mitotic death**).
    - –**Programmed cell death** may also occur (**apoptotic death**).
- –For a constant total dose, **reduced dose rates** generally **reduce cell killing.**
    - –**Sublethal damage repair** can occur when the **radiation delivery** is *protracted.*
- –The radiobiologic **LD$_{50}$** is the lethal dose that will **kill 50%** of irradiated cells.
- –**LD$_{50}$** values are generally **several Gy,** much higher than most doses encountered in diagnostic radiology.
- –**Mammalian cells** are **more radiosensitive** than **bacteria,** because they have a larger amount of DNA.
- –**Rapidly proliferating cells** (e.g., bone marrow stem cells) are most **sensitive.**
- –**Highly differentiated** and/or **nonproliferating cells** (e.g., nerve cells) are **least sensitive.**
- –**Oxygen influences** the biologic **effect** of x-rays.
- –The **oxygen enhancement ratio (OER)** is (doses of hypoxic irradiation)/(dose of aerated irradiation) that produces the same amount of biologic damage.
- –The **OER** for **x-rays** is between **2** and **3.**
    - –This means that **oxygenated cells** are therefore **two** to **three times more sensitive** when irradiated by x-rays than anoxic cells.

D. Linear energy transfer (LET) and relative biologic effectiveness (RBE)
- –**Linear energy transfer (LET)** is the energy transferred per unit length of track.
- –**LETs** for **x-rays** are **~1 keV/μm.**
    - –X- and gamma-rays are said to be sparsely ionizing, and ionizing events from x-ray interactions are well separated.
- –**Alpha particle LETs** are **~100 keV/μm.**
    - –Alpha particles are said to be densely ionizing, and ionizing events from alpha particles are close together.
- –Radiobiologists use the term **relative biologic effectiveness (RBE)** to compare the ability of different *types of radiation* to cause biologic damage.
- –Relative biologic effectiveness (RBE) of some test radiation is the ratio **D$_{250}$/D$_{test}$,** in which D$_{250}$ is the dose of 250-kV x-rays and D$_{test}$ is the dose from the test radiation.
    - –RBE pertains to a specified **biologic end point** (e.g., surviving fraction of 50%).

–For the same absorbed dose, **high LET radiations** produce *more* **biologic damage** than low LET radiation.

–RBE is close to unity for low LET (~1 keV/μm) radiation.

–**RBE increases** with **LET** to a maximum at ~100 keV/μm.

–High LET radiations can have RBE values up to eight times higher than x-rays (i.e., low LET radiation).

–**Biologic effects** of radiation depend on *both* total energy absorbed (i.e., **dose**), and radiation type (i.e., **LET**).

E. **Equivalent dose**

–**Equivalent dose (H)** quantifies biologic damage by *different types* of radiation.

  –**High LET** radiation (alpha particles) causes **more biologic damage** than low LET radiation (x-rays and beta particles).

–The **equivalent dose** is the **absorbed dose (D)** multiplied by the **radiation weighting factor (w_R)** of the radiation, or $H = D \times w_R$.

  –For **radiologic protection** purposes, w_R permits **comparisons** of effects of different types of **radiation** on a common scale.

–The radiation weighting factor w_R **depends** on the radiation **LET**.

–For **low LET** radiation sources (e.g., electrons, x-rays, gamma rays), w_R **is 1**.

–For **high LET** radiation sources (e.g., alpha particles), w_R may be as high as **20**.

–**Equivalent dose** is expressed in **sievert (Sv)**.

–In **diagnostic radiology** and **nuclear medicine**, x-rays, gamma rays, and beta particles have a **radiation weighting factor w_R** equal to **1**.

–**1 Gy** of **x-rays** corresponds to an equivalent dose of **1 Sv**.

  –1 mGy of x-rays corresponds to an equivalent dose of 1 mSv.

–**High LET** radiations have **high w_R** values.

–Alpha particles have w_R equal to 20.

  –Neutrons can also have a w_R value as high as 20.

–An absorbed dose of **1 Gy** from **alpha particles** corresponds to an equivalent dose of **20 Sv**.

–**Equivalent dose** is primarily used for **radiation protection** purposes (see Chapter 8).

–Equivalent doses are *approximate indicators* of potential **biologic harm**.

  –**Biologic effects** of **radiation** are best assessed taking into account **type** of **radiation**, as well as any temporal and spatial patterns of **dose distribution**.

II. HIGH-DOSE EFFECTS

A. **Whole-body irradiation**

–**Lethal doses** are normally associated with (approximately) *uniform whole-body exposures*.

–**LD$_{50}$** is the **uniform whole-body dose** that would **kill** half **(50%)** the population.

–The **LD$_{50}$** is **3 to 4 Gy** for young adults without medical intervention.

  –**LD$_{50}$** is likely to be **lower** for **children,** and **older individuals**.

–Symptoms at doses of ~LD$_{50}$ include **anorexia, nausea,** and **vomiting**.

–A **whole-body dose** of ~**100 Gy** will **kill in 1 to 2 days** from permeability changes in the brain blood vessels (i.e., **cerebrovascular syndrome**).

  –Fatal whole-body doses are associated with symptoms of diarrhea and low blood pressure.

–A **whole-body** dose of ~**10 Gy** kills in 5 to 10 days due to loss of epithelial lining of the gastrointestinal tract (i.e., **GI syndrome**).

–A **whole-body** dose of ~**2** to **5 Gy** sterilizes dividing precursor stem cells, which reduces circulating blood elements within 2 or 3 weeks (i.e., **hematopoietic syndrome**).

–Lethal doses of radiation are rare and occur during catastrophic accidents such as the Chernobyl Nuclear Power plant accident in Ukraine (1986).

  –About **30 fire fighters** are reported to have been **killed** during the **Chernobyl** accident because of their **high doses** of radiation.

B. **Deterministic effects**

–**Radiation doses** in diagnostic **radiology** are generally *nonuniform*.

–The magnitude of the localized (i.e., **organ) dose** is used to predict the effect of the radiation delivered to this organ.

–*A **localized dose** to a region has effects that are very **different** from the same dose delivered uniformly to the **whole body.***
    –Five Gy to a toenail is of no clinical consequence, but 5 Gy to the whole body could be lethal.
–**High organ doses** may result in **deterministic** radiation effects.
–A deterministic effect has a **threshold** dose, below which the effect does not occur.
–When the **threshold dose** is **exceeded, deterministic effects** are **possible.**
    –**Deterministic effects** are also called **harmful tissue reactions.**
–**Radiation-induced skin damage** is the most common example of a deterministic effect.
    –Deterministic effects also include **cataract induction** and **induction** of **sterility.**
–**Deterministic effects** are mainly a result of **cell killing.**
–**Severities** of **deterministic** effects **increase** with **dose.**
–The *practical threshold* dose for use in diagnostic radiology is **2 Gy.**
–**Below 2 Gy,** clinically **significant deterministic** effects are most **unlikely.**
–**Above 2 Gy,** deterministic effects are possible, and the **patient** should be **monitored** for such a possibility.
–At doses **well above 2 Gy, deterministic effects** are **likely** to occur.

C. Skin reactions
    –The most common deterministic effect in diagnostic radiology is **damaged skin.**
        –Highest skin doses occur where the x-ray beam enters the patient.
    –For skin doses >~**2 Gy, transient erythema** may occur in a matter of hours.
    –Skin **doses** of ~**6 Gy** produce **erythema** 1 to 2 weeks following the exposure.
    –Skin doses that exceed 10 Gy can produce **dry desquamation.**
        –Dry desquamation arises from the loss of clonogenic skin cells.
    –**Moist desquamation** occurs at skin doses >**15 Gy.**
    –Skin effects are reversible if the population of basal cells can recover.
    –**Epilation** is another deterministic effect that can occur in diagnostic radiology.
    –At **doses** <~**3 Gy,** there will be **no epilation.**
    –For skin **doses** of **3 to 5 Gy, temporary epilation** can occur.
    –The onset of **epilation** occurs after **2 to 3 weeks.**
        –Hair that grows after a radiation-induced epilation may be of a different color (i.e., gray).
    –At **doses** >~**7 Gy, epilation** can be **permanent.**
    –Figure 7.2 depicts how radiation affects skin erythema and hair loss.

D. Cataractogenesis
    –**Cataracts** are **opacifications** of the eye lens that is normally transparent.
        –The eye lens has no method of removing dead or damaged cells.

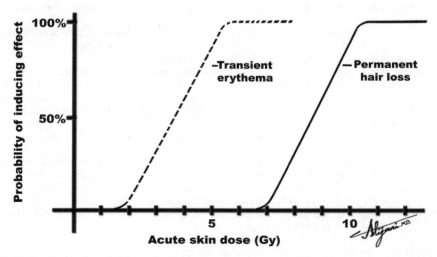

FIGURE 7.2   Idealized probability of inducing two deterministic effects (skin erythema and hair loss) as a function of the absorbed dose to skin.

–The induction of **cataracts** is an important **deterministic effect** of ionizing radiation.
   –Cataracts are a **late effect** of radiation.
–Cataracts that appear at the **posterior pole** of the lens of exposed individuals would **suggest** that the cataract has been **caused by radiation.**
–Cataract induction is a possibility for **patients** undergoing lengthy **interventional procedures.**
–There is evidence of **early cataracts** in **astronauts.**
–Cataract formation is dependent on the **total dose** and on the **time** over which this dose is delivered.
–An **acute dose** of $\sim$**2 Gy** is required to produce a cataract.
–For chronic exposure, the **threshold dose** for radiation-induced cataracts is $\sim$**5 Gy.**
–There is a **latent period** between irradiation and the subsequent appearance of cataracts.
   –**Latency** periods for cataractogenesis are reported as $\sim$**8 years** after eye lens doses of a **few Gy.**
–**Neutrons** are especially **effective** in **causing cataracts.**
   –Neutron RBE values are between 10 and 50, depending on the dose level.
E. **Sterility**
   –In the male, low doses of $\sim$0.2 Gy can produce a **diminished sperm count.**
   –Doses above 0.5 Gy can result in azoospermia (**temporary sterility**).
      –Recovery time from temporary sterility depends on dose.
   –**Sterility** requires a single dose of $\sim$**6 Gy** in **men.**
   –In males, fractionated exposure to the gonads produces *more* damage than acute exposure.
   –**Permanent sterility** can result from $\sim$**3 Gy fractionated** over a few weeks.
   –In the female, **radiation** can induce **permanent ovarian failure.**
      –The dose for female sterility is highly dependent on age.
   –The dose required for **permanent sterility** in the **female ovaries** is reported to be as high as **12 Gy** in **prepuberty.**
   –**Female** permanent **sterility** results from a dose of $\sim$**2 Gy** for **premenopausal women.**

III. CARCINOGENESIS

A. **Stochastic risks**
   –**Carcinogenesis** is the main concern following doses of ionizing radiations **below** the **threshold** for induction of **deterministic effects (i.e., <2 Gy).**
   –Carcinogenesis is a **stochastic effect** of radiation, meaning **random** or **probabilistic.**
   –The **severity** of radiation-induced **stochastic effects** is *independent* of the radiation **dose.**
   –The radiation **dose affects** only the *probability* of the **stochastic effect occurring.**
      –**Radiation** induces both **benign** and **malignant** tumors.
   –As **dose increases,** the **chance** of a **stochastic effect increases.**
   –For **radiation protection purposes, stochastic effects** have **no threshold.**
   –In addition to **carcinogenesis,** the other radiation-induced stochastic risk is the **induction** of **hereditary effects.**
   –**Stochastic risks** are dependent on **sex** and **age** at exposure.
      –Radiation-induced thyroid cancer is more likely in children and women than in men.
   –**Carcinogenesis** is the principal **radiation concern** in **diagnostic radiology.**
   –**Radiation-induced malignancies** are **similar** to **natural malignancies** of the same type, and appear at similar ages.
   –**Bone marrow, colon, lung, female breast, stomach,** and **childhood thyroid** are the organs that are **most susceptible** to **radiation-induced malignancy.**
   –**Bladder, liver,** and **esophagus** are **moderately radiosensitive.**
   –Minimizing patient radiation doses in diagnostic radiology is very important because this minimizes stochastic radiation risks.
B. **Epidemiologic studies (medical)**
   –**Epidemiologic** studies of **radiation-induced carcinogenesis** require **large cohort** size(s) and adequate **control group(s).**
      –**Long follow-up periods** (decades) are essential for observing **solid tumors.**
   –**Leukemia** has been observed in patients irradiated for **ankylosing spondylitis.**
      –Radiation induces acute and chronic myeloid leukemia but not chronic lymphocytic leukemia.

–**Radiation-induced thyroid cancer** has been observed in children irradiated to treat **enlarged thymus** or diseases of the **nasopharynx** and **tonsils.**
  –Thyroid cancers have also been observed in children where radiation was used to treat **acne, tonsillitis, tinea capitis** (ringworm), and **cancer.**
–**Breast cancer** appears in patients treated with x-rays for **postpartum mastitis.**
–Patients **fluoroscoped** repeatedly during the management of **tuberculosis** have also shown an elevated incidence of **breast cancer.**
  –Two independent studies in Nova Scotia and Massachusetts have shown similar results of increased female breast cancer.
–A significant **excess** of **cancers** has been observed **following radiotherapy** for **Hodgkin lymphoma, prostate cancer,** and carcinoma of the **cervix.**
–Excess cancers have been observed following **radiation therapy** for **breast cancer** and **carcinoma** of the **testes.**
–**Secondary cancers** have also been seen following **radiation therapy** for **childhood malignancies.**
–**Bone cancers** have been observed in patients who had injections of **radium** for **tuberculosis** or **ankylosing spondylitis.**
C. A-bomb survivors/radiation workers
  –Detrimental effects of radiation have been studied in **atomic bomb survivors** and **radiation workers.**
  –The **largest group studied** for radiation-induced cancer is the survivors of the atomic bomb survivors of **Hiroshima** and **Nagasaki.**
  –**Excess cancer deaths** depend on **dose, age** at exposure, time since exposure, and **gender.**
  –For **solid tumors,** the excess cancer incidence was found to be a **linear function** of dose.
    –**Leukemia** data were best fitted by a **linear quadratic function** of dose.
  –**Lung cancer** has been observed in **uranium miners** who were exposed to radon and radon daughter products.
    –**Excesses** of **lung cancer** have been observed in **miners** in **Colorado** (U.S.), uranium mines in **Czechoslovakia,** fluorspar mines in Newfoundland (Canada), and **Swedish** mines (nonuranium).
  –**Bone sarcomas** and **carcinomas** of the epithelial cells lining the **nasopharynx** have been observed in **dial painters** who ingested **radium.**
  –**Radiation-induced skin cancers** have also been reported in **radiologists, dentists, technologists** working in the **early 20th century** when radiation safety was lax.
  –Ongoing **studies** of **registries** of **radiation workers** show trends of **increased cancer risk** with **occupational exposures.**
D. Risk models
  –Obtaining **risk estimates** from epidemiologic data (e.g., Japanese atomic bomb survivors) requires the use of a **model** of **radiation-induced carcinogenesis.**
  –**Risks** should be **projected** for the **whole life span.**
    –Few exposed populations have yet lived out their life span.
  –**Risks** obtained by studying one population (e.g., **Japanese**) must be **transferred** to other populations (e.g., **U.S.**) that have very different patterns of cancer incidence.
  –The **absolute risk model** assumes that radiation produces a discrete number of cancers that is independent of the spontaneous level of cancer incidence.
  –The **relative risk model** assumes that radiation increases the spontaneous level of cancer incidence by a given percentage.
  –Since the natural cancer incidence increases with age, the relative risk model predicts a large number of excess cancers appearing late in life.
  –**Radiation-induced cancer risk estimates** generally **use** the **relative risk model,** not the absolute risk model.
  –**Latency** refers to the time interval between irradiation and the appearance of the malignancy.
  –Cancer induction has a **latency** of **2** to **25 years** or more for **leukemia.**
    –Leukemia incidence is age dependent, with a peak at 15 years (average).
  –**Latency** for **solid tumors** is **measured** in **decades,** with a minimum of 5 to 10 years.
E. Quantitative risks
  –Japanese atomic bomb risk estimates are primarily obtained for high acute doses delivered at a high dose rate.
  –A **dose** and **dose-rate effectiveness factor (DDREF)** converts high dose (and high dose rate) risk estimates to those applicable at low doses and chronic exposure.

TABLE 7.1   Lifetime Attributable Risk of Breast Cancer Incidence and Mortality following an Average Glandular Dose of 1 mGy per Million Exposed Females Taken from BEIR VII

Female Age (Years)	Incidence (per 10^6 per mGy)	Mortality (per 10^6 per mGy)
Newborn	120	27
10	71	17
20	43	10
40	14	3.5
60	3.1	0.9
80	0.4	0.2

–The most common **DDREF** used for radiation risk estimation is a **factor** of **two.**
  –Risk estimates used for radiation protection purposes are about half the risk estimates for the A-bomb survivors.
–The U.S. National Academy of Sciences Committee on the **Biological Effects** of **Ionizing Radiation (BEIR)** provides detailed information on radiation risks.
–**BEIR VII** report was published in **2006** and provides data on potential cancer incidence (and mortality) for males and females ranging from the newborn to 80-year-olds.
–The **age** of the **exposed individual** is the most **important** factor affecting the lifetime attributable risk of cancer incidence and cancer mortality.
  –Table 7.1 shows how radiation risk of breast cancer varies with age.
–Risk of **breast cancer varies** by over **two orders** of **magnitude** between **newborns** and **elderly women.**
–**1 Gy** of **uniform** whole-body irradiation (x-rays) is equivalent to **1 Sv.**
–For **30-year-old males,** the risk of **cancer incidence** is **6.9% per Gy** of uniform whole-body radiation, and the corresponding risk of fatal cancer is 3.8%.
  –For **newborn males,** the risk of **cancer incidence** increases to **26% per Gy** of uniform whole-body radiation, and the corresponding risk of fatal cancer is 11%.
–For **30-year-old females,** the risk of **cancer incidence** is **11% per Gy** of uniform whole-body radiation, and the corresponding risk of fatal cancer is 5.4%.
  –For **newborn females,** the risk of **cancer incidence** is **48% per Gy** of uniform whole-body radiation, and the corresponding risk of fatal cancer is 18%.
    – On average, children may be taken to be ten times more radiosensitive than retired adults.
–*Quantitative* **radiation risk** *estimates from the* **United Nations Scientific Committee on the Effects of Atomic Radiation (UNSCEAR)** *and the* **International Commission on Radiological Protection (ICRP)** *are similar to those of* **BEIR.**

IV. HEREDITARY AND TERATOGENIC EFFECTS

A. Hereditary effects
  –**Irradiation** of **germ cells** that are involved in reproduction can result in **hereditary effects.**
  –The **induction** of **hereditary effects** is a **stochastic** process with **no threshold.**
  –New, unique mutations are *not* produced by radiation.
  –**Radiation increases** the **incidence** of the **mutations** that **occur spontaneously.**
  –There is **no epidemiologic evidence** of **hereditary effects** in *exposed humans.*
    –Studies of **children** born to the **A-bomb survivors** (>40,000) have **not** shown any **significant increased hereditary effects.**
  –Information on the hereditary effects of radiation comes almost entirely from **animal experiments** combined with our current understanding of genetics.
  –**Mutation rates** have been measured in studies on the **fruit fly** (*Drosophila melanogaster*).
  –Mutation rates have also been measured in **mice,** in a study using ~7 million mice (**MegaMouse** project) at Oak Ridge National Laboratory in the late 1940s.
B. Hereditary risks
  –**Hereditary effects** depend on the **demographics** of the exposed populations.
  –**Older populations** have **lower risks** than younger populations for the same exposure.

–Before 1950, hereditary effects were considered the most important risk of radiation exposure.

–Nowadays, concern about hereditary effects is much lower.

–In the latest ICRP 103 report (2007), **hereditary effects accounted for** ~8% of the **total detriment** (i.e., induction of fatal/nonfatal cancer plus genetic effects).

–The current ICRP **hereditary risk** estimate is **0.2% per Gy** up to the second generation.

  –An absorbed dose of **1 Gy** to the **gonads** produces **one** genetic effect **per 500 live births.**

–For a **working population,** the hereditary risk factor recommended by the ICRP is **0.1% per Gy** of x-ray exposure.

  –Hereditary risks for a working population are lower than a general population because they exclude children.

–The **doubling dose** is the absorbed dose to the gonads of the whole population that would double the *spontaneous* mutation incidence.

–The current estimate of the doubling dose is ~**2 Gy.**

–Only a **few percent** of **spontaneous mutations** in **humans** may be ascribed to natural **background radiation.**

C. Radiation and the conceptus

–**Radiation effects** are *not* expected **prior** to **fertilization.**

–The fetal risk when exposing pregnant women depends on the gestation period.

–**Doses** of radiation >**100 mGy** during the **first 2 weeks postconception** could result in a **spontaneous abortion.**

–The **fetus** is considered most vulnerable to **radiation-induced congenital abnormalities** (excluding cognitive effects) during the **first trimester.**

–**Radiation-induced mental retardation** is possible **8 to 15 weeks postconception.**

–A much **smaller excess** has been reported for irradiation between **16 and 25 weeks.**

  –Mental retardation could be caused by radiation affecting brain cell migration.

–The greatest effect of **exposure** in **late pregnancy** is an **increased risk** of **childhood cancers.**

–In the United States, a **congenital abnormality** occurs in ~**5%** of **live births,** making the effect of medical x-rays difficult to evaluate.

D. Conceptus risks

–For irradiation of the human in utero, the **risk** of **severe mental retardation** as a function of dose appears to follow a **linear dose response** curve.

–The **risk coefficient** is taken to be ~**40% per Gy** of x-rays at 8 to 15 weeks after conception.

  –**Loss** of **IQ** is estimated to be about **30 points per Gy** of x-rays.

–Studies in the United Kingdom and United States have shown that **diagnostic x-rays** *in utero* **increase childhood cancers.**

  –The increased childhood cancers are **primarily leukemia.**

–**Fetal doses** that resulted in elevated childhood cancers were estimated to be ~**10 mGy.**

–The absolute risk of inducing **childhood cancer** is ~**6% per Gy** of x-rays.

–A **fetal dose** of ~**10 mGy** corresponds to a risk of **childhood cancer** of ~**0.06%.**

  –An **absolute risk** of **0.06%** of childhood cancer corresponds to an increase in the *relative risk* of ~**40%** (i.e., childhood cancers are relatively rare).

E. Exposure of pregnant patients

–**Unnecessary exposure** of a **conceptus** should be avoided.

–Before a pregnant patient is exposed to x-rays, it is essential that the magnitude of the **fetal** or **embryo dose** be quantified and the corresponding **radiation risks** estimated.

–If the x-ray beam does **not directly irradiate** the fetus or embryo, the corresponding **dose** will be very **low** and of little practical importance.

–The decision to proceed with x-ray examinations of pregnant patients requires a **risk– benefit** analysis to be performed.

–The **benefit** of the information obtained from any radiologic examination must always **exceed** any possible **risks** to the patient and an exposed conceptus.

–**Risks** of congenital abnormalities are **negligible** at radiation doses <**10 mGy.**

–For **doses up to 100 mGy,** any **radiation risks** are deemed to be **low** when **compared** with the **normal risks** of pregnancy.

–When the **conceptus dose exceeds 100 mGy** during the period **2 to 15 weeks postconception,** risks of development deficits are believed to start to appear.

TABLE 7.2   Representative Embryo Doses (mGy) in Diagnostic Radiology

Type of Examination	Embryo Dose	Comment
Chest radiograph	Negligible	PA projection
Chest CT	<0.1 mGy	Scatter radiation only
Abdominal x-ray	1 mGy	AP projection
Fluoroscopy	10 mGy/min	AP projection
CT scan	30 mGy	Abdomen + pelvis

–**After 15 weeks postconception,** the **primary concern** is an **elevated cancer risk,** which is too small to justify consideration of any medical intervention.

–Consideration of **medical intervention** needs to take into account all **clinical aspects,** as well as **social conditions** of the patient.

–Table 7.2 shows typical doses to patients undergoing a range of diagnostic examinations that use x-rays.

–Most x-ray examinations result in **embryo/fetal doses** <**100 mGy** and would not warrant consideration of any intervention.

V. PATIENT DOSIMETRY

A. Skin dose

–The **air kerma** incident on a patient undergoing an x-ray study is called the **entrance air**

–**Air kerma,** which is measured **free in air** (i.e., without the patient).

–Figure 7.3 shows how the entrance air kerma can be measured at the point where the x-ray beam would enter the patient, but in the absence of the patient.

–**Entrance air kerma** is generally **easy** to **measure.**

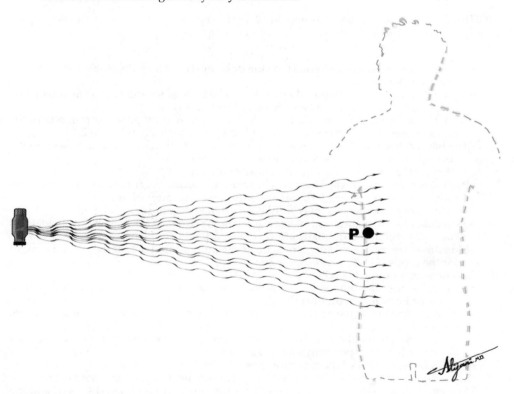

FIGURE 7.3   Entrance air kerma is a measurement made at the point P, where the x-ray beam would enter the patient, but obtained without a patient being present (i.e., free in air).

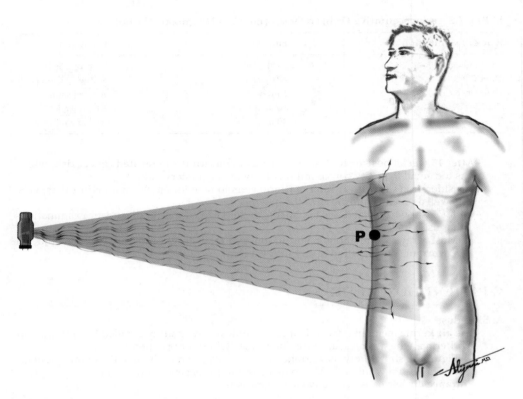

FIGURE 7.4   Backscatter factor is obtained by taking the ratio of air kerma at point P to the corresponding air kerma in the absence of the patient (see Fig. 7.3).

–Converting an **entrance air kerma** to a **skin dose** must account for the different properties of air and soft tissue.
–**Tissue doses** are ~**10% higher** than **air kerma** because of the different x-ray interaction properties of air and tissue (see Chapter 2, Section VI).
–An x-ray beam incident on a patient will also result in x-ray photons from within the patient being **backscattered** to the **skin location** as depicted in Figure 7.4.
–The **backscatter factor** is the ratio of the tissue dose in the absence of a patient, to the corresponding tissue dose with the patient present.
    –A typical backscatter factor in **diagnostic radiology** is **1.4.**
–**Skin doses** are thus *higher* than the **incident air kerma** because tissue absorbs more radiation than air **(times 1.1),** and also includes backscatter **(times 1.4).**
    –**Entrance air kerma** of **1 mGy** results in **entrance skin doses** of ~**1.5 mGy.**
–**Skin doses** for virtually all radiologic examinations are *much lower* than threshold doses **(i.e., ~2 Gy)** for **deterministic effects** (epilation, skin erythema, etc.).
–**Skin doses** are poor predictors of patient **stochastic radiation risk,** as they do not account for the exposed body region, x-ray beam area, and x-ray beam penetration.
B. **Air kerma–area product (KAP)**
    –A quantity that takes into account the *total* amount of radiation incident on the patient is the **air kerma–area product (KAP).**
    –KAP is the product of the **entrance air kerma** and **cross-sectional area** of the x-ray beam (exposed area).
    –Figure 7.5 shows that the air kerma–area product can be obtained by multiplying the air kerma by the corresponding x-ray beam area.
    –**KAP** is **independent** of the **measurement** location because increases in beam area are exactly compensated for by the reduction of beam intensity (inverse square law).
    –The entrance air kerma for an adult chest x-ray (PA projection) is ~0.1 mGy, and the corresponding x-ray beam area is ~1,000 cm^2
        –An **adult chest KAP** is thus **0.1 Gy-cm^2.**

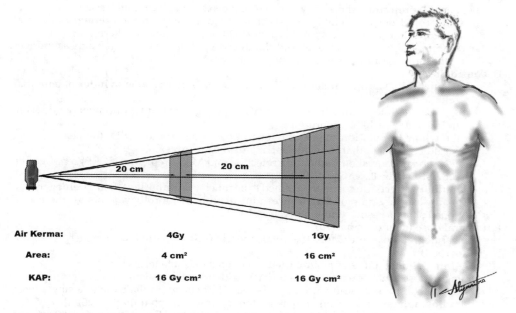

Air Kerma: 4Gy   1Gy

Area: 4 cm²   16 cm²

KAP: 16 Gy cm²   16 Gy cm²

FIGURE 7.5   Air kerma area product is obtained by multiplying the air kerma by the corresponding x-ray beam area, showing that this parameter is a constant at all locations.

–**KAP** values may also be computed for **CT examinations.**
–A single **head CT** scan has a KAP of ∼**13 Gy-cm²,** and a single **abdomen CT** scan has a KAP of ∼**25 Gy-cm².**
–**KAP** can be used to **compare doses** from different imaging systems (or facilities) for similar types of examinations on similar-sized patients.
  –**KAP** values indicate **relative radiation risks** for similar types of examinations performed on similar-sized patients.
–Table 7.3 shows typical values of KAP in diagnostic and interventional radiology.
C. Organ doses
–Entrance air kerma data can be converted into an estimate of **organ dose.**
  –**Organ doses** are **lower** than the **skin dose.**
–Organ doses depend on the **x-ray beam quality** (half-value layer or penetrating power), as well as the **x-ray beam area.**
  –Organ doses also depend on the **location, size,** and **fraction** of the **organ being irradiated.**
–**Organs** that are **not** in the **direct field of view** are only subject to scatter radiation and will generally receive very **low radiation** doses.
–When a pregnant patient undergoes a radiologic examination, an estimate needs to be made of the embryo or fetal dose.
–When the x-ray **beam** *directly irradiates* the **embryo,** the projection is an important factor in determining the embryo dose.

TABLE 7.3   Representative KAP for Diagnostic and Interventional X-ray Examinations

Radiologic Examination	Typical Air Kerma–Area Product (KAP) Gy-cm²
Radiography: head or chest	1
Radiography: abdomen	5
Radiography/fluoroscopy: barium study	20
Radiography/fluoroscopy: interventional	100

-For an **AP projection,** the **embryo dose** is about **1/3** the **entrance air kerma.**
  -**PA projections** have embryo doses about **1/6** of the **entrance air kerma,** and **lateral projections** have embryo doses about **1/20** of the entrance air kerma.
-In mammography, the **average glandular dose (AGD)** is obtained from a measurement of the entrance air kerma using a breast phantom.

D. Gonad doses
  -The **genetically significant dose (GSD)** is a dose parameter that is an **index** of **potential genetic damage.**
  -The GSD takes into account the **dose** received by the **gonads** and the number of **offspring** an **individual** is likely to **produce.**
  -If the **whole population** received a gonad dose equal to the **GSD,** the genetic harm would be equal to that from current **medical exposures.**
  -The National Council on Radiation Protection and Measurements (NCRP) reported the **U.S. GSD** to be **0.3 mGy** in 1980.
  -**Hereditary effects** are currently deemed to be much **less important** than **carcinogenesis.**
  -**Gonad doses** are now of **little concern** in **diagnostic radiology,** although the use of gonad shields is still common practice.

E. Integral dose (energy imparted)
  -The **integral dose** measures the **total energy (mJ)** imparted to a patient (i.e., absorbed).
  -**Integral dose** and **energy imparted** are interchangeable terms.
  -Integral dose can be **calculated** from **KAP** incident on the patient.
  -A single **chest x-ray** radiograph imparts ~**2 mJ** of energy to the patient, a single **head radiograph** imparts ~**5 mJ,** and an **abdominal radiograph** imparts ~**20 mJ.**
  -A **head CT** scan imparts ~**150 mJ** of energy, and a **body CT** scan imparts ~**500 mJ.**
  -A **500-W microwave imparts 500,000 mJ every second** to the food in the microwave oven (heat).
    -**Microwaves** are not ionizing radiation and raise the food temperature, whereas x-rays are ionizing and can break apart molecules such as DNA.
  -**Energy imparted** may be used as a (crude) indicator of **relative risks** for patients of the **same size** undergoing **similar types** of radiologic **examinations.**

VI. EFFECTIVE DOSE

A. Effective dose
  -Most **radiologic examinations** result in a *nonuniform* **dose distribution** within the patient.
    -An **AP abdominal x-ray** results in an **entrance skin dose** of ~**3 mGy,** exit skin dose of ~**0.1 mGy,** and (scatter) **thyroid dose** <**0.003 mGy.**
  -The **effective dose (E)** is obtained by **taking into account** the **equivalent dose** to *all* **exposed organs,** as well as **each organ's relative radiosensitivity.**
  -**E** is obtained by multiplying **equivalent dose (H)** to an organ by the organ **weighting factor (w),** and summed for all irradiated organs.
    -**E** is $\Sigma(H\,w)$ for all irradiated organs.
  -The organ **weighting factor w** is a measure of the *relative organ radiosensitivity* for the induction of stochastic effects.
    -Table 7.4 lists the tissue weighting factors currently recommended by the ICRP.

TABLE 7.4 Tissue Weighting Factors Recommended by the International Commission on Radiological Protection in Publication 103 (2008)

Tissue	Weighting Factor w
Bone marrow, colon, lung, breast, stomach, remainder	0.12
Gonads	0.08
Bladder, esophagus, liver, thyroid	0.04
Bone surfaces, brain, salivary glands, skin	0.01

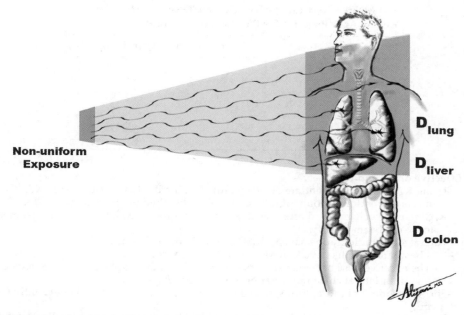

FIGURE 7.6   The effective dose is the *uniform whole-body equivalent dose* resulting in the same stochastic risk that would occur for a *nonuniform pattern of dose* as shown above.

–The **most radiosensitive** organs are the **red bone marrow, colon, lung, breast,** and **stomach.**

–Moderately sensitive organs are the bladder, esophagus, liver, and thyroid.

–**Lower-sensitivity** organs include the **skin, bone surfaces, brain,** and **salivary glands.**

–The "remainder" organs include the adrenals, gall bladder, heart, kidney, pancreas, prostate, small intestine, spleen, thymus, and uterus/cervix.

–The **effective dose** is expressed in terms of the **equivalent dose (mSv)** and is related to the patient **stochastic risk.**

   –**Equivalent doses** to individual **organs** and patient **effective dose** both use the same **dosimetric quantity (i.e., mSv),** which is often a source of confusion. (To minimize confusion, all effective doses in this book are expressed in mSv, whereas organ doses are given in mGy.)

–The **effective dose E** is the **uniform whole-body dose** that results in the **same stochastic risk** as any **nonuniform pattern** of **dose** such as depicted in Figure 7.6.

–A major benefit of the **effective dose** is that it **permits all radiologic examinations** that use ionizing radiations to be **directly compared** using a single common scale.

B. **Effective dose and skin dose**

–**Skin dose** may be converted to **effective dose** by taking into account **irradiation geometry** and **x-ray beam characteristics (i.e., area** and **quality).**

–For adults, **lateral skull** radiographs have an effective dose per unit skin dose of ∼**0.01 mSv/mGy.**

–**Adult PA chest radiographs** have effective dose per unit skin doses of ∼**0.2 mSv/mGy.**

   –Chest conversion factors are much higher than skull radiographs because the chest contains many more radiosensitive organs and a larger area is exposed.

–The adult effective dose per unit skin dose value for **AP chest radiographs** is ∼**0.25 mSv/mGy,** and for **lateral chest** radiographs is ∼**0.1 mSv/mGy.**

   –AP chest radiographs have a higher E/(skin dose) conversion factor because the breast dose is higher.

–For adult **AP abdominal radiographs,** effective dose per unit skin dose is ∼**0.15 mSv/mGy.**

–**Beam quality** (e.g., kV) also **impacts** on the **mSv/mGy conversion factors.**

–Reducing the x-ray tube voltage in chest radiography from **120** to **80 kV reduces** the **mSv/mGy** conversion factor ∼**25%.**

TABLE 7.5   Representative Effective Dose per Unit Air Kerma Area Product for PA Chest Radiographs

Patient Age	E/KAP (mSv/Gy-cm^2)
Newborn	2.5
1 year	1.0
5 years	0.70
10 years	0.45
15 years	0.3
Adult	0.25

C. Effective doses and KAP
  –Using **KAP** helps **differentiate** between **radiation incident** on a patient (i.e., KAP), and the corresponding amount of radiation that is **absorbed** by the patient (**i.e., E**).
  –**KAP** may be converted to **effective dose** by taking into account **irradiation geometry** and **x-ray beam quality.**
  –**Lateral skull radiographs** have E/KAP of $\sim$**0.035 mSv/Gy-cm^2.**
  –**PA chest radiographs** have E/KAP of $\sim$**0.2 mSv/Gy-cm^2.**
    –The effective dose per unit skin dose for **AP chest radiographs** is $\sim$**0.3 mSv/Gy–cm^2** and for **lateral chest radiographs** is $\sim$**0.15 mSv/Gy–cm^2.**
  –For **AP abdominal radiographs,** the effective dose per unit skin dose is $\sim$**0.2 mSv/Gy–cm^2.**
  –Patient size is an important determinant of E/KAP conversion factor, as illustrated by the data in Table 7.5.
    –**E/KAP conversion** factors for **newborns** are an **order** of **magnitude higher** than those for **adults.**
D. Effective dose and energy imparted
  –A normal-sized adult (**70 kg**) who is irradiated to a **uniform whole-body dose** of **1 Gy absorbs 70 J** of energy (energy = dose × mass).
  –A uniform **whole-body dose** of **1 Gy** of x-rays corresponds to an **effective dose** of **1 Sv.**
  –For uniform **whole-body** x-ray irradiation, **70 J** of energy can correspond to **1 Sv (1,000 mSv).**
    –For adults uniformly exposed, **each joule** of imparted energy corresponds to an effective dose of **14 mSv** (i.e., 1,000 mSv/70 J).
  –Effective dose per unit energy imparted conversion factors (E/ε) are available for most common radiologic examinations.
  –**Skull radiographs** have E/ε values of $\sim$**5 mSv/J,** and **head CT** scans have E/ε values of $\sim$**9 mSv/J.**
  –**Body radiographs** have E/ε values $\sim$**18 mSv/J,** and exposure of the **extremities** $\sim$**3 mSv/J.**
  –A **newborn (3.5 kg)** uniformly irradiated to **1 Gy** absorbs **3.5 J** of energy and receives an **effective dose** of **1 Sv.**
  –For newborns undergoing uniform irradiation, **each joule** absorbed corresponds to an **effective dose** of **290 mSv** (1,000 mSv/3.5 J).
    –E/ε conversion factors for **newborns** are **35 times higher** than for **adults.**
  –**Effective dose per unit energy imparted** conversion factors are **inversely proportional** to the **patient weight.**
    –For a given type of examination, the same energy absorbed by a patient with half the mass will double the effective dose.
E. Effective dose and dose length product (DLP)
  –CT **DLP** doses can be converted into an **effective dose** using **E/DLP conversion factors.**
  –**Adult head** and **neck** scans use **DLP** measured in **16-cm**-diameter phantoms, whereas **body** scans use **DLP** measured in **32-cm**-diameter phantoms.
    –E/DLP values for 32-cm-diameter phantoms are generally twice as high as E/DLP values for 16-cm-diameter phantoms.
  –Table 7.6 show E/DLP conversion factors for normal-sized adult patients undergoing a range of CT examinations.
    –**Patient size–specific E/DLP** conversion factors need to be used.
  –**Head CT E/DLP** conversion factors are $\sim$**4.0 μSv/mGy-cm** for a **5-year-old** and $\sim$**11 μSv/mGy-cm for** a **newborn** (16-cm phantom).

TABLE 7.6   E/DLP Conversion Factors for CT Scans of Normal Size Adults (120 kV)

CT Examination	E/DLP Conversion Factor (μSv/mGy-cm)	Diameter of Acrylic Phantom in Which DLP Is Measured (cm)
Head	2.2	16
Neck	5.4	16
Chest	17	32
Heart	19	32
Abdomen	16	32
Pelvis	19	32

–**Body CT E/DLP** conversion factors are ~**19** μ**Sv/mGy-cm for** a **5-year-old** and ~**44** μ**Sv/mGy-cm for** a **newborn** (16-cm phantom).

–Head **E/DLP** conversion factors are **independent** of x-ray tube **voltage (kV).**

–Increasing the CT x-ray tube voltage from **80** to **140 kV increases E/DLP** for body CT examinations by ~**25%.**

F. **Effective dose and risk**

–The **International Commission of Radiological Protection (ICRP)** publishes estimates of risk and detriment associated with any effective dose exposure (mSv).

–The most recent risk estimates were published in **Publication 103 (2008),** which replace the estimates published in Publication 60 (1990).

–ICRP risk estimates are averaged over both gender and age and are provided for (a) fatal cancer risks, (b) all cancer risks, and (c) all stochastic risks (cancer plus hereditary).

–The incidence of **fatal cancer** from radiation is estimated at ~**4% per Sv.**

–ICRP estimates radiation detriment by making adjustments for lethality and impact on quality of life.

–The nominal **cancer detriment** is ~**5.5% per Sv.**

–ICRP estimates of total detriment also include the induction of hereditary effects.

–**Total radiation detriment (cancer plus hereditary effects)** is ~**6% per Sv.**

   –Current risk estimates are slightly lower than those provided in 1990.

–For **radiation protection** purposes, the ICRP considers a risk coefficient of ~**0.00005 per mSv** (i.e., 5% per Sv) to be reasonable.

REVIEW TEST

7.1   What fraction of cell damage most likely results from direct action of x-ray radiation?
a. 1/6
b. 1/3
c. 1/2
d. 2/3
e. 5/6

7.2   How many cells exposed to an LD_{50} dose are most likely to be killed (%)?
a. 5
b. 25
c. 50
d. 75
e. 95

7.3   Which cells are likely to be the most resistant to ionizing radiation?
a. Marrow cells
b. Neuronal cells
c. Lymphoid tissues
d. Spermatids
e. Skin cells

7.4   The energy lost per unit length along the track of charged particles is most likely a measure of:
a. ionization
b. scintillation
c. linear attenuation coefficient
d. mass energy absorption
e. linear energy transfer

7.5   The radiation weighting factor (w_R) is used to convert absorbed dose into:
a. exposure
b. air kerma
c. equivalent dose
d. effective dose
e. collective dose

7.6   If the absorbed dose to lungs from radon daughters (i.e., alpha emitters) is 10 mGy, the lung equivalent dose (mSv) is:
a. 10
b. 20
c. 50
d. 100
e. 200

7.7   After an acute whole-body dose of 1 Gy, which effect is most likely to be observed?
a. Reduced lymphocytes
b. Skin erythema
c. Patient diarrhea
d. Eye cataracts
e. Hair epilation

7.8   The threshold dose (Gy) for the induction of deterministic effects in interventional radiology is likely to be taken as:
a. 0.5
b. 1
c. 2
d. 3
e. 5

7.9   The threshold dose (Gy) for temporary epilation is most likely:
a. 1
b. 3
c. 5
d. 7
e. 10

7.10   The time (days) before radiation-induced skin necrosis will manifest is most likely:
a. 0.5
b. 1
c. 2
d. 5
e. 10

7.11   The acute threshold dose (Gy) for cataract induction is most likely:
a. 1
b. 2
c. 5
d. 10
e. >10

7.12   The fractionated dose (Gy) that can induce permanent sterility in males is most likely:
a. 0.5
b. 1
c. 3
d. 5
e. 10

7.13   Stochastic effects of radiation include:
a. epilation
b. sterility
c. carcinogenesis
d. cataracts
e. erythema

7.14   Which of the following is *least* likely to show evidence of radiation-induced cancers?
a. Radiation therapy patient
b. Lung fluoroscopy patient
c. Radium dial painter
d. Nuclear medicine (NM) imaging patient
e. A-bomb survivor

7.15 Which of the following is most sensitive to radiation-induced carcinogenesis?
a. Heart muscle
b. Brain tissue
c. Gall bladder
d. Adrenal gland
e. Thyroid gland

7.16 Which radiation-induced cancers have the shortest latency period in exposed adults?
a. Breast
b. Colon
c. Leukemia
d. Lung
e. Stomach

7.17 The dose and dose-rate effectiveness factor (DDREF) is most likely:
a. 0.5
b. 2
c. 3
d. 5
e. 10

7.18 The relative cancer radiosensitivity of a child compared to 70-year-olds is most likely:
a. 1:1
b. 3:1
c. 10:1
d. 30:1
e. 100:1

7.19 Which group of irradiated individuals have demonstrated hereditary effects of radiation?
a. A-bomb survivors
b. Radiotherapy patients
c. Uranium miners
d. ^{131}I therapy patients
e. No human data

7.20 The average number of hereditary effects in the first two generations following an exposure of 1 mGy to the gonads is most likely:
a. 1 in 50
b. 1 in 500
c. 1 in 5,000
d. 1 in 50,000
e. 1 in 500,000

7.21 Gross malformation is most likely to occur:
a. preimplantation
b. early organogenesis
c. late organogenesis
d. early fetal period
e. late fetal period

7.22 The conceptus dose (mGy) that triggers consideration of medical intervention is likely:
a. 1

b. 3
c. 10
d. 30
e. 100

7.23 A fetal dose of 10 mGy likely increases the incidence (%) of childhood cancer by about:
a. 0 (no risk)
b. 0.5
c. 2.5
d. 10
e. 40

7.24 The backscatter factor in diagnostic radiology is most likely:
a. 1.1
b. 1.4
c. 1.8
d. 2.5
e. >2.5

7.25 An air kerma of 1 mGy will most likely result in a skin dose (mGy) of:
a. 0.5
b. 1.5
c. 3
d. 10
e. 20

7.26 If the entrance air kerma in an adult PA chest x-ray is 0.1 mGy, the air kerma–area product (Gy-cm^2) is most likely:
a. 0.1
b. 1
c. 10
d. 100
e. 1,000

7.27 If the skin dose in a lateral abdominal examination is 100%, the embryo dose (%) is most likely:
a. 50
b. 20
c. 5
d. 1
e. 0.2

7.28 Which of the following is *least* likely to affect the fetal dose in a radiographic examination?
a. Beam area
b. Beam HVL
c. Focal spot
d. Projection
e. Skin dose

7.29 All of the following organs have a tissue weighting factor (w) of 0.04 except:
a. bladder
b. esophagus
c. brain
d. liver
e. thyroid

7.30 For radiation protection purposes, an effective dose of 1 mSv corresponds to an average patient detriment (%) of about:
a. 50
b. 5

c. 0.5
d. 0.05
e. 0.005

ANSWERS AND EXPLANATIONS

7.1b. One third is direct, and the remaining 2/3 is indirect damage.

7.2c. LD_{50} kills 50% of the exposed cells (by definition).

7.3b. Neuronal cells are resistant to radiation because they are highly differentiated and nondividing.

7.4e. The energy lost (keV) per micron is the linear energy transfer.

7.5c. The radiation weighting factor (w_R) converts absorbed dose into equivalent dose.

7.6e. An alpha dose of 10 mGy corresponds to an equivalent dose of 200 mSv, since the alpha particle radiation weighting factor is 20.

7.7a. A whole body dose of 1 Gy will reduce the number of lymphocytes.

7.8c. Two Gy is the practical skin dose below which deterministic effects will not occur.

7.9b. Three Gy is the threshold dose for temporary epilation.

7.10e. Serious burns become visible ~10 days after the exposure occurs.

7.11b. Two Gy is the acute threshold dose for inducing eye cataracts.

7.12c. Three Gy (fractionated) could produce male sterility.

7.13c. Carcinogenesis is one of the two important stochastic radiation risks (hereditary effects is the other one).

7.14d. NM imaging patients have not been shown to have elevated risks of any type of cancer.

7.15e. The (young) thyroid is relatively sensitive to radiation. (The cancer fatality rate is relatively low [~5%], which explains why the thyroid weighting factor w is only 0.04.)

7.16c. Leukemia has a much shorter latency period than all solid tumors.

7.17b. Two is the DDREF factor used by the ICRP.

7.18c. Newborns are taken to be ~10 times more sensitive than 70-year-olds.

7.19e. There are no human data for the induction of hereditary effects by ionizing radiation.

7.20e. One in 500,000 (i.e., 0.2% per Gy).

7.21b. Gross malformation occurs in early organogenesis.

7.22e. The ICRP states that below 100 mGy, no medical intervention would be warranted.

7.23e. Forty percent, although the absolute risk is much lower at only ~0.06% (i.e., natural background incidence of childhood cancer is very low).

7.24b. A common backscatter value used in radiology is 1.4.

7.25b. The skin dose is 1.5 mGy after accounting for differences in dose to air/tissue (10%) and backscatter (40%).

7.26a. A KAP of 0.1 Gy-cm^2, since the exposed area at the patient entrance is ~1,000 cm^2.

7.27c. The fetal dose is ~5% of the skin dose for a lateral projection in abdominal radiography.

7.28c. The size of the focal spot has negligible effect on any patient (or operator) dose.

7.29c. The brain tissue weighting factor is 0.01.

7.30e. A determinant of 0.005%, or 5×10^{-5}, is the most likely risk of detriment (harm) from 1 mSv (i.e., ~5% per Sv).

Chapter 8

RADIATION PROTECTION

I. MEASURING RADIATION

A. Film dosimetry
  –**Film** can be used to measure **radiation doses** received by radiation **workers.**
  –**Film sensitivity,** however, depends on **x-ray photon** *energy.*
  –**Silver** in film, which has a **25 keV K-shell binding energy,** absorbs 30-keV photons very
    well but would absorb far fewer 300-keV photons.
      –For the *same* air kerma, the **blackening** of film at **30 keV** is much **greater** than for
        300-keV photons.
  –Film badges consist of a small case with a piece of film placed between different **fil-
    ters.**
      –Filters are little squares of **Cu, Sn, Al,** and **plastic.**
  –The pattern of blackening behind the filters provides evidence of the energies of the
    photons responsible for the operator's exposure.
      –**More uniform blackening** behind the filters implies a **higher photon energy.**
  –The **film** is **processed** and the optical **density measured** to estimate air kerma.
  –The **minimum air kerma** film badges can detect is ~**0.2 mGy.**
  –One advantage of film badges is that they provide a permanent record of operator dose.
  –**Film** badges have **limited accuracy** because of their strong energy dependence.
  –The accuracy of the reading can also be affected by heat and chemicals.
  –For all these reasons, **film badges** have been **largely replaced** by alternative devices (e.g.,
    thermoluminescent dosimeters [TLD]).
B. Thermoluminescent dosimeters
  –**Solid-state** materials can **store energy absorbed** during x-ray exposure in electron traps.
      –The stored energy is in the form of electrons trapped in high-energy imperfections in
        the crystal.
  –In **thermoluminescent dosimeters (TLDs),** these energetic electrons are released by the
    application of **heat.**
  –The **released electrons** result in the emission of **visible light.**
  –Heating TLDs after exposure results in a **light output** that is **proportional** to the radiation
    air kerma incident on the material.
  –**Lithium fluoride (LiF)** is the TLD used in diagnostic radiology because it **simulates** the
    absorption of x-rays by **soft tissues.**
      –LiF has an atomic number ($Z = 8.3$), close to that of soft **tissue** ($Z = 7.7$), which makes
        it **tissue equivalent.**
  –The response of **TLD** does **not** depend on photon **energy,** and similar signals would be
    obtained at both 30 keV and 300 keV (same air kerma).
      –The energy response of **LiF** is thus far **superior** to that of **film.**
  –TLDs materials are available that can measure doses as low as **0.01 mGy** or as high as
    10,000 mGy (10 Gy).
  –**TLDs** are frequently used to measure **patient** doses during radiographic examinations
    and may be used for **personnel dosimetry.**
  –The **detection limit** of a **TLD** used to monitor workers in radiology is ~**0.2 mGy.**

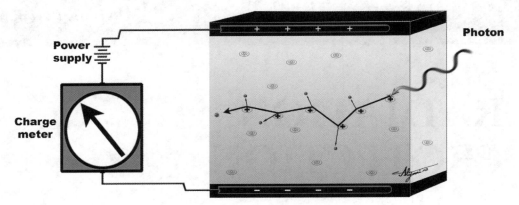

FIGURE 8.1   Schematic of the essential parts of ionization chambers that measure the electrons produced by x-rays interacting with air atoms.

C. Ionization chambers

–**Ionization chambers** detect ionizing radiation by measuring the **charge (electrons) liberated** when x-ray photons ionize the gas inside.

–Ionization chambers need a **positive voltage** at the collecting electrode (**anode**), which **attracts** the **liberated electrons.**

–The **applied voltage** should be **high** enough to collect all the liberated electrons.

–Figure 8.1 shows a schematic of the components of an ionization chamber.

–Charge liberated in the chamber is collected and used to determine the **air kerma.**

–**Ionization chambers** are *accurate* dosimetry devices.

–**X-ray tube output** is measured using **ionization chambers.**

–X-ray tube output is the air kerma (mGy/mAs) at a specified distance and voltage.

–A typical **x-ray tube output** is ~**0.1 mGy/mAs** at a **distance** of **1 m (80 kV).**

–**Ionization chambers** are **not very sensitive,** and would be **useless** for detecting small amounts of **radioactive contamination** in a nuclear medicine (NM) department.

D. Geiger counters

–A **Geiger counter** is an ionization chamber with a **very high voltage** across the chamber.

–An incident **photon** interacting in this chamber produces a **small number** of **free electrons.**

–These electrons are **accelerated** by the large positive voltage and **gain energy.**

–These energetic electrons will cause more electrons to be ejected from gas atoms in the chamber, which are further accelerated and produce even more electrons.

–As a result, there is an **electron avalanche** corresponding to a large amplification of the initial charge liberated by the incident electron.

–The large amplified output results in the **"click"** heard when using a **Geiger counter.**

–**Quenching gases** are added to Geiger counters to improve stability.

–**Geiger counters** are **sensitive** and are used to detect **low levels** of **radioactive contamination.**

–Geiger counters are far too sensitive to measure diagnostic x-ray beams.

–The number of **photons** in **x-ray beams** is ~10^7 **photons/mm^2** (i.e., huge).

–Geiger counters *cannot differentiate* between different types of radiation.

–Any beta particle or individual photon results in the same signal (electron avalanche).

–**Geiger counters** are **not** *accurate* radiation dosimeters.

–A Geiger counter provides "counts per minute", not mGy/minute.

E. Pocket dosimeters

–**Pocket dosimeters** are ionization chambers that look like **large pens.**

–A typical analog dosimeter uses a **positively charged quartz fiber** suspended in an air-filled chamber.

–**X-rays** incident on the chamber will **produce ions** that neutralize the charge and **cause** the **fiber** to **move.**

–The x-ray photon energy must exceed 20 keV to penetrate the wall of the dosimeter.

–The typical range of a pocket ionization chamber is **0 to 2 mGy.**

–Pocket ionization chambers are also available that work up to 50 mGy.

–**Pocket ionization chambers** are **easily recharged** and **reused.**

–Pocket ionization chambers are **frail** and may be damaged if dropped on the floor.
–Digital pocket dosimeters can be obtained that use radiation-sensitive diodes coupled to solid-state electrons to measure and display the dose.
–The principal **benefit** of pocket dosimeters is that they **provide** *immediate* **readings.**
–Pocket dosimeters are used to assess the **dose** to a **parent** who **holds** a **child** or infant during a radiologic examination.
  –Doses to parents holding children will be low (scatter radiation is 0.1% of the entrance air kerma at 1 m).
–**Pocket ionization chambers** can confirm low doses, and **reassure parents** who hold children.

II. DOSE LIMITS

A. Organizations
–The **International Commission** on **Radiological Protection (ICRP)** was founded in 1928 and issues periodic recommendations on radiation protection.
–**ICRP Publication 103 (2007)** is the latest publication from the ICRP that provides recommendations for radiation workers, patients, and members of the public.
  –ICRP Publication 103 replaces **Publication 60 (1990).**
–The **International Commission on Radiological Units and Measurements (ICRU)** advises on issues such as measurement units in radiology.
  –The **ICRU** was responsible for **replacing exposure (R)** with **air kerma (Gy).**
–In the United States, the foremost radiation protection body is the **National Council** on **Radiation Protection and Measurements (NCRP).**
–The NCRP advises federal and state regulators on radiation protection.
–In the United States, the **federal government** is primarily responsible for **regulating radioactive materials.**
–The **Nuclear Regulatory Commission (NRC)** is responsible for the rules and regulations regarding nuclear materials.
  –Specific rules and regulations are compiled in Parts 19 and 20 in Chapter 10 of the *Code of Federal Regulation (CFR).*
–Some states are known as **agreement states** and arrange with the NRC to self-regulate medically related licensing and inspection requirements for nuclear materials.
–Other states (i.e., **non–agreement states**) are **regulated** directly by the **NRC.**
–**U.S. states** are responsible for **regulating x-ray emitting devices.**
–States coordinate their x-ray protection activities through the **Conference of Radiation Control Program Directors (CRCPD),** which meets annually.

B. Occupational (whole body)
–**Occupational dose limits** *exclude* doses from **medical** procedures and natural **background** radiation.
–The **ICRP** recommends an effective dose limit of **20 mSv per year,** when averaged over 5 years.
–The **NCRP** recommends a lifetime cumulative effective dose limit of **ten times** the **individual's age (mSv).**
–Both ICRP and NCRP limit occupational exposure *in any year* to 50 mSv.
  –ICRP and NCRP philosophy is to balance operational flexibility with an adequate level of safety over a longer time frame.
–In the **United States,** the **regulatory** (i.e., legal) effective dose limit for radiation workers is **50 mSv/year.**
–Regulatory dose limits are similar at the federal and state levels.
  –Federal laws generally apply to exposures from radioactive materials (NM), whereas state regulations cover exposures from x-ray devices including CT.
–The most highly exposed workers are unlikely to receive regular annual effective doses >~**5 mSv** (2008).
–People who are **occupationally exposed** to radiation should be monitored using **personnel dosimeter** such as film badges or TLDs (see Section I).
–Emergency occupational exposures can exceed these dose limits if lifesaving actions are involved.
  –Older workers with low lifetime accumulated effective doses should volunteer for emergencies where high exposures are expected (up to 500 mSv).

–If an **emergency exposure exceeds 500 mSv,** possible **acute** and **long-term risks** need to be **addressed.**

C. **Public**
  –**Dose limits** for **members** of the **public** are much **lower** than those for occupational exposure.
  –The **ICRP** recommends a whole-body dose limit for members of the **public** of **1 mSv/year.**
    –ICRP Publication 103 (2007) maintained the public dose limit set in ICRP Publication 60 (1990).
  –ICRP dose limits may be exceeded in any 1 year provided the 5-year average dose does not exceed 1 mSv/year.
  –In the United States, the regulatory dose limit for members of the public is **1 mSv/year (2008).**
  –**X-ray facilities** must be designed to ensure that exposure to members of the **public does not exceed 1 mSv/year.**
  –**Dose limits** to members of the **public** *exclude* **natural background radiation.**
  –For regulatory purposes, **medical doses** are also **excluded** when determining doses for a member of the public.
    –Exclusion of medical x-rays is justified because diagnostic information from radiologic examination will confer a benefit to the exposed individual.
  –**Public exposures** from **radiologic** activities are normally **negligible.**

D. **Pregnant workers**
  –The ICRP recommends a limit of **1 mSv** from declaration of a **pregnancy** by a radiation worker to the subsequent birth of a child.
    –The **ICRP** considers the **fetus** to be a **member** of the **public** for radiation protection purposes.
  –Once a pregnancy is declared, the **NCRP** recommends a **monthly limit** of **0.5 mSv** to the embryo or fetus of a radiation worker.
  –The limitation on the *rate* at which the fetus is exposed helps ensure that any radiation risks to the fetus are kept to a minimum.
  –In the United States, the **regulatory dose limit** for the **fetus** of a radiation worker is **0.5 mSv/month,** which implies a total **dose limit** of **5 mSv.**
    –This fetal dose limit is *higher* than that of members of the public (1 mSv).
  –*This higher **fetus legal** dose limit **permits women** of reproductive capacity to seek employment as **radiation workers** (e.g., nuclear medicine technologists).*
    –Setting the fetal dose limit at 1 mSv would have deprived women of reproductive capacity employment as radiation workers.
  –**Pregnant radiation workers** are monitored by a **dosimeter worn** on the **abdomen** to ensure fetal dose limits are not exceeded.
  –Figure 8.2 shows a pregnant radiation worker wearing two dosimeters, one (A) worn outside the lead apron, and the other (B) that is worn under the lead apron.
    –Dosimeter A is used to estimate the worker effective dose and dosimeter B is used to estimate the embryo/fetus dose.
  –The **dose** to the **fetus** may be taken to be **half** the **skin dose** to account for attenuation by soft tissues between the fetus and skin surface.

E. **Miscellaneous**
  –The dose limit to the **eye lens** of an **occupational worker** is **150 mSv per year.**
  –The special eye lens dose limit is to **prevent** the induction of **eye cataracts** over a working lifetime.
  –The **dose limit** to the **skin** of a radiation worker is **500 mSv per year.**
  –Skin doses are to be averaged over the most highly exposed 1 cm^2.
  –The **skin dose limit** is designed to **prevent** the induction of **deterministic effects.**
    –Radiation therapy shows that skin tolerates fractionated doses of 20 Sv (20 Gy); 20 Sv divided by 40 working years corresponds to 500 mSv/year.
  –The dose limit for the **hands** and **feet** of **radiation workers** is also **500 mSv/year.**
  –Dose limits to **members** of the **public** are **15 mSv/year** for the **eye lens** and **50 mSv/year** for **skin.**
  –Dose limits for member of the public have historically been 1/10th of those of radiation workers.
  –Public dose limits are **conservative** to account for the possibility of **multiple sources** of **exposure.**

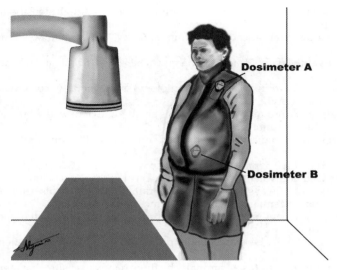

FIGURE 8.2   Monitoring the doses to a pregnant radiation worker.

III. PROTECTING WORKERS

A. Protection in radiology
  –One important objective of radiation protection is to **prevent significant deterministic effects.**
  –Deterministic effects can be prevented by keeping doses below the threshold dose of ~2 Gy.
  –A second objective of protection practice is to **minimize stochastic risk (cancer** and **hereditary effects).**
  –Minimization of stochastic risks needs to be reasonable and take into account any benefits gained by the radiation workers.
  –**Personnel monitoring devices** are worn to ensure that workers receive doses below the appropriate **dose limit** and to **monitor radiation safety practices.**
  –X-ray personnel receive significant exposures only when they are standing close to the patient undergoing the x-ray examination (i.e., in the same room).
  –Sources of exposure to x-ray personnel include **patient scatter** and **leakage radiation** from the x-ray tube.
  –As a general rule, the scatter dose level from patients at **1 m** is ~**0.1%** of the **entrance skin dose.**
  –Table 8.1 illustrates the scatter radiation exposures for common radiologic examinations.
  –Leakage radiation from the tube housing is very low.
  –Regulatory limits specify that **leakage radiation** must be <**1 mGy/hour** at a distance of **1 m.**
B. Lead aprons
  –**Lead** is an effective **protective barrier** with a very **high attenuation** coefficient.

TABLE 8.1   Representative Scatter Radiation Air Kerma Levels in Radiology

Examination	Air Kerma at 1 m (μGy)
PA chest x-ray	0.1
Lateral skull x-ray	1.5
AP abdominal x-ray	3
CT scan	30
Fluoroscopy (1 min)	20

–Attenuation of x-rays by lead is high because of its high density and high atomic number.

–The **half-value layer** of lead is ~0.1 mm at 60 kV, ~0.2 mm at 80 kV, and ~0.3 mm at 130 kV.

–The **tenth-value layer** of lead is ~0.35 mm at 60 kV, ~0.65 mm at 80 kV, and ~0.9 mm at 130 kV.

–**Lead aprons** used in diagnostic radiology are generally constructed from **lead-impregnated vinyl.**

  –**Tin impregnation** may also be used as an alternative to lead, as it has a more appropriate K-absorption edge.

–**Lead aprons** used in diagnostic radiology should have **0.25 mm** or **0.5 mm equivalents** of lead.

–A lead apron with 0.5 mm lead equivalence weighs about **5 kg** (10 lb).

–A 0.5-mm lead-equivalent apron attenuates most of the x-ray beam in diagnostic radiology and should always be worn when working close to patients being irradiated.

  –**Lead aprons attenuate at least 90%** of most x-ray beams.

–Individual organs not protected by lead aprons may receive much higher doses during fluoroscopy.

–Lead aprons should be stored on appropriate racks, as folding them can produce cracks.

–**Lead aprons** need to be **tested annually** by **fluoroscopy** to ensure that they do not contain any cracks.

C. Room shielding

–The design of **barriers** in radiology departments depends on the **workload (W),** which is how often the machine is in operation **(mA-minute/week).**

  –The workload can be combined with the x-ray tube output (mGy/mAs) to determine the radiation intensity at the patient location.

–The **source** to the **barrier distance** is used to estimate exposures outside the x-ray facilities by means of the **inverse square law.**

–Room shielding also depends on the use factor and occupancy factor.

–The **use factor (U)** is the fraction of time that radiation points toward a specific barrier.

  –For primary barriers, the use factor is 1 for the floor, 1/16 for the walls, and 0 for the ceiling.

–The **occupancy factor (T)** is fraction of time people work on the other side of the barrier.

  –Occupancy factors are 1 for offices and laboratories, 1/5 for corridors and employee lounges, and 1/20 for restrooms and storage areas.

–**Primary protective barriers** absorb primary radiation.

–**Secondary barriers** protect workers from scattered and leakage radiation.

–In practice, the shielding used for most x-ray installations is **1.6 mm (1/16 inch)** of **lead** in the walls.

–X-ray facilities need to ensure that there are no gaps between doors and that shielding extends at least **2 m** from the **floor.**

–Figure 8.3 shows a schematic of an x-ray facility.

D. Operator doses

–**Shielding** of x-ray rooms and booths housing the x-ray controls offers a **high degree** of **attenuation** of the x-ray beams.

–As a result, most **x-ray technologists** receive relatively **low effective doses.**

–Doses to 90% of x-ray technologists will be below the detection limit of the radiation badges used.

–**Significant doses** to operators occur when **operators are** in the **room** when the x-ray beam is activated.

–The most likely sources of **operator doses** in diagnostic radiology are **fluoroscopy** examinations and **interventional radiology.**

–**Radiologists** and **technologists** who routinely work **inside x-ray rooms** are likely to receive annual effective doses of ~**5 mSv.**

–Dosimeters worn **outside** the **lead apron** (obviously) **overestimate** the operator effective dose.

–**Effective doses** can be obtained from dosimeters worn over a protective lead apron by use of a **correction factor** that accounts for the additional **attenuation** of **lead aprons.**

–Dosimeters worn above the lead apron may be used to estimate the dose to **unshielded body parts** such as the lens of the eye.

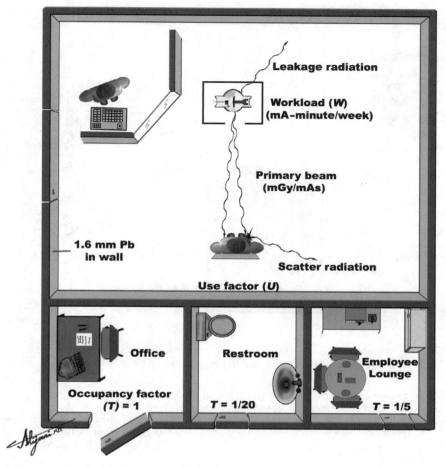

FIGURE 8.3   Schematic depiction of the most important factors taken into account when designing shielding for x-ray facilities.

- –The lifetime eye lens dose for interventional radiologists can approach the threshold dose for the induction of cataracts (5 Gy for chronic exposures).
- –Interventional radiology (IR) personnel should consider using **leaded prescription glasses** to increase their *safety margin* (i.e., [cataract threshold dose] minus [operator lifetime eye lens dose]).
    - –**Leaded glasses** might attenuate ~50% of an incident x-ray beam.
- –**Extremity doses** in radiology are likely to be well below the regulatory dose limits of **500 mSv/year.**
E. **Minimizing operator doses**
    - –During **fluoroscopy,** workers should **not** be in the **room** if not **necessary.**
    - –**Operator doses** are directly **proportional** to **patient doses.**
    - –Scattered radiation is dependent on the x-ray beam area, which should be minimized without sacrificing the diagnostic information provided by the study.
    - –Radiation workers should never hold a patient for a study.
        - –A parent or relative should position the patient and be given a lead apron to wear.
    - –Methods of **controlling radiation dose** are **decreasing exposure time, increasing distance** from the radiation source, and using appropriate **shielding.**
    - –**Fluoroscopy time,** and the number of **photospot images,** should always be **minimized.**
    - –Because radiation intensity falls off as the inverse square of the distance, **doubling** the **distance** reduces doses **fourfold.**
    - –Operators should maximize the distance between them and the patient without impeding patient safety or the diagnostic information provided by the x-ray examination.
        - –For **portable examinations,** operator should stand at least **2 m** from patients.

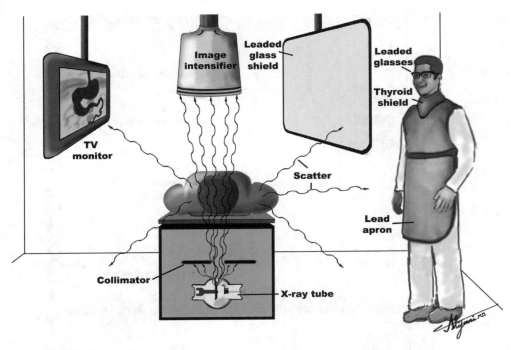

FIGURE 8.4 Scattered radiation in fluoroscopy, and protective devices (i.e., lead apron, thyroid shield, leaded glasses, leaded glass shields) used to minimize the radiation worker doses.

–**Lead aprons** *must* be worn at **all times** during **fluoroscopy** examinations.
–A **neck shield** can significantly reduce the dose to the thyroid.
–**Protective gloves** have a lead equivalence of 0.25 mm and may be used to minimize extremity doses when the hands are placed into the direct x-ray beam.
–Figure 8.4 shows how operator doses from scattered radiation in fluoroscopy should be minimized.

IV. PATIENT DOSES

A. Radiography
–Entrance **skin doses** in conventional radiography are very **low.**
–There is no possibility of inducing deterministic effects in any common radiographic examination.
–The **entrance skin dose** in a single **PA chest radiograph** is ∼0.2 mGy.
    –A **lateral chest x-ray** has a **skin dose** of ∼0.5 mGy.
–Table 8.2 shows typical skin doses in projection radiography and CT.
–Pediatric patients are smaller and the skin doses will generally be lower than those for adults.

TABLE 8.2   Representative Skin Doses in Radiology

Examination	Skin Dose (mGy)
Chest radiograph (AP)	0.2
Skull radiograph (AP)	1.5
Abdominal radiograph	3
Lumbar spine (lateral)	10
Fluoroscopy (1 min)	20
Body CT	30
Head CT	60

TABLE 8.3   Representative Effective Doses to Adult Patients Undergoing Radiographic Examinations of the Spine, Hip, and Extremities

Examination (Complete)	Effective Dose (mSv)
Cervical spine	0.3
Thoracic spine	1.5
Lumbar spine	2.0
Pelvis and hips	1.0
Limbs and joints	0.05

–The **effective dose** of a **chest** radiographic examination (PA plus lateral views) is typically **0.05 mSv.**
–The **effective dose** of a complete **skull** radiographic examination is ∼**0.1 mSv.**
–The **effective dose** of a complete **abdominal** radiographic examination is ∼**0.5 mSv.**
–Table 8.3 shows typical effective doses for examinations of the spine, hip, and extremities.
–**Radiation doses** in **projection radiography** are **low** in comparison to **gastrointestinal (GI) studies, interventional radiology,** and **CT.**

B. Fluoroscopy
  –**Entrance air kerma rates** in fluoroscopy typically range from **10** to **100 mGy/minute.**
  –A typical entrance skin air kerma rate in fluoroscopy for **normal-sized adults** is **30 mGy/minute.**
  –In the United States, the **legal limit** for entrance skin air kerma rate is **100 mGy/minute.**
  –**No regulatory limits** apply when a fluoroscopy imaging chain acquires *diagnostic images.*
      –Diagnostic images include **cardiac cine, digital subtraction angiography (DSA),** and **photospot.**
  –Modern fluoroscopy systems provide the option of either **continuous** or **pulsed fluoroscopy.**
  –**Patient doses** can be **reduced** by up to ∼**50%** using **pulsed mode.**
  –**Larger patients** require more radiation in fluoroscopy, which is achieved either by **increasing** the **x-ray tube voltage (kV)** and/or **increasing** the **tube current (mA).**
      –Table 8.4 shows how the fluoroscopy entrance air kerma rate varies with patient size.
  –Increasing the **tube voltage (kV)** in fluoroscopy **reduces patient doses** but also **reduces image contrast.**
  –Increasing the **tube current (mA)** in fluoroscopy **increases patient doses** but **maintains image contrast.**
  –**High-dose modes** in fluoroscopy may be activated to maintain image quality in very large patients.
      –Special activation mechanisms, as well as visible or audible indicators, indicate high-dose mode is being used.
      –The **maximum air kerma rate** in high-dose mode is ∼**200 mGy/minute.**
  –**Extended fluoroscopy** may result in **high doses** and produce skin damage or epilation.

C. Mammography
  –**Average glandular doses (AGD)** are obtained from entrance skin air kerma when imaging an ACR phantom that simulates a **4.2-cm breast with 50% glandularity.**

TABLE 8.4   Entrance Air Kerma Rates in Fluoroscopy as a Function of Patient Size, Where 23 cm Corresponds to a Normal-sized Adult Abdomen (AP Projection)

Patient Thickness (cm)	Entrance Air Kerma Rate (mGy/min)
10	1
15	3
20	10
23	30
25	50
30	200

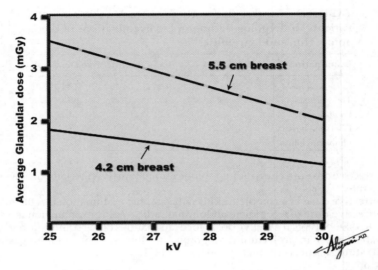

FIGURE 8.5   Average glandular dose in screen–film mammography as a function of x-ray tube voltage.

- –The **AGD** depends on x-ray beam techniques **(kV** and **mAs), beam filtration,** and **breast thickness** and **composition.**
- –Figure 8.5 shows that increasing the x-ray tube voltage (at a constant image receptor exposure) reduces the AGD because the beam becomes more penetrating.
- –**AGD** values are ~**1.8 mGy** per image in **screen–film.**
- –In **digital mammography, AGD** values are ~**1.5 mGy** per image.
    - –**Digital mammography** uses **higher beam qualities** (i.e., increased kV and filtration) resulting in reduced doses.
- –Breast doses to **patients** also depend on **breast characteristics** and the selected radiographic **techniques.**
    - –Actual patient doses can differ markedly from the AGD obtained using a breast dosimetry phantom.
- **D. GI studies/interventional radiology**
    - –Effective doses in GI studies depend on total fluoroscopy time as well as the number of photospot images.
    - –**Barium swallow** examinations have effective doses of **1** to **2 mSv.**
    - –Effective doses from **barium meal** examinations generally range between **2** and **8 mSv.**
    - –**Barium enemas** have effective doses that range between **5** and **15 mSv.**
    - –Double contrast enema studies doses are ~20% higher than single contrast.
    - –Effective doses for a **cardiac catheterization** examinations are ~**7 mSv.**
        - –Therapeutic catheterizations of the heart vessels are likely to result in higher radiation doses.
    - –**Cerebral angiography** has effective doses that range from **1** to **10 mSv.**
    - –Abdominal interventional radiography includes hepatic, renal mesenteric studies, as well as those of the aorta.
    - –Typical effective doses in **abdominal angiography** are ~**20 mSv.**
    - –**Peripheral angiography** studies have effective doses of ~**5 mSv.**
    - –Interventional radiology may result in deterministic effects.
        - –It is estimated that fewer than **1** in **10,000** patients undergoing interventional radiology *by qualified personnel* suffer from **serious deterministic** effects.
- **E. Computed tomography (CT)**
    - –Doses in **head CT examination are** ~**60 mGy** and well below the threshold for inducing eye cataracts.
    - –Doses in **body CT** examination are ~**25 mGy.**
    - –Skin doses in CT are well below the threshold dose for the induction of erythema.
        - –In **CT fluoroscopy,** higher skin doses are possible and are proportional to the fluoroscopy time and the selected technique (mA).
    - –If the **embryo/fetus** is directly exposed in CT, the **embryo dose** will likely to be ~**25 mGy** per single examination (phase).

TABLE 8.5   Representative Effective Doses to Adult Patients Undergoing CT Examinations

Type of Examination	Effective Dose from a Single Scan of the Specified Region (mSv)
Head	1–2
Chest	5–10
Abdomen/pelvis	5–10
Lower extremities	<1

–If the **embryo** is **8 cm** from the **directly irradiated** region, the mean dose will be no more than **10%** of the dose in the directly irradiated region.

–Table 8.5 shows typical effective doses to adults undergoing CT examinations.

–The effective dose for **head CT examinations** in **infants** and young children can be up to **four times higher** than for **adults** when performed using the same techniques.

–**Body CT examinations** in **infants** and young children can be **double** those of **adults** when performed using the same techniques.

  –Effective doses are higher in children than adults because of smaller organ sizes.

–The high doses associated with CT examinations prompted the **FDA** to issue an **advisory** in 2001 to **reduce radiation doses** to **pediatric patients.**

V. PROTECTING PATIENTS

A. Patient risks

–**Deterministic effects** are very **rare** and occur only in high-dose procedures such as interventional radiology.

–**Deterministic** effects can be **prevented** by keeping the organ **doses below 2 Gy.**

  –**Deterministic** effect occur ∼**10 days** after the exposure, and patients who may develop such effects must be adequately advised and monitored.

–A low-dose radiographic examination, with an **effective dose** of **0.2 mSv,** has a nominal **fatal cancer risk** of ∼**1** in **100,000** (population average).

–A high-dose CT examination, with an **effective dose** of ∼**20 mSv,** has a nominal **fatal cancer risk** of ∼**1** in **1,000** (population average).

–There are **large uncertainties** (and controversies) associated with all **patient radiation risk estimates.**

–**Epidemiologic studies** of radiation-induced **breast cancer** have breast doses on the order of a few **Gy,** whereas a **screening mammogram** results in an **AGD** of ∼**4 mGy.**

  –Patients may differ from a general population in terms of their sensitivity to radiation and their life expectancy.

–Figure 8.6 shows the **linear no threshold (LNT)** model used to extrapolate radiation risks from high to low doses.

–Controversies regarding radiation risks at low doses are unlikely to be resolved by epidemiologic studies because of the high background incidence of cancer.

  –In the United States, **42%** of the **population will get cancer during their lifetime.**

–**Difficulties** of detecting **radiation-induced cancers** from diagnostic **x-rays** would suggest that any **radiation risks** must be **small.**

B. Justification

–It is considered **prudent** to assume that radiation **risks** are **real** at doses encountered in diagnostic radiology (precautionary principle).

–**UNSCEAR, BEIR, NCRP,** and **ICRP** have all recently stated that the **LNT model** is a **reasonable** for **radiation protection purposes.**

–Assuming that all exposures are associated with possible radiation risk means that **radiologic examinations** need to be **justified.**

–Referring physicians should practice. **DAM (Don't order tests** that **don't affect management)** (coined by Dr. George S Bisset III of Duke University).

–**No patient** should be exposed to x-ray radiation unless he or she will obtain a **net benefit** from the **radiologic examination.**

  –A **net benefit** requires that the **diagnostic information** obtained is **greater than any radiation risks.**

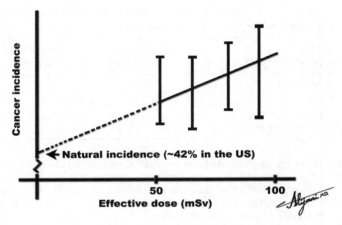

FIGURE 8.6   Linear no threshold (LNT) model showing how epidemiologic cancer incidence data are extrapolated (*dashed line*) to lower doses where no data are presently available.

–Justification requires that practitioners understand the magnitude of radiation risks and the corresponding uncertainties.
  –Practitioners also need to understand the benefits from alterative diagnostic examinations that could also be used to solve clinical problems.
–**Diagnostic radiologists** are knowledgeable about **radiation risks** and **diagnostic imaging** and can therefore *determine whether exams are justified.*

C. **Risk/benefit (screening mammography)**
  –A **two-view screening examination** will likely have an **AGD** that is below ~4 mGy for women with an average sized breast.
  –A breast dose of 4 mGy to 1 million examined 50-year-old women corresponds to an estimated risk of inducing **eight fatal breast cancers.**
  –This mammogram radiation risk is equivalent to the risk of dying in an accident when traveling 600 miles by car.
  –**Screening one million women** is expected to **identify 4,000** cases of **breast cancer.**
  –Without a screening program, the breast cancer fatality rate is ~25%.
  –**Screening programs** should **reduce** the **average fatality rate** by ~**25%,** or save ~**250 lives.**
  –*The benefit to risk ratio associated with **mammography screening** is therefore **very high.***
  –It is also important to note that the **benefits** of screening have been **demonstrated** in epidemiologic studies, which show benefits ranging from 15% to 35%.
  –The **radiation risks** at low doses on the order of a few mGy are **theoretical** and mainly based on extrapolations of observed effects at doses of a few Gy.
  –**Radiation doses (risks)** in **mammography** are very **low** and should **not deter** any women from having a **screening examination.**

D. **As low as reasonably achievable (ALARA)**
  –Assuming that all radiation exposures may carry some radiation risk requires that **patient doses** be **minimized.**
  –Minimizing patient doses means that no more radiation should be used than is technically required to obtain the required diagnostic information.
  –Minimizing patient doses in this way is known as **ALARA (as low as reasonably achievable).**
  –**Image quality** should be just **sufficient** to generate accurate **diagnostic information.**
    –Above a certain level, **higher doses** do **not improve diagnostic performance.**
  –**ALARA** requires **tailoring techniques** to the **diagnostic task.**
  –Radiation used for performing **follow-up scoliosis** studies in young patients with scoliosis can be more than **ten times lower** than conventional radiographs.
  –In CT, **reduced x-ray tube voltages (e.g., 80 kV)** may offer substantial improvements in the **visibility** of iodinated **contrast** material.
  –**Chest CT** for detecting **lung cancer** in asymptomatic patients (**i.e.,** *screening*) can use substantially reduced doses.

TABLE 8.6   Relative Techniques (mAs) for Performing Body CT Normalized to 100% for a Normal-sized Adult Abdomen

Patient Size	Chest	Abdomen
Newborn	40	45
1-year-old	45	50
5-year-old	55	60
10-year-old	60	65
Adult (normal size)	80	100
Adult (large)	130	160

–Follow up examinations for previously diagnosed lung nodules can often be performed with reduced radiation.
–Techniques in CT always need to be adjusted to take into account the size of the patient.
–Table 8.6 shows a typical technique chart for use when performing CT body scans of different-sized patients.
–Adult heads vary very little with patient age or size, and constant techniques are appropriate.
  –X-ray beam intensity **(mAs)** in head CT should be **reduced** by ~15% for a **1-year-**old and by ~25% for a **newborn.**
E. **Reducing patient doses**
  –The eye lens, gonads, and breasts may be shielded for specific examinations.
  –**Breast shields** are generally used during scoliosis examination since they will protect the breast without affecting the diagnostic information (spine curvature).
  –**Gonad shields** should be considered for patients of reproductive capacity.
  –Use of shielding may be appropriate when the gonads are in the direct x-ray beam and when this does not interfere with obtaining a satisfactory diagnosis.
  –The **number** of **radiographic exposures** obtained should be kept to a **minimum.**
  –Minimizing the exposure time in fluoroscopy is very important.
    –Exposure times in fluoroscopy can be reduced by the use of **last image hold (LIH).**
  –The **scan length** in **CT** should always be **minimized,** providing the anatomic area of interest has been adequately covered.
  –The need for **CT multiphase studies** should be carefully reviewed.
    –A **four-phase abdominal** CT scan (precontrast; arterial; venous; delayed) can **quadruple** the patient effective **dose.**
  –In multiphase CT scans, radiation techniques for *each component* need to be individually optimized.

VI. POPULATION DOSES

A. **Background radiation**
  –Contributions to natural background come from **cosmic radiation, terrestrial radioactivity,** and **radionuclides** incorporated in the **body.**
  –Cosmic rays are energetic charged particles that originate in galaxies.
  –Most cosmic rays interact with the atmosphere, with <0.05% reaching sea level.
  –In the United States, **cosmic rays** deliver ~**0.3 mSv/year.**
    –Leadville, Colorado, has an additional 0.9 mSv per year attributed to higher cosmic radiation (3,000 m elevation).
  –A **transcontinental U.S. flight** results in a dose of ~**0.03 mSv.**
  –**Air crews** receive an additional **5 mSv each year** flying ~1,000 hours at ~30,000 feet. **Space travel** results in ~**0.01 mSv/hour.**
  –In the United States, **external radiation (gamma rays)** from naturally occurring radionuclides in the soil delivers ~**0.3 mSv/year.**
    –Leadville also has elevated levels of terrestrial radioactivity, which results in an additional dose of ~0.7 mSv per year.

–**Internal radionuclides** include ^{40}K and ^{14}C, which have been present since the birth of our planet.
–The average dose from these primordial radionuclides is ~0.4 mSv/year.
–**Each year,** cosmic radiation, terrestrial radioactivity, and primordial radionuclides contribute an average annual effective dose of ~**1 mSv** *to everyone* in the **United States.**

B. Radon
–The biggest contribution to natural background radiation is from **domestic radon.**
–**Radon (^{222}Rn)** is a radioactive gas formed during the decay of radium.
–**Radium (^{226}Ra)** is a decay product of uranium found in the soil.
–**Radon** is an **alpha emitter,** which has a half-life of ~4 days.
–The **progeny** of **radon** are also radioactive and include two short-lived beta emitters and two short-lived alpha emitters.
–**Radon daughters** attach to aerosols and are deposited in the **lungs,** thereby permitting the bronchial mucosa to be irradiated and inducing bronchogenic cancer.
–The average concentration of radon outdoors is 4 to 8 Becquerel (Bq)/m^3 (0.1 to 0.2 pCi/L).
–Indoors, the average radon concentration is 40 Bq/m^3 (1 pCi/L).
–Average annual **effective doses** from **radon** are ~**2 mSv/year.**
–There are *very wide* variations in radon exposure.
–Radon levels in high-rise buildings are very low but can be high in poorly ventilated basements.
–Indoor radon is an important problem involving radiation exposure of the general public.
–Many homes are tested for radon levels when bought and sold.
–**Remedial action** is recommended at levels in **excess** of **160 Bq/m^3 (4 pCi/L).**
    –Practical remedial steps using improved ventilation can often be taken to reduce radon levels at modest costs (<$1k).

C. Average patient doses (United States)
–In 2006, ~**500 million diagnostic examinations** were performed in the **United States.**
    –Table 8.7 shows the types of examinations that were performed, together with the average effective dose per patient examination.
–Patient **effective doses** per examination in **radiography** are modest (**0.7 mSv**).
–Average effective doses are low in **mammography (0.1 mSv)** and **extremely low** in **dental radiography (<0.1 mSv).**
–Average patient effective doses are relatively high in **interventional radiology (8.6 mSv)** and in **CT (6.6 mSv).**
–Average patient effective doses in **NM (11.6 mSv)** are the highest encountered in all of diagnostic radiology.
–**Nuclear cardiology** accounts for nearly **60%** of **all nuclear studies.**

D. Population medical doses
–Table 8.8 shows the per capita doses in the United States for 2006 from diagnostic radiologic examinations.
    –**The per capita medical dose** is the collective medical dose divided by the U.S. population.
    –**The collective medical dose** is the average effective dose times the number of examinations.
–Per capita doses from mammography and dental radiography are negligible.

TABLE 8.7   Approximate Number of Radiologic Examinations Performed in the United States in 2006

Type of Examination	Examinations Performed (Millions)	Average Effective Dose per Patient Examination (mSv)
Radiography	280	0.7
Interventional radiology	15	8.6
Computed tomography	70	6.6
Mammography	35	0.1
Dental x-rays	125	<0.1
Nuclear medicine	20	11.6

TABLE 8.8   U.S. Population Average (i.e., per Capita)
Effective Doses from Diagnostic Medical Examinations
(2006)

Type of Examination	Per Capita Effective Dose (mSv)
Radiography	0.6
Interventional radiology	0.4
Computed tomography	1.5
Nuclear medicine	0.7

–In **2006,** the **U.S.** population average **dose** from diagnostic **medical** examinations was **3.2 mSv.**
   –In **1980,** the U.S. population average dose from diagnostic medical examinations was only **0.6 mSv.**
–*Per capita doses from diagnostic radiology have increased sixfold in one generation.*
–Diagnostic **medical imaging** now accounts for most of the **U.S. population dose** and exceeds doses from all sources of natural background combined.
–The most important reason for increased medical doses is increased use of CT.
–In the United States, **12%** of all **diagnostic exams** are **CT** scans, but this modality is responsible for nearly **half** the **population dose** from diagnostic imaging.
–In the United Kingdom in the 1990s, CT accounted for 4% of all radiologic examinations but accounted for 40% of the collective medical dose.
–Use of **CT** has been increasing at a rate of ∼**10% per year** over the last decade.
   –Population growth over the same period has been <1% per year.
–On average, **western** countries had ∼**14 CT scanners per million** inhabitants in 2005, with marked differences between countries.
   –For each **million** inhabitants, **Canada** has **11 CT scanners,** the **United States** has **32 CT** scanners, and **Japan** has **93 CT** scanners.
E. **Man-made (nonmedical) radiation exposure**
   –Major sources of exposure from consumer products are **building materials** and the **water supply.**
   –Other sources of exposure from consumer products include **luminous watches,** airport inspection systems, and **smoke detectors.**
   –Public radiation exposure from **consumer** products is ∼**0.1 mSv per year.**
   –Occupational exposure includes workers in medicine, the nuclear fuel cycle, and industry.
   –Most individuals who are classified as **radiation workers,** however, receive no measurable amount of radiation exposure.
   –Exposed workers in **medicine** have **average doses** of ∼**1.5 mSv/year.**
      –Average doses in **industry** are ∼**2.5 mSv/year,** and for **nuclear power workers,** average doses are ∼**5 mSv/year.**
   –The **nuclear fuel cycle** contributes ∼**0.004 mSv per year** to the U.S. population dose.
   –The contribution of **occupational doses** to the total exposure of the U.S. population is very low (∼**0.01 mSv/year).**
   –Nowadays, **fallout (e.g., ^{137}Cs)** from nuclear weapon testing in the 1950s contributes very little to U.S. population doses (<**0.01 mSv/year).**

REVIEW TEST

8.1 Which is *least* likely to be categorized as an x-ray detector?
a. Ionization chamber
b. Scintillation detector
c. Geiger-Muller counter
d. Photostimulable phosphor
e. Photomultiplier tube

8.2 Absorbed x-ray doses may be quantified by heating thermoluminescent dosimeters and measuring the emitted:
a. radio waves
b. microwaves
c. infrared
d. visible light
e. ultraviolet

8.3 When ionization chambers absorb x-rays, they most likely measure the resultant:
a. charge
b. heat
c. light
d. photons
e. voltage

8.4 Which of the following works on the principle of air ionization?
a. Intensifying screen
b. Thermoluminescent dosimeter
c. Photostimulable phosphor
d. Radiographic film
e. Geiger counter

8.5 Which dosimeter would likely be used when a parent holds a child for an x-ray examination?
a. Ionization chamber
b. Geiger counter
c. TLD
d. Film badge
e. Pocket dosimeter

8.6 Who coordinates the radiation control programs in all 50 states in the United States?
a. CRCPD
b. ICRP
c. BEIR
d. NCRP
e. NRC

8.7 The regulatory (2008) effective dose limit (mSv/year) for U.S. x-ray technologists is:
a. 1
b. 5
c. 10
d. 20
e. 50

8.8 The regulatory (2008) effective dose limit (mSv) for a patient chest CT scan is:
a. 1
b. 5
c. 20
d. 50
e. no limit

8.9 Regulatory dose limits for the public include only doses received from:
a. dental radiographs
b. airplane flight
c. terrestrial radioactivity
d. screening radiographs
e. radiology cafeterias

8.10 The regulatory (2008) dose limit (mSv/year) to a member of the public is:
a. 0.25
b. 0.5
c. 1
d. 2
e. 5

8.11 Scattered radiation intensities at 1 m in diagnostic examination, expressed as a percentage (%) of the patient skin dose, is most likely:
a. 0.01
b. 0.03
c. 0.1
d. 0.3
e. 1

8.12 Leakage radiation (mGy per hour) at 1 m from an x-ray tube must not exceed:
a. 0.01
b. 0.1
c. 1
d. 10
e. 100

8.13 The transmission of x-rays (%) by a 0.5-mm Pb apron in diagnostic radiology is most likely:
a. 5
b. 15
c. 25
d. 35
e. 45

8.14 Which is *least* likely to be required in designing the shielding for an x-ray room?
a. Beam filtration
b. Occupancy factor
c. Room dimensions
d. Use factor
e. Workload

8.15 The annual effective dose (mSv) received by a nuclear medicine technologist is most likely:
a. 0.3
b. 1
c. 3
d. 10
e. 30

8.16 If a radiologist were to increase the distance to a fluoroscopy patient from 1 to 2 m, his or her radiation dose would likely be:
a. 1/2
b. 1/3
c. 1/4
d. 1/5
e. 1/8

8.17 Entrance skin dose (mGy) for an AP abdominal x-ray examination is most likely:
a. 0.1
b. 0.5
c. 2
d. 10
e. >10

8.18 The patient exposure rate during fluoroscopy is *least* likely to be affected by the:
a. exposure time
b. grid ratio
c. patient thickness
d. tube current
e. tube voltage

8.19 The average glandular dose per film (mGy) in screening mammography is most likely:
a. 0.5
b. 1.5
c. 3
d. 5
e. 10

8.20 The chance (%) that a patient undergoing an IR procedure in a radiology department will suffer a serious deterministic injury is likely:
a. 10
b. 1
c. 0.1
d. 0.01
e. 0.001

8.21 Fetal doses in CT would likely be *reduced* with increasing:
a. patient size
b. tube voltage
c. tube current
d. scan time
e. scan length

8.22 The most likely patient effective dose (mSv) from a four-phase abdominal CT examination is most likely:
a. 5
b. 10
c. 25
d. 75
e. 150

8.23 The benefit–risk ratio of screening mammography is most likely:
a. 2:1
b. 4:1
c. 8:1
d. 16:1
e. >16:1

8.24 The average effective dose (mSv/year) from background radiation in the United States, excluding radon, is likely:
a. 0.1
b. 0.3
c. 1
d. 3
e. 10

8.25 Which are the most damaging emissions from the decay of ^{222}Rn (radon) and its daughters?
a. Alpha
b. Beta plus
c. Beta minus
d. Neutrino
e. Gamma ray

8.26 The largest exposure to the U.S. population from man-made radiation is the result of:
a. A-bomb fallout
b. diagnostic x-rays
c. industrial radiography
d. nuclear power plants
e. nuclear waste sites

8.27 The average effective dose to the U.S. population from diagnostic imaging in 2006 was most likely:
a. 0.5
b. 1
c. 2
d. 3
e. 5

8.28 The average patient effective dose (mSv) in NM imaging (2006) was most likely:
a. 0.5
b. 1
c. 2.5
d. 5
e. 10

8.29 The number of diagnostic x-ray examinations (millions) performed in the United States in 2006 was most likely:
a. 100
b. 250
c. 500
d. 1,000
e. 2,000

8.30 The contribution (%) of medical imaging to the U.S. population dose from all man-made radiation exposure is most likely:
a. 50
b. 75
c. 90
d. 95
e. >95

ANSWERS AND EXPLANATIONS

8.1e. Photomultiplier tubes detect light, not x-rays.

8.2d. TLDs emit visible light when heated.

8.3a. Ionization chambers collect and measure charge (or charge per second in fluoroscopy).

8.4e. Geiger counters are essentially (air) ionization chambers, but operated at a high voltage.

8.5e. Pocket ionization chamber because it is so easy to read (just point at the window, and read off the exposure that was received).

8.6a. Conference of Radiation Control Program Directors (CRCPD).

8.7e. Fifty mSv per year is the legal limit in the United States for radiation workers.

8.8e. There are no dose limits in radiology (except for fluoroscopy and mammography).

8.9e. Imaging center cafeteria since the dose received comes from the (shielded) CT facility and must not exceed 1 mSv.

8.10c. One mSv is the current regulatory dose limit to members of the public.

8.11c. The scattered intensity is likely 0.1% of what the patient gets; at 1 m from a fluoroscopy patient, the radiologist is exposed to 0.02 mGy/minute since the patient receives 20 mGy/minute.

8.12c. One mGy per hour is the current regulatory limit in the United States (100 mR/hour).

8.13a. Five percent is likely to get through a lead apron, and the remaining 95% absorbed.

8.14a. Beam filtration is not used in shielding calculations.

8.15c. Three mSv per year is a typical NM operator dose.

8.16c. One fourth by the inverse square law.

8.17c. Two mGy is a typical skin dose in abdominal radiography for an AP projection.

8.18a. Exposure time is relevant only for the total exposure, not the exposure rate.

8.19b. For an average-sized breast, 1.5 mGy per image is typical (3 mGy is the ACR/MQSA limit).

8.20d. The chance is 0.01% or 1 in 10,000 patients for a serious injury.

8.21a. Larger patient size will reduce fetal dose because of additional attenuation (dilution) of the x-ray beam.

8.22c. The most likely dose would be 25 mSv (6 mSv/scan would be typical).

8.23e. A ratio of >16:1 (a value of 30:1 was obtained in this book).

8.24c. One mSv per year in the United States, with an additional 2 mSv from radon.

8.25a. Alpha particles are emitted by radon and its daughters.

8.26b. Diagnostic x-rays are the dominant contributor to man-made radiation exposures in the United States.

8.27d. Three mSv is the average dose to the U.S. population from diagnostic imaging.

8.28e. Ten mSv (NM is the imaging modality with the highest average patient doses).

8.29c. About 500 million examinations were performed in the United States in 2006, including dental x-rays.

8.30e. More than 95% of man-made exposures are from diagnostic imaging.

Chapter 9

NUCLEAR MEDICINE

I. RADIONUCLIDES

A. Stable nuclei
  –Atomic **nuclei** contain **protons** and **neutrons** (i.e., nucleons).
  –Nucleons are held together by the **strong force.**
  –Energy required to remove a nucleon from a nucleus is **nucleon binding energy.**
  –Nuclide **mass number A** is the sum of the number of protons (Z) and neutrons (N).
    –For each nuclide, **A = Z + N.**
  –Stable ^{127}I has 127 nucleons (Z = 53 and N = 74).
  –Nuclides having the same mass number **A** are called **isobars.**
  –Nuclides having the same **atomic number** (protons) are called **isotopes.**
    –Table 9.1 lists the three isotopes of hydrogen.
  –Nuclides having the same number of **neutrons** are called **isotones.**
  –An **isomer** is the **excited state** of a **nucleus.**
  –**Stable low mass** number nuclides have approximately **equal** numbers of **neutrons (N)** and **protons (Z).**
    –The most common carbon nucleus (^{12}C) has six protons and six neutrons, and the most common oxygen nucleus (^{16}O) has eight protons and eight neutrons.
  –**Stable high mass number** nuclides have more **neutrons** than **protons.**
    –The most common tungsten nucleus (^{184}W) has 74 protons and 110 neutrons.
  –Figure 9.1 graphically shows the number of neutrons and protons in stable nuclei found in nature.

B. Unstable nuclei
  –**Unstable nuclides** are called **radionuclides.**
  –Very heavy nuclei **(Z > 82)** tend to be **unstable.**
  –The transformation of an unstable nuclide is called **radioactive decay.**
  –The original nuclide is the **parent,** and the nuclides resulting from the nuclear transformation are **daughters.**
  –Unstable nuclides undergo nuclear transformation as summarized in Table 9.2.
  –In all nuclear transformations, the **total energy** is always **conserved.**
  –**Mass number** and **electric charge** are also **conserved** when nuclei decay.
  –The **ground state** is the lowest energy state of a nucleus.
    –Nuclear ground states are the most stable arrangement of nucleons.
  –**Higher energy levels (excited states)** are known as **isomeric** states.
    –Isomeric states are always unstable.
  –Excited states will transform into a lower energy level, emitting a **gamma ray or internal conversion electron.**
    –A gamma ray is **electromagnetic radiation** originating in a nuclear transformation.
  –The excess energy may be transferred to an orbital electron, which is then emitted from the atom as an **internal conversion electron.**
    –After an **isomeric** transition, both **parent** and **daughter nuclei** have the **same mass number** and **atomic number.**
  –Isomeric states that have long lifetimes are called **metastable.**
    –To be called **metastable,** the half-life must be longer than 10^{-9} **second.**
  –The metastable state of an atom is denoted by a lower case m following the mass number (e.g., ^{99m}Tc).

TABLE 9.1   Isotopes of Hydrogen

				Name	
Symbol	Protons (Z)	Neutrons (N)	Number A	Nucleus	Atom
^{1}H	1	0	1	Proton	Hydrogen
^{2}H	1	1	2	Deuteron	Deuterium
^{3}H	1	2	3	Triton	Tritium

C. Alpha decay

–In **alpha decay,** a radionuclide emits an **alpha particle** consisting of **two neutrons** and **two protons.**

–An alpha particle is the **nucleus** of a **helium atom.**

–Alpha decay is most common in atoms with a high **atomic number (Z>82).**

–^{226}**Ra** is a common alpha emitter found in nature.

–^{226}**Ra decays** to ^{222}**Rn (radon),** which is another alpha emitter.

–In alpha decay, the atomic number decreases by two and the mass number decreases by four.

–**Energies** of alpha particles are generally between **4** and **7 MeV.**

–Alpha particle energies are **discrete** and well defined for a given alpha emitter.

–**Alpha particles** travel **<0.1 mm** in **tissue,** losing their energy by ionizing atoms along the track length.

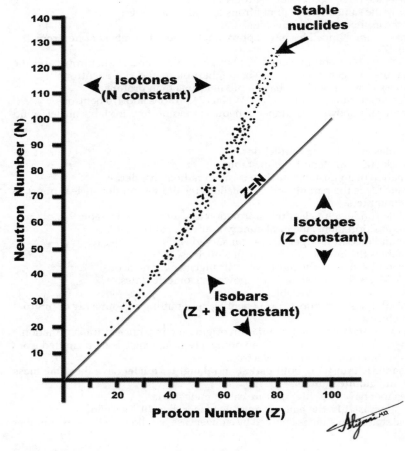

FIGURE 9.1   Each dot represents a stable nucleus found in nature.

TABLE 9.2   Radioactive Decay Modes for Unstable Nuclei Containing Protons (Z), Neutrons (N), and mass number A = Z + N

| Decay Mode | Daughter Nucleus Value | | | Comments |
	Mass No.	Atomic No.	Neutron No.	
Isomeric transition	A	Z	N	Metastable if half-life $> 10^{-9}$ s
Beta minus (β^-)	A	Z + 1	N − 1	Emits electrons and antineutrinos
Beta plus (β^+)	A	Z − 1	N + 1	Emits positrons and neutrinos
Electron capture	A	Z − 1	N + 1	Emits neutrinos (and x-rays[a])
Alpha decay	A − 4	Z − 2	N − 2	Dominant decay mode for $Z > 82$

[a] Characteristic x-rays emitted when the inner shell vacancies are filled.

–Alpha particles pose **little risk** as an **external radiation** source as they cannot penetrate through the skin.
–Alpha particles may pose a **high risk** if **ingested, inhaled,** or **injected.**
    –Radioactive **radon (plus daughters)** is hazardous because radioactivity is deposited in the lung, with a subsequent risk of **lung cancer** (Chapter 8, Section VI).
D. Beta minus decay
    –In **beta minus (β^-) decay,** a **neutron** inside the nucleus is converted into a **proton.**
    –**Beta minus** decay occurs in nuclei with an **excess** of **neutrons** (i.e., too few protons).
        –The excess energy is released as an **energetic electron,** called a **beta particle.**
    –Beta minus decay also results in the emission of an **antineutrino.**
        –**Antineutrinos** have **no rest mass** or **electric charge** and rarely interact with matter.
    –In **beta minus** decay, the **atomic number increases** by **one,** but the mass number remains constant.
    –**Beta particles (electrons)** emitted during beta minus decay have a **range** of energies up to a **maximum** energy.
        –Plotting the number of electrons at each energy against the energy shows the electron **spectrum.**
    –The **maximum energy** in this spectrum is denoted E_{max}.
    –The average energy of beta emitters is approximately one third the maximum.
        –**Average beta particle energy is** $\sim E_{max}/3$.
    –The **energy difference** between E_{max} and any given beta particle energy is carried away by the **antineutrino.**
    –^{32}P is a pure beta emitter with maximum beta particle energy of 1.71 MeV.
        –The mean beta particle energy of ^{32}P is $\sim$0.570 MeV.
    –^{3}**H (tritium)** (E_{max} = 18 keV) and ^{14}**C** (E_{max} = 156 keV) are **low energy** β^- emitters that are ubiquitous in biomedical research.
    –Figure 9.2A shows the beta minus decay of tritium.
E. Beta plus decay
    –In **beta plus (β^+) decay,** a **proton** inside the nucleus is **converted** into a **neutron.**
    –The excess energy is emitted as a positively charged electron called a **positron.**
        –Positrons have the same properties as electrons, except that their **charge** is **positive** (electrons have negative charges).
    –**Beta plus decay** (positron emission) occurs in **neutron-deficient nuclei (i.e., too many protons).**
    –**Beta plus** decay also results in the emission of a **neutrino.**
    –**A neutrino** has **no electric charge** or **rest mass** and is similar to an **antineutrino.**
        –**Beta plus** decay is also known as **positron emission.**
    –In **beta plus** decay, the **atomic number decreases** by **one** and the **mass number** stays the same.
    –Energetic **positrons lose** their **energy** by **ionization** and **excitation** of atomic electrons.
    –When the positron loses all of its kinetic energy, it **annihilates** with an **electron.**
    –The **mass** of the positron and electron (511 keV each) are converted into two **511-keV photons** that are emitted in opposite directions (i.e., **180 degrees apart**).
    –Many common positron emitters have very short half-lives.
        –^{11}**C** half-life is **20 minutes** (Fig. 9.2B), and ^{15}**O** half-life is **2 minutes.**

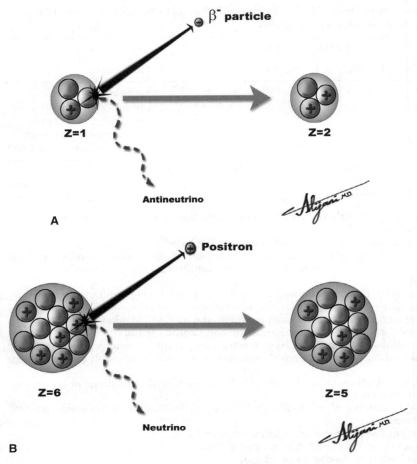

FIGURE 9.2   Beta decay. **A:** Beta minus decay of tritium **(left),** which decays by emitting an electron (i.e., beta minus particle) and an antineutrino and is thereby transformed into ^{3}He **(right); B:** Beta plus (positron emitter) of ^{11}C **(left),** which decays by emitting a positron and neutrino and is thereby transformed to ^{11}Boron **(right).**

   –The most popular positron emitter used in nuclear medicine is ^{18}F with a half-life of **110 minutes.**
   –The **maximum energy** of the ^{18}F **positron is 0.63 MeV,** and the average positron energy is one third the maximum (i.e., 0.21 MeV).
   –The **distance (range)** that the average ^{18}F positron travels in soft tissue is ~**0.4 mm.**
      –Positron ranges will increase in lower density tissues (e.g., lung).
F. **Electron capture**
   –In **electron capture,** a **proton** inside the nucleus is converted into a **neutron** by **capturing** an **atomic electron.**
   –The electron that is captured most likely originates in the **K-shell.**
   –A **neutrino** is emitted during **electron capture.**
   –**Electron capture** occurs in nuclei **deficient** in **neutrons** (too many protons).
   –In **electron capture,** the **atomic number decreases** by **one** and the mass number stays the same.
   –If the captured electron is from the K-shell, the resultant **K-shell vacancy** is filled by an outer shell electron.
   –The excess energy is emitted either as a **characteristic x-ray** or **Auger electron** (see Chapter 1).
   –**Electron capture** may **compete** with **beta plus decay.**

–Important electron capture radionuclides used in nuclear medicine are ^{67}Ga, ^{111}In, ^{123}I, and ^{201}Tl.

–^{57}Co is also an electron capture radionuclide used for **quality control** of scintillation camera uniformity.

II. RADIOPHARMACEUTICALS

A. Production of radioactivity

–**Radionuclides** may be produced in a **nuclear reactor** by **adding neutrons** to a stable nuclide.

–^{59}Co + neutron → ^{60}Co, which is called **neutron activation.**

–**Neutron activation** products **cannot** be **chemically separated.**

–**Reactor-produced radionuclides** generally decay by a **beta minus** process.

–**Radionuclides** may be produced in **cyclotrons** where **charged particles** (e.g., protons or deuterons) are added to stable nuclides.

–^{201}Hg + deuteron → ^{201}Tl + two neutrons.

–**Cyclotron-produced radionuclides** can decay by a **beta plus** process.

–^{15}O is produced in a cyclotron and is a **positron emitter.**

–Cyclotron-produced radionuclides may also decay by electron capture.

–^{123}I is produced in cyclotrons and decays via **electron capture.**

–Radionuclides may also be produced as **fission products** when heavy nuclides break up.

–In nuclear medicine, **generators** are used to produce radionuclides that are short lived.

–In a **generator,** the useful radionuclide **(daughter)** is continuously produced by the radioactive decay of a *longer-lived* **(parent)** radionuclide.

–In generators, the parent half-life is longer than that of the daughter.

–**Technetium-99m** and **rubidium-82** are obtained from NM **generators.**

–^{99m}Tc is obtained from ^{99}Mo and emits gamma rays **(isomeric transition),** and ^{82}Rb is obtained from ^{82}Sr and is a **positron emitter.**

–Table 9.3 lists the modes of production, as well as key characteristics, of common radionuclides used in nuclear medicine.

B. Measuring radioactivity

–**Activity** is the number of **transformations per unit time.**

–The **SI** unit of activity is the **becquerel (Bq).**

–**One becquerel** is **one transformation per second.**

–The **non-SI** unit is the **curie (Ci).**

–**One curie** is **3.7 × 10^{10} transformations per second.**

–An activity of **1 mCi** is equivalent to **37 MBq.**

–**Physical half-life (T$_{1/2}$)** is the time required for a half of the radionuclide present to decay.

–The fractional activity remaining after **n half-lives** is **1/2^n** (Fig. 9.3).

–After **ten half-lives,** only **0.1%** of the initial activity remains (1/2^{10} is ~1/1,000).

–**Radioactivity decays exponentially** and is characterized by the decay constant λ.

–**Activity** is **N × λ,** where N is the number of atoms in the sample.

–The fractional activity of a source remaining at time t is **e$^{-\lambda \times t}$.**

–The relationship between λ and half life **T$_{1/2}$** is given by **T$_{1/2}$ = 0.693/λ.**

TABLE 9.3   Characteristics of Common Radionuclides

Nuclide	Photons (keV)	Production Mode	Decay Mode	Half-life (T$_{1/2}$)
^{67}Ga	93, 185, 300	Cyclotron	EC	78 hours
^{99m}Tc	140	Generator	IT	6 hours
^{111}In	173, 247	Cyclotron	EC	68 hours
^{123}I	159	Cyclotron	EC	13 hours
^{131}I	364	Fission product	β	8 days
^{133}Xe	80	Fission product	β	5.3 days
^{201}Tl	70, 167	Cyclotron	EC	73 hours

EC, electron capture; IT, isomeric transition; β, beta decay.

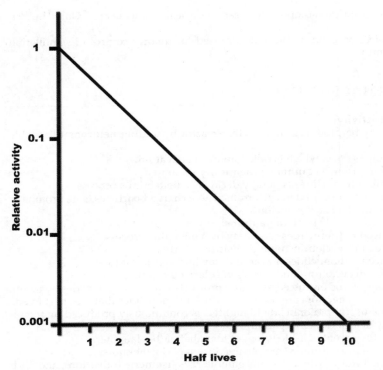

FIGURE 9.3 Plot of relative activity as a function of half-life (time), showing that the remaining activity after ten half-lives is only 0.1% of the initial activity.

C. ^{99}Mo/^{99m}Tc generators

– Technetium (^{99m}Tc) is readily available from a generator used in ~**80%** of all **nuclear medicine** examinations.
   – ^{99m}Tc has a gamma ray energy of **140 keV** that is ideal for imaging and a **half-life** of **6 hours** that is convenient.
– Pertechnetate (^{99m}TcO$_4$) is produced directly from ^{99}Mo using a **saline eluant.**
– The technetium generator is shielded with lead and consists of an **alumina column** loaded with ^{99}Mo.
– ^{99}Mo decays to ^{99m}Tc, and saline is added to the generator when ^{99m}Tc is needed.
– Saline passes through the column to elute (wash off) the ^{99m}Tc in the form of **sodium pertechnetate.**
– The ^{99}Mo is **not soluble** in saline and remains in the column.
– ^{99m}Tc decays by **isomeric transition** where **88% of nuclear transformations** result in emission of a **140-keV gamma ray.**
   – Energy is also emitted in the form of **internal conversion electrons, characteristic x-rays,** and **Auger electrons.**
– The **half-life** of ^{99}Mo is **66 hours,** which allows the generator to remain useful for approximately **1 week** (~2.5 half-lives).
– A ^{99m}Tc generator is normally eluted daily over the course of a week (Fig. 9.4) and then replaced.

D. Generator equilibrium

– A brand new ^{99}Mo/^{99m}Tc generator has only ^{99}Mo activity but no ^{99m}Tc activity.
   – A typical generator initially starts with ~37 GBq (1 Ci) of ^{99}Mo.
– As ^{99}Mo decays, ^{99m}Tc activity is **produced.**
– The **daughter** (^{99m}Tc) activity increases until equilibrium is reached.
– For practical purposes, at **equilibrium** the **activities** of **parent** and **daughter** may be taken to be approximately **equal.**
   – In equilibrium, a **1 Ci ^{99}Mo** generator also has **approximately 1 Ci of ^{99m}Tc.**

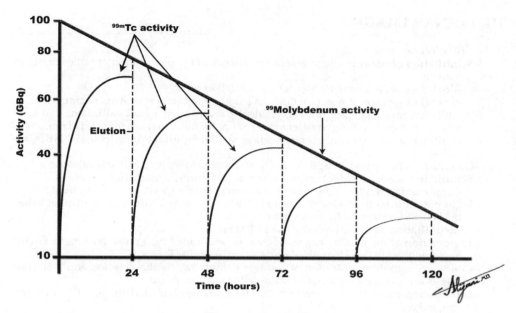

FIGURE 9.4   Idealized plot of parent ^{99}Mo and daughter ^{99m}Tc activities as a function of time, where the ^{99}Mo/^{99m}Tc generator is eluted at intervals of 24 hours.

–It takes approximately four **daughter half-lives** to reach **equilibrium**.
  –A ^{99}**Mo** generator thus takes approximately **24 hours** to reach **equilibrium**.
–Figure 9.4 shows an idealized schematic of the activity of the parent ^{99}Mo and the daughter ^{99m}Tc.
  –In equilibrium, the activity of ^{99m}Tc is ~90% of the ^{99}Mo activity.
–**Transient equilibrium** is the name given when the **parent** radionuclide is **short lived**.
  –**Secular equilibrium** is the name given when the **parent** is long **lived**.
–The *essential physics* of **secular** and **transient equilibrium** are **identical**.
  –Both **secular** and **transient** equilibrium occur after **four daughter half-lives** with both **parent** and **daughter activities** being approximately **equal**.
E. **Radiopharmaceuticals**
–Radionuclides should have a **short half-life** to **minimize** the patient **radiation dose**.
–Ideal gamma rays have energies between **100** and **300 keV**.
  –The gamma ray must have enough energy to get out of the patient, but not so high that it is difficult to detect.
–Radionuclides should have **minimal particulate radiations** (e.g., beta particles) to minimize patient dose.
–Evaluation of **function, not anatomy,** sets **nuclear medicine** studies apart.
–**Radiopharmaceuticals** are designed to mimic a natural **physiologic process.**
–The design of a radiopharmaceutical should ensure that it will **localize** in the **organ** or tissue of interest.
–Important characteristics of radiopharmaceuticals are that they be **nontoxic,** and contain **no contaminants.**
  –Contaminants of radiopharmaceuticals include chemicals and radionuclides.
–There are a number of radiopharmaceutical localization mechanisms.
–**Active transport** such as thyroid uptake scanning with **iodine.**
–**Compartmental localization** such as blood pool scanning with **human serum albumin,** plasma, or **red blood cells.**
–Simple **exchange** or **diffusion** such as bone scanning with **pyrophosphates.**
–**Phagocytosis** such as liver, spleen, and bone marrow scanning with **radiocolloids.**
–**Capillary blockade** such as lung scanning with **macroaggregate** (8–75 μm) or **organ perfusion** studies with intra-arterial injection of macroaggregates.
–**Cell sequestration** such as spleen scanning with **damaged red blood cells.**

III. PLANAR IMAGING

A. Scintillation cameras
–**Scintillation cameras** produce **projection images** of the distribution of radioactivity in patients.
–Figure 9.5 shows a schematic view of a scintillation camera.
  –Scintillation cameras are sometimes called **gamma cameras** or **Anger cameras.**
–Scintillation rays emerging from the patient pass through a **lead collimator** that only allows photons traveling **parallel to** the collimator holes to reach the **scintillator.**
  –**Collimators** are essential for providing **spatial information** in planar NM imaging.
–Gamma rays that pass through the collimator are incident on a **NaI scintillator.**
–**Scintillators** absorb incident gamma photons and **produce** many **light photons.**
  –**Approximately 10%** of the absorbed **gamma ray energy** is converted to **light.**
–**Light** output from the NaI scintillator is detected by an array of **photomultiplier tubes (PMTs)** and converted to an electrical signal.
  –**Scintillation cameras** typically use **55 PMTs.**
–The **position** of the **gamma ray** interaction is determined by a **pulse arithmetic circuit** based on the relative strength of signals from each PMT.
–**Count** refers to the registration of a **single gamma ray** by the detector, and ∼**500,000** counts are acquired for a typical scintillation camera image.
–**Scintillation cameras** use computers to **store, manipulate,** and **display** the acquired image data.

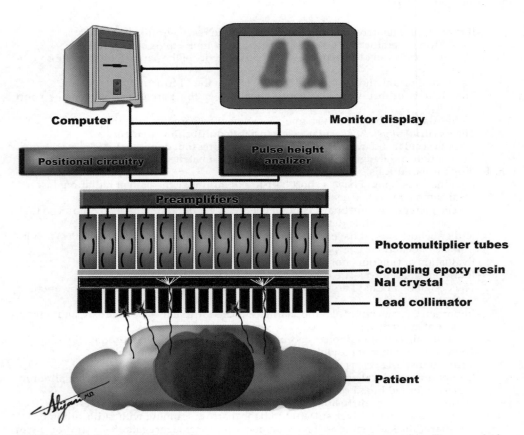

FIGURE 9.5   Schematic of a scintillating camera showing the key components of a collimator which include the NaI detector, an array of light detectors (i.e., photomultiplier tube), and light analysis circuits (i.e., PHA + positional circuitry).

–Scintillation cameras have corrections made to the acquired image data that correct for system **spatial nonlinearity** and **nonuniformities.**
  –**Energy corrections** are also incorporated to account for differences in the response of individual photomultiplier tubes.
–Scintillation cameras have **lead shielding** to prevent unwanted background radiation from the room or other areas of the patient from contributing to the image information.

B. Collimators
  –**Collimators** are typically made of **lead** and contain multiple holes (Fig. 9.5).
    –The lead strips between the holes are called **septa.**
  –**Parallel-hole** collimators project the same object size onto the camera, and the **field of view (FOV)** does not change with distance.
  –**Converging collimators** produce a magnified image, and FOV decreases with distance.
  –**Diverging collimators** project an image size that is smaller than the object size, and FOV increases with distance.
  –**Pinhole collimators** are cone shaped with a single hole at the apex.
  –Images generated using a **pinhole** collimator are normally **magnified** and **inverted.**
    –Figure 9.6 shows a pinhole collimator used to obtain magnified images of the thyroid.
  –**Collimator sensitivity** is the fraction of gamma rays reaching it from all directions that pass through the holes.
  –Collimator **sensitivity** is **low** with approximately 10^{-4}, or **only 0.01%,** of the emitted photons being detected.
  –**High-sensitivity collimators** have larger holes and lower resolution.
  –**High-resolution collimators** have smaller holes and lower sensitivity.
  –Table 9.4 summarizes the collimator resolution performance.
    –**Resolution** is degraded with increasing distance from the collimator.
  –**Low-energy** collimators used with ^{99m}Tc and ^{201}Tl have thin septa.
    –**Low-energy high-resolution (LEHR)** collimators are most frequently used.
  –**Medium-energy collimators** used with ^{67}Ga and ^{111}In have thicker septa and therefore fewer holes and lower sensitivity.
  –**High-energy collimators** are required for ^{131}I imaging and have the thickest septa.

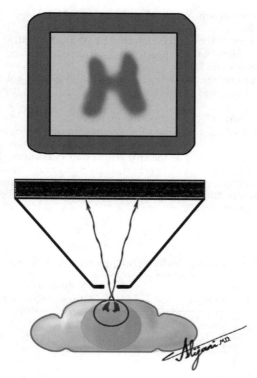

FIGURE 9.6   Pinhole collimator used to generate thyroid images.

TABLE 9.4   Representative Full Width Half Maximum (FWHM) Resolution

Distance from Collimator (cm)	Spatial Resolution FWHM (mm)		
	High Resolution	All-purpose Collimator	High Sensitivity
0	2	3	5
5	5	7	10
10	8	10	15
15	12	14	20

C. NaI crystal
- **NaI** scintillators detect gamma rays emerging from patients and are generally **rectangular.**
- **NaI** crystals are very **fragile** and easily damaged.
- For gamma ray imaging, **NaI scintillators** are ~**10 mm thick.**
- As scintillator **thickness increases,** sensitivity improves but **resolution** gets worse.
- A **photopeak** is when an incident gamma ray is *completely* absorbed **(photoelectric effect).**
- The **detection efficiency** is the **percentage** of incident **gamma rays** absorbed in the scintillator.
- Table 9.5 shows how NaI detection efficiency varies with photon energy.
  - **Increasing** the photon **energy** from 100 to 500 keV **reduces** detection **efficiency** from 100% to 6%.
- An iodine **escape peak** occurs at approximately 30 keV below the photopeak and is the result of characteristic K-shell x-rays from iodine that escape the crystal.
- **Scatter events** in the NaI crystals occur where the energy of a **Compton electron** is absorbed in the crystal but the **Compton scattered photon** escapes.

D. Energy resolution
- When the gamma ray is completely **absorbed** by the **NaI,** some of this energy (~10%) is converted to light.
- Light output from the NaI crystal is detected by **photomultiplier tubes (PMTs).**
- The output voltage from PMTs is directly proportional to the amount of energy absorbed by the scintillating material.
- The average amount of light detected is proportional to the photopeak energy.
  - Light produced by 140-keV photons would be half the light produced by 280-keV photons.
- There is a **distribution** of light around the mean value.
  - Some photons produce more than the average amount of light, whereas others produce less.
- **Photopeak width** is measured as the **full width half maximum (FWHM).**
- The broadening of the photopeak (FWHM) is termed **energy resolution.**
- Photopeak broadening is expressed as a percentage of the photopeak energy.
  - A **measured width** (broadening) of **28 keV** for ^{99m}Tc **(140 keV)** corresponds to an **energy resolution** of **20%.**

TABLE 9.5   Sodium Iodide (NaI) Detection Efficiency

Photon Energy (keV)	% Photons Detected by 10-mm-Thick NaI Crystal
100	100
140(^{99m}Tc)	92
200	54
300	22
500	6

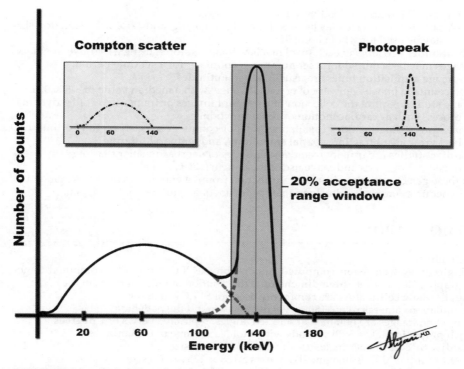

FIGURE 9.7   Pulse height analysis (PHA) used to process the total amount of light generated by a gamma ray photon detected in a scintillator camera.

E. Pulse height analysis
- –A **pulse height analyzer (PHA)** is an electronic device used to determine which portion of the detected spectrum is used to create images (Fig. 9.7).
- –The **PHA** can be set to allow only **selected energies** to be counted, and **reduce** the number of **Compton scatter** photons in the image.
- –PHA analysis *maximizes* the number of photopeak events while *minimizing* the detected photons that would degrade image quality (i.e., **Compton scatter**).
- –The PHA allows the operator either to set the **upper** and **lower energy limits** or to set a peak energy level and associated window.
- –The **window,** measured by percent, determines the **acceptable range** of **energies** around the peak for subsequent counting.
- –A **peak** of **140 keV** with a **20% window** (±10%) accepts photon energy levels ranging from **126 to 154 keV** (see Fig. 9.7).
- –A 20% window will include many photons that have been Compton scattered within the patient.
  - –The energy of a photon scattered through 53 degrees is 126 keV, which would be included in a 20% ^{99m}Tc window.
  - –Only photons scattered through angles greater than 53 degrees would fall outside a 20% window for ^{99m}Tc.
- –**Wide windows** accept more photons and produce images in a **shorter time** but include **more scatter** photons that degrade image quality.
- –Some radionuclides such as ^{67}Ga require that **multiple windows** be set since these emit several gamma rays (Table 9.3).

F. Planar NM imaging
- –NM images can be viewed in **real time** on a display monitor during the acquisition.
- –A **long persistence screen** on which each count remains on the screen for a prolonged period can be used to help patient positioning.
- –**Analog** to **digital converters** are used to generate the digital information.

–A typical NM matrix size is **128 × 128.**
  –A 64 × 64 matrix size may be used for cardiac imaging, and 1,024 × 1,024 matrix size may be used for whole-body imaging.
–The **number** of counts in each **pixel** in a NM image is stored using a **two-byte** memory.
–Images may be acquired for a **set number** of **counts** or for a **set time period.**
  –**Image acquisition** times are usually **several minutes.**
–The **counts** in images can vary over a wide range, with a **median value** of ~**500,000.**
–Some studies require the collection of a series of images or frames to record a dynamic process such as **cardiac motion** or **renal function.**
–Image processing includes calculating plots of **counts** in selected **regions** of **interest, background subtraction, spatial smoothing,** and **temporal filtering.**
–**Cardiac studies** are usually recorded in a series of short acquisitions lasting only a few dozen milliseconds and make use of the patient's **ECG** signal.
–In these gated cardiac studies, the information from several hundred frames is added to generate a **composite cine loop** that has an adequate number of total counts.

IV. TOMOGRAPHY

A. SPECT physics
  –**Single photon emission computed tomography (SPECT)** provides computed tomographic views of the **three-dimensional** distribution of **radioisotopes** in the body.
  –**Parallel-hole collimators** are commonly used for SPECT imaging.
  –Scintillation cameras rotate **180 or 360 degrees** around the patient.
  –Projection images are obtained at selected angles, typically every **3** or **6 degrees.**
  –Each **projection** takes ~**30 seconds** with a total scan time of ~**15 minutes.**
  –**Cardiac SPECT** images make use of a **64 × 64** matrix size.
    –Noncardiac SPECT imaging likely uses a 128 × 128 matrix size.
  –In cardiac SPECT, at each camera angle there will be **64 projections,** with each projection containing 64 data points, permitting reconstruction of **64 tomographs.**
  –**Scan projections** were originally used as inputs for **filtered-back projection reconstruction algorithms** to compute tomographic images.
  –**Iterative reconstruction** algorithms are now used.
    –**Iterative reconstruction** is more **accurate** and **minimizes artifacts.**
  –**SPECT** generates an **isotropic volume data** set that permits **transverse, sagittal,** and **coronal** views to be generated.
  –**Rotating three-dimensional** representations can also be created and displayed.
  –*Quantitative* information from SPECT imaging requires **corrections** for **scatter** and **attenuation.**
B. SPECT imaging
  –**Multiheaded cameras** are used to increase system sensitivity and **reduce scan times.**
  –The use of **elliptical orbits (i.e., body contouring)** for scintillation camera traveling around the patient allows the distance to the patient to be minimized.
  –Most SPECT equipment uses two scintillation camera heads.
  –The major benefit of SPECT is the **improved contrast** that results from the elimination of **overlapping structures.**
  –Common clinical SPECT applications include **myocardial ischemia** or **infarctions** and evaluation of abnormalities seen on planar bone scans.
  –SPECT studies are also performed with [111]In **octreotide** for neuroendocrine imaging, ^{111}In labeled **ProstaScint** for prostate imaging, and ^{67}Ga for infections.
  –A **SPECT/CT** system contains separate SPECT and x-ray CT imaging systems, with a patient bed passing through both systems.
  –In SPECT/CT, the **CT scan** can be a **low-dose scan** for image **coregistration** and **attenuation correction** only.
    –Higher-dose CT scans may be acquired for **diagnostic** imaging.
C. Positron emission tomography (PET) physics
  –A **PET camera** contains rings of detectors (scintillators) surrounding the patient.
  –Detectors are coupled to **photomultiplier tubes (PMTs)** to detect light produced in each detector.
  –Electronic analysis of the output of these PMTs provides **positional information** and permits **pulse height analysis.**

–Most early-generation PET scanners had detectors made of **bismuth germanate (BGO).**
–Modern PET scanners use detectors made of **lutetium oxyorthosilicate (LSO)** or **gadolinium oxyorthosilicate (GSO).**
  –**Lutetium yttrium oxyorthosilicate (LYSO)** is also used, which is **LSO** doped with a small amount of **yttrium.**
–BGO and LSO have similar gamma ray absorption properties, but **GSO** is a markedly **poorer absorber** of **511-keV gamma rays.**
–GSO and LSO are **inorganic scintillators** that **emit more light than BGO.**
  –**Increased light** output of GSO and LSO **improves energy resolution.**
–**Organic scintillators** emit their light much **faster than those of BGO.**
  –Shorter **decay times** improve count rate performance (reduced dead time).
  –Shorter decay times reduce **coincidence timing windows** and lower **random coincidences.**
–To efficiently **detect 511-keV** annihilation photons, thick detectors are used (i.e., **20–30 mm**).

D. Image formation
  –Figure 9.8 shows detection of **annihilation radiation** in a PET scanner.
  –Two interactions occurring within a specified time interval τ **(coincidence timing window)** are called a **coincidence event.**
  –There are three types of coincidences: a. **true coincidences,** b. **scatter coincidences,** and c. **random (accidental) coincidences.**
  –A **true coincidence** is the **simultaneous detection** of two **511-keV** annihilation photons (Fig. 9.8).
  –**Scatter** and **random coincidences degrade image** quality.
  –Simultaneous detection using coincidence circuitry allows identification of the **line** of **response.**
  –Line of response data are used to create a **sinogram,** which may be reconstructed using **filtered back projection algorithms** (i.e., as in CT).
    –**Filtered back projection** was popular in the early days of PET but is now rarely used.
  –Image reconstruction in PET corrects for **attenuation** of **511-keV** photons within the patient.

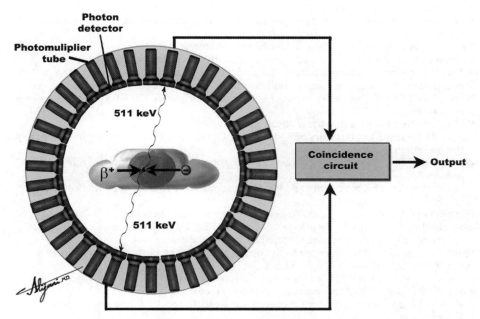

FIGURE 9.8   Schematic depiction of a positron emission tomography (PET) imaging system showing how *positional* information is obtained by detecting annihilation photons in coincidence.

–**Attenuation** in PET is **depth independent** and depends only on the total thickness of tissue traveled.

–**CT images** are used to generate **attenuation correction** factors for use in PET.

–Images are reconstructed using **statistically based algorithms** such as **ordered-subset expectation maximization (OSEM)**.

–Measuring the difference in arrival times of the two annihilation photons from an annihilation is used in **time** of **flight (TOF) PET**.

–**TOF** information can be used in the reconstruction process to improve image quality including **improved spatial resolution** as well as **enhanced lesion contrast.**

–**TOF PET** can identify the location of an annihilation event with an **uncertainty** that corresponds to a Full Width Half Maximum of ~**7.5 cm.**

E. **PET imaging**

–**PET images** typically have **several million counts.**

–The most common positron emitter used for PET imaging is ^{18}F ($T_{1/2} =$ **110 minutes**).

–^{18}F in the form of **fluorodeoxyglucose** is the most commonly used agent.

–**Rubidium** (^{82}Rb, $T_{1/2} =$ **75 s**) and **gallium** (^{68}Ga, $T_{1/2} =$ **68 min**) can be obtained from generators.

–**PET** systems have rings that extend over an **axial length** up to **22 cm,** which permit several **transverse image slices** to be **simultaneously** acquired.

–**Shadow shields (septa)** may be used to **define planes** and limit the number of coincidence counts (2D mode).

–**Septal** collimators are **not needed** for **localization** of **photons.**

–In **2D mode,** coincidences are detected within each individual ring of detectors, or between adjacent rings.

–In **3D mode, septal collimator rings** are **not used** and coincidences are detected among many or all rings of detectors.

–For **3D** systems, coincidences are detected in the **complete imaged volume.**

–Three-dimensional data sets have to **rebin** the data for reconstruction.

–**FORE (Fourier rebinning)** can accurately rebin 3D data into 2D data sets.

–Three-dimensional scanner **sensitivity** (without septa) is **six** times **higher** than 2D scanner sensitivity (with septa).

–The fraction of **scattered coincidences** and increased random counts are much higher in 3D mode.

–Modern PET scanners generally operate in **3D mode,** allowing **smaller activities** to be administered to patients.

–**PET** studies can produce **absolute quantitative** data (perfusion and metabolism).

F. **PET/CT**

–**Nuclear medicine** images often **lack** sufficient **anatomic detail.**

–**Coregistration** of the nuclear medicine image with CT improves lesion localization.

–A **PET/CT** system contains separate PET and x-ray CT imaging systems, with a patient bed passing through the bores of both systems.

–Nearly **2,000 PET/CT systems** have been installed worldwide **(2008),** and these systems now account for *all* PET sales.

–PET/CT systems normally offer a **70-cm gantry** aperture.

–Activity (^{18}F) in PET is typically **555 MBq (15 mCi)** and is administered 60 to 90 minutes before imaging is to commence.

–**Low-dose CT** scans may be performed for attenuation correction only (e.g., **40–80 mAs**).

–Low-dose CT images can also be used as a **scout view** to define the anatomic region for PET scanning.

–**High-dose CT** scans can be used to generate diagnostic images (e.g., **150–200 mAs**).

–**Sixteen-slice CT** scanners are adequate for most **PET/CT** applications.

–**Sixty-four-slice** scanners are targeted for **cardiac** applications.

–Spiral CT scanning from the **eyes to** the **upper thigh** can be performed in **15 to 20 s.**

–Axial coverage in PET is 15 cm to 22 cm.

–Current clinical PET scans use about **five detector positions** to cover the body.

–Typical PET scans take **2 to 3 minutes** at **each detector position.**

–Up to **11 positions** would be required for **head to toe PET** imaging of melanoma patients.

–**PET/CT** is primarily used for **staging** of **malignant disease** to **monitor patient response** to therapy.

V. QUALITY CONTROL

A. Generator quality control
–A damaged technetium generator may permit ^{99}**Mo** to break into the **saline** elute.
   –^{99}**Mo** has gamma ray energy levels of **181, 740** and **780 keV.**
–^{99}**Mo breakthrough** results in an unnecessary and high radiation dose to the patient.
   –Breakthrough ^{99}Mo degrades image quality because of **septal penetration.**
–A **dose calibrator** is used to determine the content of ^{99}Mo each time the generator is eluted.
–A **lead** shield **blocks** the ^{99m}**Tc gamma rays,** allowing ^{99}Mo gamma rays to be counted.
–The legal limit for molybdenum breakthrough is **5.5 kBq** of ^{99}**Mo** per **37 MBq** of ^{99m}**Tc.**
   –In non-SI units, this legal limit is **0.15 μCi** of ^{99}**Mo** per **mCi** of ^{99m}**Tc.**
–**Alumina** can also break through into the saline.
–Alumina interferes with the proper formation of ^{99m}Tc radiopharmaceutical kits.
–**Color indicator** paper is used to test for **alumina breakthrough.**

B. Radiopharmaceutical quality control
–**Radionuclide purity** relates to the presence of unwanted radionuclides in the sample.
–**Contaminant radionuclides** are identified by their (distinctive) photopeak energies using **gamma ray spectroscopy.**
–An example of a radionuclide impurity is the presence of ^{99}**Mo** in ^{99m}**Tc.**
   –^{201}**Tl** may contain ^{202}**Tl.**
–**Radionuclide purity** is mainly checked by the manufacturer.
–Radiochemical purity is the chemical purity of the isotope.
   –**Thin-layer chromatography** is used to check **radiochemical purity.**
–Free pertechnetate in ^{99m}Tc labeled DTPA is a **radiochemical contaminant.**
–**Chromatography** separates compounds that are soluble in saline.
–**Chemical purity** refers to the amount of unwanted chemical contaminants in the agent.
–**Sterility** means that the radiopharmaceutical is free of any microbial contamination.
–Even if a preparation is sterile, it may still contain **pyrogens,** which may cause a reaction if administered to a patient.
–**Sterility** and **pyrogenicity** tests should be performed before the agent is administered to a patient.
–Sterility and pyrogenicity tests are performed on each **batch** of short-lived radionuclides (e.g., ^{99m}Tc), because testing is not feasible for each individual dose.

C. Scintillation camera quality control
–The **photopeak window** of the PHA is evaluated by using a source that radiates the whole crystal.
   –Irradiation of the whole crystal may be achieved using a **sheet source,** or a **point source** at a distance.
–**The photopeak window** is checked daily.
–**Field uniformity** is the ability of the scintillation camera to reproduce a uniform distribution of activity.
   –Differences in the PMT response and transmission of light in the crystal contribute to nonuniformity.
   –**Nonuniformities** of greater than $\pm$**5%** from the mean are unacceptable for clinical imaging.
–Modern cameras have a **uniformity** of better than **2%** between adjacent areas.
–**Field uniformity** is commonly checked daily by placing a large-area disc made of ^{57}**Co** in front of the camera.
   –^{57}Co discs have a size that is comparable to the scintillation camera dimensions.
–^{57}**Co** emits **122 keV** photons and has a half-life of **270 days.**
   –Sources of ^{57}Co require replacement every year or so.
–**Extrinsic flood images** are obtained with the **collimator** in place and will assess the system performance including the collimator.
   –**Intrinsic floods** are performed **without** the **collimator** and assess the performance of NaI crystal and associated light detectors.
–**Resolution** (i.e., the ability to separate two points) is checked using a **quadrant bar phantom.**
   –Quadrant bar phantoms have **four sets** of **parallel bars,** with each rotated through 90 degrees, with dimensions of **3.5, 3.0, 2.5,** and **2.0 mm.**
–**Bar pattern** phantoms also check for **linearity** (i.e., ability to image straight lines).

D. Dose calibrator quality control
   –A **dose calibrator** is an **ionization chamber** used to measure the activity of a radioisotope dose.
   –**Dose calibrators** make measurements in **MBq** or **mCi.**
   –**Each dose** must be **determined** *before* **injection** into the patient.
   –Measurements can be made in a dose calibrator, or a decay calculation can be performed of the activity measured at a nuclear pharmacy at a reference time.
   –**Constancy** is checked daily by measuring the same standard source that has a long half-life.
   –^{137}Cs has a half-life of **30 years** and is therefore ideal for measuring calibrator constancy.
   –Day to day measurements should vary by **less than 5%.**
   –**Accuracy** is checked at installation and **annually** using **calibrated sources.**
   –**Linearity** is checked quarterly by measuring the decay of ^{99m}Tc over **72** hours or more.
      –**Linearity** can also be checked by using a source placed into a calibrated cylinder of lead that attenuates the source by a known amount.

VI. IMAGE QUALITY

A. Contrast
   –**Contrast** is the difference in intensity (counts) in any abnormality compared to the intensity in the surrounding normal anatomy (background).
   –**Subject contrast** is the difference in activities in the abnormality and surrounding normal anatomy.
   –**Image contrast** is the corresponding difference in image counts in the abnormality and normal anatomy.
   –Contrast in nuclear medicine images is high when **radiopharmaceuticals localize** well in the organ of interest.
      –**Excellent localization** in an organ of interest is known as **"hot spot"** imaging.
   –Some radioactivity is always found in other tissues, and photons from this activity generate undesirable **background** counts.
   –**Background** counts **degrade** image **contrast.**
   –The ratio of organ-specific uptake to unwanted uptake in other tissues is called the **target to background ratio.**
   –Contrast is affected by **septal penetration** and **scatter.**
B. Spatial resolution
   –Nuclear medicine **resolution** is the ability to distinguish two adjacent radioactive sources.
   –An image of a **line source** of activity will be larger (i.e., blurred) than the line itself.
   –An **image** of a **line** is known as the **line spread function.**
   –Measurement of the **full width half maximum (FWHM)** of the line spread function is the most common measure of resolution in nuclear medicine.
   –**Intrinsic resolution** refers to the performance of the camera without the collimator.
      –Intrinsic resolution assesses the performance of the NaI crystal, light detectors (PMTs) and associated electronics.
   –**Intrinsic resolution** of a scintillation camera is typically between **3** and **5 mm.**
      –**Increasing** the NaI detector **thickness** will **degrade resolution** because of increased light diffusion in the detector.
   –**System resolution (R)** depends on the intrinsic resolution of the scintillation camera (R_i) and resolution of the collimator (R_c).
   –System resolution is given by $R = (R_i^2 + R_c^2)^{0.5}$.
   –**FWHM** in NM is generally ~**8 mm** with the **low-energy high-resolution (LEHR)** collimator most commonly used in clinical imaging.
      –A **FWHM** of **8 mm** corresponds to a limiting spatial resolution of $1/(2 \times 8)$ lp/mm, or **0.06 lp/mm.**
   –The spatial **resolution** of **SPECT** is *always* **poorer than** that of **planar imaging.**
   –**Spatial resolution** of commercial PET systems can approach **5 mm FWHM** when imaging a line source of activity.
C. Noise
   –**Noise** is any unwanted counts in a nuclear medicine image that can interfere with the detection of abnormalities.
   –**Noise** may be classified as random or structured.

–**Random noise** results from statistical variation in pixel counts and is called **quantum mottle.**
–**Quantum mottle** in nuclear medicine is much higher than in x-ray imaging because the number of photons used to generate an image is low.
–A **lung NM image** with **600,000** counts covering an area of 250 mm × 250 mm has a count intensity of ~**10 photons/mm^2.**
  –A **chest radiograph** has **20,000 x-ray photons incident** on **every mm^2** of the image receptor.
–**Quantum mottle** can be **reduced** only by **increasing** the number of **counts** in the image.
–Ways of increasing image counts include **increasing** the **administered activity, increasing imaging time,** or using a **higher-sensitivity collimator.**
–**Quantum mottle** is a major factor in SPECT due to the **low** number of **photons** used to reconstruct each voxel.
–**PET images** have high **counts** and lower levels of image mottle.
  –Collimators are not used in PET, which markedly increases their sensitivity.
–**Structured noise** includes nonuniformities in the scintillation camera.
–**Energy, linearity,** and **uniformity corrections** are applied to scintillation camera images.
  –Nonuniformities are a minor contributor in planar imaging.
–**Overlying objects** in the patient can also result in **structured noise.**
  –Uptake in the **gastrointestinal tract** when **imaging** the **kidneys** is an example of **structured noise.**
D. Artifacts
  –Patient **motion** is one of the most common sources of artifacts in all NM imaging.
  –**Damaged collimators** can cause significant uniformity problems.
  –**Cracked crystals** produce defects in the image, whose characteristics reflect the shape of the crack.
  –**PMT failure** may also produce a cold defect and shows up well on a flood image.
  –**Edge packing** refers to the increased brightness at the edge of the crystal.
    –**Internal reflection** of light at the edge of the crystal and absence of PMTs beyond the crystal edge are the cause of edge packing.
  –**Crystals** are deliberately made **larger** than the imaged **field of view** to **minimize edge packing.**
  –Off-peak images on the low side of the photopeak contain excessive **Compton scatter.**
    –Off-peak images (low energy) have decreased contrast and resolution.
  –Metal objects worn by the patient produce **photopenic areas** that may mimic pathologic cold lesions.
  –SPECT studies are susceptible to **image artifacts** caused by **nonuniformities** and by **axis** of **rotation misalignment.**
    –The **image reconstruction** algorithm **amplifies** the detrimental effects of image **noise** and nonuniformities.
  –Contrast material (e.g., barium) and implanted metal objects may cause **"hot" artifacts** in *CT attenuation-corrected* PET images.

VII. RADIATION DOSES

A. Effective half-life
  –The **physical half-life (T$_{1/2}$)** is an intrinsic characteristic of each radionuclide.
    –**T$_{1/2}$** is given by the expression **0.693/λ,** where λ is the radionuclide decay constant.
  –Most radiopharmaceuticals are also **cleared** from **organs** by various **physiologic** processes.
  –**Biologic clearance** of material (radioactivity) from the body can be modeled as being **exponential.**
  –The **biologic clearance** will be characterized by a **biologic half-life (T$_b$).**
  –The **effective half-life (T$_e$)** of a radionuclide in any organ encompasses both **radioactive decay** and **biologic clearance.**
  –**Effective half-lives** must always be **shorter** than the physical or biologic half-life.
  –The relation between T$_{1/2}$, T$_b$, and T$_e$ is **1/T$_e$ = 1/T$_b$ + 1/T$_{1/2}$.**
  –If a radionuclide has a physical half-life of 6 hours and a biologic half-life of 3 hours, then $1/T_e = 1/6 + 1/3$, and T$_e$ = 2 hours.

–When the **biologic half life** is much longer than the physical half-life, the **effective half-life** is equal to the **physical half-life.**

–When the **physical half-life** is much longer than the biologic half life, the **effective half-life** is equal to the **biologic half-life.**

B. Cumulative activity

–The total **number** of **nuclear transformations** in an organ is called **cumulative activity (A_∞).**

–The cumulative activity is one of two key data required to generate organ doses in NM.

–The other key datum is the **S factor** (see next section).

–**Cumulative activity** is the **area under** the **curve** when activity in an organ or tissue is plotted as a function of time.

–When the **organ activity** is **constant,** the **time–activity curve** is a **horizontal line.**

–For constant activity in an organ, the area is obtained from the area of a rectangle (i.e., constant activity multiplied by the time).

–A constant activity of 10 Bq in a time of 100 seconds results in a cumulative active of 1,000 nuclear transformations.

–When the activity in the organ is **decaying exponentially,** the area under the curve is more difficult to determine (i.e., requires **integration** of an **exponential** function).

–Figure 9.9 shows a typical exponential curve.

–For **exponential decay,** cumulative activity A_∞ is **$1.44 \times A \times T_e$** where A is the initial activity in the organ and T_e is the **effective half-life.**

–Values of **cumulative activity** are obtained by monitoring the **time** course of **activity** in **organs** of interest for dosimetry.

–**Cumulative activities** may differ for **normal patients** and patients with certain **diseases.**

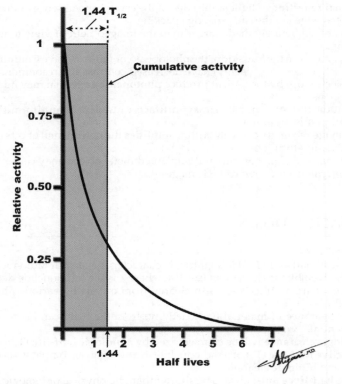

FIGURE 9.9 Integration of an exponential decay of radioactivity (*curved line*) yields the cumulative activity that is mathematically equivalent to the product of the initial activity and a time of $1.44\,T_{1/2}$ (i.e., area under the exponential curve equals the area of the shaded rectangle).

TABLE 9.6   S Factors for ^{99m}Tc Activity Normalized to Unity for Uniform Whole-Body Activity Irradiating the Whole Body (i.e., S$_{\text{whole body}\rightarrow\text{whole body}}$ equal to 1)

Source Organ	Target Organ	Relative S Factor
Whole body	Whole body	1
Liver	Liver	23
Thyroid	Thyroid	2,300
Thyroid	Liver	0.08

C. S factor
- –The **radiation dose to any organ** or tissue is obtained by dividing the total energy absorbed in the organ by the organ mass.
- –**Energy absorbed** in a target organ per nuclear emission in the source organ depends on three factors.
  - –The first is the **number** of **emissions** per **transformation.**
  - –The second is the **energy** associated with each **emission.**
  - –The third is the **fraction** of emitted **energy** deposited in the target **organ.**
- –The total energy deposited in the target organ is then obtained by **summing over all** the **radiations** emitted by the nuclide in the source organ.
- –Dividing the **absorbed energy** by the target organ **mass** gives the **S factor.**
- –The **S factor** is thus the absorbed dose in a target organ per unit cumulative activity in a source organ (i.e., S$_{\text{source}\rightarrow\text{target}}$).
- –S-factor data are obtained from **reference books,** and use units of **mGy/Bq-s** in the SI system.
  - –S-factor are given in **rad/μCi-hr** in the non-SI system.
- –Table 9.6 shows S factors for ^{99m}Tc for different source and target organs.
- –**Uniform** distribution of ^{99m}Tc in the **whole body** results in an average whole-body dose of **1.6×10^{-13} mGy/Bq-s.**
- –**S factors** generally **increase** as the **size** of the organ **decreases** (see Table 9.6).
- –**Small organs** taking up radioactivity are likely to receive **high doses.**
- –**Doses** to **distant target organs** are always **low.**
  - –Liver doses from activity in the thyroid are generally very low.
- –Beta emitters always result in high doses.
  - –**S$_{\text{thyroid}\rightarrow\text{thyroid}}$** is **ten times higher** for ^{131}I **(beta emitter)** than for ^{99m}Tc **(gamma emitter).**

D. Diagnostic NM doses
- –The dose to a **target organ,** from activity in one **source organ,** is obtained by multiplying the source organ **cumulative (A$_{\infty}$)** and the **source** to **target S factor.**
- –In general, **organ dose D $=$ A$_{\infty} \times$ S$_{\text{source}\rightarrow\text{target}}$.**
- –The **total dose** to an **organ** is obtained by summing the doses from all source organs that contain radioactivity.
- –**Organs** that take up **radiopharmaceuticals** will receive the **highest doses.**
  - –The lung receives the highest dose from a ventilation or perfusion examination.
- –**Highest organ doses** from diagnostic nuclear medicine procedures are $\sim$**50 mGy.**
- –Several organs are irradiated in most nuclear medicine studies.
- –The **effective dose** takes into account the absorbed doses to *all* organs, as well as their relative radiosensitivity.
  - –As in radiology, the **effective dose** is the best indicator of **patient risk** in **NM.**
- –Effective doses for common NM examinations are listed in Table 9.7.
  - –The **average effective dose** for the 14 listed procedures is **5 mSv.**
- –**Effective doses** in **PET** imaging are $\sim$**10 mSv.**
- –In **PET/CT,** the CT component of the imaging procedure $\sim$**15 mSv** when the **CT** scan is acquired for **diagnostic** purposes.
- –**CT scans** performed for **attenuation correction** and **fusion purposes** alone use lower techniques with reduced effective doses of $\sim$**5 mSv.**

E. Therapeutic NM dose
- –**Radionuclides** are sometimes used for **therapeutic** (not diagnostic) applications.
- –**Beta emitters** are **ideal** for therapy applications because the beta particle energy is primarily deposited in the organ taking up the radionuclide.
- –**Target organ doses** in ^{131}I **therapy** applications are extremely **high.**

TABLE 9.7   Effective Doses in Nuclear Medicine

Procedure	Radiopharmaceutical	Administered Activity MBq (mCi)	E per Procedure mSv
Brain	^{99m}Tc HMPAO	1,110 (30)	10
Bone	^{99m}Tc pyrophosphate	750 (20)	6
Liver/spleen	^{99m}Tc sulphur colloid	200 (5)	2
Biliary	^{99m}Tc HIDA	200 (5)	4.5
Cardiac (MUGA)	^{99m}Tc red blood cells	750 (20)	5.5
Cardiac	^{99m}Tc sestamibi	750 (20)	6.5
Cardiac	^{201}Tl thallus chloride	75 (2)	7
Lung	^{99m}Tc MAA	150 (4)	2.5
Renal	^{99m}Tc DTPA	600 (15)	6
Inflammation	^{67}Ga gallium citrate	200 (5)	20
Thyroid scan	^{99m}Tc pertechnetate	200 (5)	2.5
Thyroid uptake	^{123}I sodium iodide	7.5 (0.2)	0.55
Infection	^{111}In leukocytes	2 (0.05)	1.2

HIDA, hepatoiminodiacetic acid; MUGA, multiple-gated acquisition; MAA, macroaggregated albumin; DTPA, diethylenetriaminepentaacetic acid.

–Administration of **370 MBq (10 mCi)** of ^{131}I can result in a high thyroid dose.
–If half of this administered activity is taken up by the thyroid, the initial thyroid activity (A) is thus 185 MBq (5 mCi).
–The physical and biologic half lives of iodine are both 8 days, so the effective half-life is 4 days (i.e., $1/T_e = 1/8 + 1/8$).
–The **effective half-life** of ^{131}I in the patient's thyroid is **4 days**.
–The cumulative activity A_∞ (i.e., total number of nuclear transformations) in the patient's thyroid is **1.44 × A × T_e.**
–A_∞ is 1.44 × 185 × 10^6 × 4 × 24 × 60 × 60 Bq-s.
–$A_\infty = 9.2 \times 10^{13}$ Bq-s
–$S_{thyroid \rightarrow thyroid}$ for ^{131}I is **1.7 × 10^{-9} mGy/Bq-s,** which was obtained from a standard text.
–The **thyroid dose** from ^{131}I in the thyroid is $S_{thyroid \rightarrow thyroid} \times A_\infty$, or 9.2×10^{13} mGy/Bq-s × 1.7 × 10^{-9} Bq-s.
–The **thyroid dose** to a patient receiving **370 MBq (10 mCi)** of ^{131}I with a **50% thyroid uptake** is thus **160,000 mGy** (i.e., 160 Gy).

F. **Radiation protection**
   –**NM technologists** are surrounded by patients full of radioactivity and receive a significant dose during **injection** of **radiopharmaceuticals.**
      –**Operator doses** during injection are **0.01 to 0.02 mSv/hour.**
   –Handling of radionuclides requires the use of **leaded syringes** to minimize extremity doses.
   –**Extremity doses** need to be monitored using **ring dosimeters** which are worn on a finger.
      –NM operators risk **intakes** of **radionuclides** such as ^{131}I and undergo **mandatory bioassay** (e.g., thyroid monitoring for iodine uptakes).
   –**Protective clothing** and handling precautions are required to **minimize contamination.**
   –**Volatile radionuclides** (^{131}I and ^{133}Xe) should be stored in **fume hoods.**
   –Personnel should wear **gloves** when handling radionuclides, and dispose of them in radioactive waste receptors after use.
   –**Wipe tests** should be performed of radionuclide use areas using a small piece of filter paper is wiped on an area and checked in a NaI well counter.
   –**Radioactive waste** can be stored for **ten half-lives** prior to being surveyed and disposed of as regular waste.
   –**Annual effective doses** for **NM** technologists range between **1** and **5 mSv.**
   –PET poses considerable challenges because of the high energies of the annihilation photons (511 keV), where *two* photons are emitted for every nuclear decay.
   –In PET, very **thick vial shields, syringe shields,** and **shadow shields** are used to protect staff handling and administering PET radiopharmaceuticals.
   –**PET imaging rooms** and **PET uptake** rooms commonly have much **thicker lead** shielding than x-ray facilities.

REVIEW TEST

9.1 ^{15}O and ^{16}O are examples of:
  a. isotopes
  b. isotones
  c. isomers
  d. isobars
  e. metastable states

9.2 37 MBq is equal to (mCi):
  a. 0.1
  b. 1
  c. 10
  d. 100
  e. 1,000

9.3 Which of the following decay modes most likely changes the mass number (A) of an unstable nucleus?
  a. Beta minus decay
  b. Beta plus decay
  c. Alpha decay
  d. Isomeric transition
  e. Electron capture

9.4 ^{60}Co (Z = 27) decaying to ^{60}Ni (Z = 28) is an example of:
  a. β^+ decay
  b. β^- decay
  c. electron capture
  d. alpha decay
  e. isomeric transition

9.5 Electron capture nuclei are most likely to produce:
  a. antineutrinos
  b. internal conversion electrons
  c. characteristic x-rays
  d. β^+ particles
  e. β^- particles

9.6 A radionuclide produced in a nuclear reactor is most likely to decay by:
  a. beta minus decay
  b. beta plus decay
  c. alpha decay
  d. isomeric transition
  e. electron capture

9.7 After ten half-lives, the fraction of activity remaining is:
  a. depends on the initial activity
  b. 1/10
  c. $(1/10)^2$
  d. $(1/2)^{10}$
  e. $(1/10)^{10}$

9.8 After one day, the remaining activity (%) of a ^{123}I source will most likely to be about:
  a. 50
  b. 25
  c. 12.5
  d. 6.3
  e. 3.2

9.9 The time (hour) when a daughter radionuclide ($T_{1/2} = 1$ hour) reaches approximate equilibrium with its long-lived parent is most likely:
  a. 1
  b. 2
  c. 4
  d. 8
  e. 16

9.10 Which type of collimator will likely result in the highest resolution for imaging the thyroid?
  a. High sensitivity
  b. Diverging
  c. High energy
  d. All purpose
  e. Pinhole

9.11 Scintillation camera detectors are most likely made of:
  a. CsI
  b. NaI
  c. Na
  d. Cs
  e. NaCl

9.12 The percentage (%) of 140-keV photons absorbed in a scintillating camera crystal is most likely:
  a. 20
  b. 40
  c. 60
  d. 80
  e. >80

9.13 A pulse height analyzer window width of 20% used with ^{99m}Tc would likely reject energies (keV) that are less than:
  a. 140
  b. 136
  c. 126
  d. 120
  e. 112

9.14 The most likely number of counts (k) in a scintillation camera image is most likely:
  a. 5
  b. 50
  c. 500
  d. 5,000
  e. 50,000

9.15 The most likely image matrix size for cardiac SPECT imaging is:
  a. 32 × 32
  b. 64 × 64
  c. 128 × 128
  d. 256 × 256
  e. 512 × 512

9.16 Pixel values in SPECT images represent:
a. physical densities
b. gamma ray absorption
c. clearance rates
d. radioisotope concentrations
e. effective half-lives

9.17 Which is *least* likely to be used as a detector material in PET imaging?
a. BGO
b. GSO
c. LSO
d. HCO
e. YSO

9.18 The amount of ^{18}F (mCi) most likely to be administered in a PET/CT scan is:
a. 1
b. 4
c. 16
d. 64
e. 256

9.19 The standard limit for ^{99}Mo breakthrough (μCi ^{99}Mo per mCi ^{99m}Tc) is most likely:
a. 0.15
b. 0.3
c. 0.5
d. 1.0
e. 1.5

9.20 The most likely radionuclide for performing a scintillation camera flood uniformity test is:
a. ^{57}Co
b. ^{60}Co
c. ^{137}Cs
d. ^{131}I
e. ^{226}Ra

9.21 The most likely radionuclide used to check the constancy of a dose calibrator is:
a. ^{14}C
b. ^{51}Cr
c. ^{137}Cs
d. ^{131}I
e. ^{32}P

9.22 Radionuclides with a higher photon energy would likely increase scintillation camera:
a. detection efficiency
b. septal penetration
c. radionuclide sensitivity
d. spatial resolution
e. image magnification

9.23 The full width half maximum width (mm) of a line source that is achieved by scintillation cameras is most likely:
a. 1
b. 2

c. 4
d. 8
e. 16

9.24 The variance (i.e., σ^2) of a NM image pixel with an average of 100 counts would likely be:
a. 10
b. 20
c. 30
d. 50
e. 100

9.25 A single circular cold spot artifact in a scintillation camera image would likely be the result of a:
a. cracked crystal
b. damaged collimator
c. defective PMT
d. faulty PHA
e. high count rate

9.26 For ^{99m}Tc, which of the following is least likely to contribute to the patient dose?
a. Auger electrons
b. Beta particles
c. Internal conversion electrons
d. Gamma rays
e. Characteristic x-rays

9.27 If both physical and biologic half lives are 2 hours, the effective half life (hour) is:
a. 0.5
b. 1
c. 2
d. 3
e. 4

9.28 Cumulative activity in an organ is *least* likely to depend on the:
a. administered activity
b. organ uptake
c. organ mass
d. physical half-life
e. biologic clearance

9.29 Adult effective doses (mSv) for a ^{99m}Tc labeled radiopharmaceutical are most likely:
a. <1
b. 1
c. 2.5
d. 5
e. 10

9.30 Adult effective doses (mSv) in PET imaging are most likely:
a. 0.3
b. 1
c. 3
d. 10
e. 30

ANSWERS AND EXPLANATIONS

9.1a. Isotopes since both ^{15}O and ^{16}O have 8 protons.

9.2b. One mCi is 37 MBq.

9.3c. Alpha decay will reduce the radionuclide atomic number by two and mass number by four.

9.4b. β^- decay since the daughter radionuclide atomic number has increased by one by emitting a β^- particle.

9.5c. Electron capture always results in characteristic x-rays, since the inner shell vacancy will be filled by an outer shell electron resulting in characteristic x-ray emission.

9.6a. Radionuclides produced in a nuclear reactor are neutron rich and therefore decay via beta minus emission.

9.7d. $(1/2)^{10}$, or 1/1,024 which is ~0.1%.

9.8b. the half-life of ^{123}I is 13 hours, so after a day (~2 half-lives), about 25% will remain.

9.9c. Four hours, since equilibrium is always established after four daughter half-lives.

9.10e. Pinhole collimators offer the highest resolution for thyroid imaging.

9.11b. NaI is the scintillator material in most current scintillation cameras.

9.12e. A scintillation camera crystal will absorb most (i.e., >80%) of incident 140-keV gamma rays.

9.13c. A PHA window width of 20% selected for ^{99m}Tc gamma rays would reject energies that are less than 126 keV and more than 156 keV.

9.14c. A scintillation camera image is most likely to have ~500k counts.

9.15b. The normal cardiac SPECT image matrix size is 64×64 (most SPECT studies are cardiac examinations).

9.16d. Pixel values in SPECT images represent radioisotope concentrations.

9.17d. HCO, which consists of hydrogen (H), carbon (C), and oxygen (O), and which would therefore be useless for detecting 511-keV photons because of their low atomic numbers.

9.18c. A typical administered activity for a PET/CT scan is 16 mCi of ^{18}F.

9.19a. The limit for ^{99}Mo breakthrough is 0.15 μCi ^{99}Mo per mCi ^{99m}Tc.

9.20a. ^{57}Co would be used for a flood uniformity test because its photon energy (122 keV) is close to that of ^{99m}Tc (140 keV).

9.21c. ^{137}Cs, which is a long-lived (30 year half-life) gamma emitter (661 keV).

9.22b. Higher photon energies increase collimator septal penetration.

9.23d. Eight mm is a typical full width half maximum width of an image of a line source obtained using a scintillation camera using a low-energy high-resolution (LEHR) collimator.

9.24e. The variance (σ^2) is 100 when a NM image pixel has an average of 100 counts (i.e., σ is 10).

9.25c. A defective PMT would likely result in a single circular cold spot in a scintillation camera image.

9.26b. Beta particles, since these are not emitted by ^{99m}Tc.

9.27b. One, since the effective half-life is given by the relationship $1/T_{effective} = 1/T_{physical} + 1/T_{biologic}$.

9.28c. Organ mass has no direct relationship to any cumulative activity.

9.29d. Five mSv is a representative adult effective dose for a ^{99m}Tc labeled radiopharmaceutical.

9.30d. Ten mSv is a representative adult effective dose for a PET study.

Chapter 10

ULTRASOUND

I. PROPERTIES

A. Sound waves
- –**Sound waves** are **pressure disturbance** that propagates through a material (e.g., tissue).
- –**Changes** in **pressure** are made by forces acting on the material molecules.
  - –**Molecules oscillate** about their unperturbed location.
- –The **amplitude** of a wave is the **size** of **pressure** difference from the equilibrium value.
- –Larger **pressure amplitudes** produce denser compressions and hence higher **intensities** of sound.
- –**Wavelength (λ)** is the distance between successive wave crests.
- –**Frequency (f)** is the number of **oscillations** in **each second.**
  - –Frequency is also the number of wavelengths that pass a given point each second.
- –Ultrasound waves are transmitted through tissue as **longitudinal waves** of alternating compression and rarefaction.
- –**Longitudinal waves** have vibrations **along** their travel direction.
  - –**Transverse** waves have vibrations **perpendicular** to the travel direction.
- –Ultrasound waves propagate in material at **velocity (v).**
  - –Sound waves **transmit energy** through the material.

B. Ultrasound frequency and wavelength
- –**Frequencies** are measured in **hertz (Hz),** where 1 Hz is one oscillation per second.
- –The **period** is the time between successive oscillations.
- –The **period** is the **reciprocal** of the **frequency (i.e., 1/f).**
  - –When the frequency is 10 Hz, the period is 0.1 second (i.e., 1/10).
- –**Audible sound** has frequencies ranging from **15 Hz** to **20,000 Hz.**
  - –1,000 Hz equals 1 kHz; 1,000 kHz equals 1 MHz (1,000,000 Hz)
- –**Ultrasound frequencies** are greater than 20 kHz.
- –**Diagnostic ultrasound** uses **transducers** with frequencies ranging from **1 to 20 MHz.**
- –At **2 MHz,** the ultrasound **wavelength** in soft **tissue** is **0.77 mm.**
- –Ultrasound wavelengths depend on the **material compressibility.**
  - –At 2 MHz, the ultrasound wavelength is 0.17 mm in air and 1.7 mm in bone.
- –Ultrasound wavelength **decreases** with increasing **frequency.**
  - –In soft tissue, the ultrasound wavelength is 0.39 mm at 4 MHz and 0.15 mm at 10 MHz.

C. Sound velocity
- –For sound waves, the relation between velocity (v) measured in m/s, frequency (f), and wavelength is $v = f \times \lambda$ **(m/s).**
- –In any material (i.e., constant v), frequency and wavelength are inversely related.
- –For a given material, **sound velocity** is **independent** of **frequency.**
  - –Different instruments in an orchestra (or rock band) produce different frequencies but travel through a concert hall at *exactly* the same speed.
- –Sound velocity depends on type of material or tissue.
  - –Velocity is inversely proportional to the square root of the **material compressibility.**
- –Materials that are not particularly compressible (e.g., bone) have high sound velocities.
  - –Compressible materials (e.g., air) have the lowest sound velocities.
- –The **average velocity** of sound in **soft tissue** is **1,540 m/s.**
  - –This velocity is *assumed* by all ultrasound scanners used to image patients.

TABLE 10.1   Ultrasound Velocities of Interest in Ultrasound Imaging

Material	Ultrasound Velocity (m/s)
Air	330
Fat	1,460
Soft tissue (average)	1,540
Bone	3,300
PZT (piezoelectric crystal)	4,000

–Sound velocities are **slightly lower** in **fat** than tissue.

  –Reduced sound velocities in fat result in imaging artifacts **(displacement artifact).**

–Table 10.1 lists sound velocities for materials and tissues of interest in ultrasound imaging.

D. Intensity

–The ultrasound **intensity** is a measure of the **energy flowing** through a given cross-sectional area each second.

–**Ultrasound intensities** are normally expressed in **milliwatts per cm^2 (mW/cm^2).**

–The total **power** in the ultrasound beam is the product of the ultrasound intensity and the beam area.

  –**Power is intensity times area.**

–The total **energy** transmitted is the product of the power and the time the beam is on.

  –**Energy is power times time.**

–**Relative sound intensity** is measured on a *logarithmic scale* and may be expressed in **decibel (dB).**

–**Decibels** are equal to **$10 \times \log_{10}(I/I_0)$,** where I_0 is the original intensity and I is the measured intensity.

–**Negative decibel** values correspond to signal **attenuation.**

  –**Positive decibel** values correspond to signal **amplification.**

–Intensity reduced to **10%** is **−10 dB,** to **1%** is **−20 dB,** and to **0.1%** is **−30 dB,** and so on.

  –**A 50% reduction** of sound intensity corresponds to **−3 dB.**

–Intensity increases of **+10 dB** correspond to a **10-fold increase, +20 dB** to a **100-fold increase, +30 dB** to a **1,000-fold increase,** and so on.

  –**Doubling** of the sound intensity corresponds to **+3 dB.**

E. Acoustic impedance

–**Acoustic impedance** is an important ultrasound property of any material or tissue.

–The **acoustic impedance (Z)** of a material is the product of the **density (ρ)** and the **sound velocity (v)** in the material.

  –Acoustic impedance **$Z = \rho \times v$**

–The acoustic impedance unit is called the **Rayl.**

–**Acoustic impedance** is **independent** of **frequency** in the diagnostic range.

–**Air** and **lung** have **low acoustic impedances.**

  –Air and lung have low physical densities as well as low sound velocities.

–**Bone** has a **high acoustic impedance.**

  –Bone has a high physical density and high sound velocity.

–Piezoelectric crystals have *very* high acoustic impedances.

–Most **tissues** have acoustic impedance values of ~**1.6×10^6 Rayl.**

–Table 10.2 lists relative values of acoustic impedance values for materials and tissues of interest in ultrasound imaging.

–**Differences** between **acoustic impedances** at interfaces determine the amount of **energy reflected** at the interface.

II. INTERACTIONS

A. Reflections

–A portion of the ultrasound beam is **reflected** at tissue **interfaces.**

–**Nonspecular reflections** are diffuse scatter from **rough surfaces** where the irregular contours are bigger than the ultrasound wavelength.

TABLE 10.2   Relative Impedances of Materials of Interest in Ultrasound Imaging

Material	Acoustic Impedance Relative to Soft Tissue
Air	<0.01
Fat	0.9
Soft tissue (average)	1
Bone	5
PZT (piezoelectric crystal)	20

–Only a **very small fraction** of energy from **nonspecular reflections** returns to the transducer.

–**Specular reflections** occur from large **smooth surfaces** (Fig. 10.1).

　–Specular reflection intensity is independent of frequency.

–The **sound reflected** back toward the transducer is called an **echo.**

　–**Specular reflection echoes** are used to generate ultrasound **images.**

–The fraction of ultrasound reflected depends on the **acoustic impedance** of the **tissues.**

–At normal incidence (90 degrees), the fraction of ultrasound intensity reflected at an interface between material Z_1 and Z_2 is $[(Z_2 - Z_1)/(Z_2 + Z_1)]^2$.

–The sum of the **transmitted** and **reflected** intensities must always **equal 1.**

　–Intensity transmitted is $(4Z_1 \times Z_2)/(Z_1 + Z_2)^2$.

–Table 10.3 lists values of reflected intensities for a range of interfaces encountered in diagnostic ultrasound.

–**Tissue/air** interfaces reflect ~**100%** of incident ultrasound beam.

–**Gel** is applied between the transducer and skin to displace the air and **minimize large reflections** that would interfere with ultrasound transmission into the patient.

–**Bone/tissue** interfaces also **reflect substantial** fractions of the incident intensity.

–In imaging the abdomen, the strongest echoes are likely to arise from gas bubbles.

–Imaging through air or bone is generally not possible.

　–**Lack** of **transmissions** beyond these interfaces results in areas void of echoes called **shadowing.**

B. Scattering

–**Scattering** occurs when ultrasound encounters objects that are **smaller** than the **ultrasound wavelength.**

–In scattering, most of the wave passes unperturbed, and a scattered wave is generated that travels outward in all directions from the scatter.

–Organs such as the **kidney, pancreas, spleen,** and **liver** are composed of complex tissue structures that **contain many scattering sites.**

　–These organs give rise to a signature that is characteristic of each tissue.

–**Hyperechoic** means a higher scatter amplitude relative to the background signal.

　–More scatter can occur because of larger number of scatters, larger acoustic impedance differences, or larger scatterers.

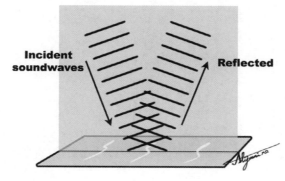

FIGURE 10.1 Specular reflection from a smooth reflector, with the angle of incidence equal to the angle of reflection.

TABLE 10.3   Reflection Intensities at an Interface between Soft Tissue and the Specified Material

Material Adjacent to Soft Tissue	Reflected Intensity
Air	>99%
Lung	50%
Bone	40%
Fat	0.8%
Muscle	<0.1%

–**Hypoechoic** means that there is a lower acoustic scatter intensity relative to the average background signal.
–Organs that contain **fluids,** such as the **bladder,** and **cysts** have no internal structure and almost **no echoes (i.e., show black).**

C. Refraction
–**Refraction** is the **change** in **direction** of an ultrasound beam when passing from one tissue to another having a different speed of sound.
–When ultrasound passes from one tissue to another having a different speed of sound, the **frequency** remains the **same,** but the **wavelength changes.**
–The change of wavelength occurs to accommodate the different velocity of sound in the second tissue and **shortens** when the **velocity** is **reduced.**
–Refraction is described by **Snell's law: $\sin\theta_i/\sin\theta_t = v_1/v_2$,** where θ_i is the angle of incidence, θ_t is the transmitted angle, v_1 is the velocity in tissue 1, and v_2 is the velocity in tissue 2.
–Figure 10.2 shows the refraction (i.e., bending) of an ultrasound beam.
  –When the velocity of sound in tissue 2 is greater than that of tissue 1, the transmission angle is greater than the angle of incidence (and vice versa).
–**Ultrasound** machines assume **straight line propagation,** and any **refraction** effects result in image **artifacts.**

D. Attenuation
–**Attenuation** is a composite effect of loss by **scatter** and **absorption.**
  –The **absorbed sound** wave energy is converted into **heat.**

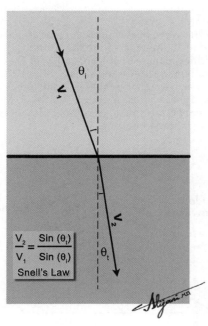

FIGURE 10.2   Refraction of an ultrasound beam when it passes from a medium with velocity v_1 to another with velocity $v_2 (v_2 < v_1)$.

–The **attenuation** of **ultrasound** in a homogeneous tissue is **exponential.**
–**Attenuation** is normally expressed in terms of **dB** and depends on the distance the ultrasound beam has traveled in tissue.
–**Attenuation increases** with **increasing frequency.**
–In soft tissues, there is a nearly linear relation between the frequency and attenuation of ultrasound.
  –For water and bone, attenuation increases approximately as frequency squared.
–Due to its high frequency, **ultrasound** is **attenuated more** readily than **audible sound.**
–Each tissue has an **attenuation coefficient dB/cm per MHz.**
–Ultrasound has an attenuation in soft tissue of ~0.5 dB/cm per MHz.
–The value of an attenuation coefficient of 0.5 dB/cm per MHz is an approximation commonly used to quantify the loss of power in ultrasound beams for clinical imaging.
  –Attenuation in soft tissue is ~0.5 dB/cm at 1 MHz and ~10 dB/cm at 10 MHz.
–**Little absorption** occurs in **fluids.**
–In ultrasound imaging, pulses travel to the reflector and back to the transducer.
  –**Distance traveled,** and consequently the attenuation, is **twice** the **penetration depth.**
E. **Depth gain compensation (DGC)**
  –An **echo** from a perfect reflector (e.g., air bubble) at the surface travels no distance and undergoes no attenuation.
  –An echo from the *same* reflector at a depth of 1 cm will be weaker because the ultrasound echo has traveled 2 cm round trip and undergone **attenuation.**
  –Echoes from this reflector at a depth of 10 cm will be extremely weak because of attenuation in traveling a round trip distance of 20 cm.
  –**Uncorrected echo data** would thus show distant echoes as being much weaker than superficial echoes.
  –Ultrasound scanners **compensate** for increased **attenuation** with image **depth.**
  –This is accomplished by increasing the signal gain as the echo return time increases.
  –Correcting for echo attenuation in this manner is known as **depth gain compensation (DGC).**
    –DGC is also known as **time gain compensation (TGC), time varied gain (TVG),** and **swept gain.**
  –DGC makes equal reflectors have the same brightness in the resultant ultrasound image.
  –**DGC controls** are usually adjusted by the **operator** during the imaging procedures.

III. TRANSDUCERS

A. **Function**
  –A **transducer** is a device that can convert one form of energy into another.
  –**Piezoelectric transducers** convert **electrical energy** into **ultrasonic energy,** and vice versa.
    –Piezoelectric means **pressure electricity.**
  –Ultrasound transducer materials include **lead-zirconate-titanate (PZT), plastic polyvinylidene difluoride (PVDF),** and the new **monocrystalline transducers.**
  –The piezoelectric effect of a transducer is destroyed if heated above its **Curie temperature.**
  –High-frequency **voltage oscillations** are produced by the scanner's front end and sent to the ultrasound transducer over coaxial cables.
  –Transducer crystals *do not conduct electricity,* but each side is coated with a thin layer of silver that acts as an electrode.
  –The electrical energy causes the crystal to momentarily change shape (i.e., expand and contract).
  –The nonconducting crystal **changes shape** in response to a **voltage** placed on its electrodes.
  –This change in shape of the crystal increases and decreases the pressure in front of the transducer, thus **producing ultrasound waves (transmitter).**
  –When the crystal is subjected to pressure changes by the returning ultrasound echoes, the **pressure changes** are converted back into **electrical energy** signals.
  –**Voltage signals** from returning **echoes** are transferred from the receiver to a computer, which are then used to create ultrasound images.
  –Transducers may be operated in either pulsed or continuous-wave mode.
    –Virtually all of medical ultrasound makes use of pulsed transducers.

B. Frequency
–The **thickness** of a piezoelectric **crystal** determines the resonant **frequency** of the transducer.
–Transducer crystals are normally manufactured so that their **thickness (t)** is **equal** to **one-half** of the **wavelength (λ)** (i.e., **t = λ/2**).
–Changing the thickness of the crystal changes the frequency but not the ultrasound amplitude or velocity.
–A **thickness** to **1 mm** and a velocity of sound of 4,000 m/s has a resonant frequency $f = v/λ = v/(2 \times t)$, or **2 MHz.**
–**High-frequency** transducers are **thin,** and **low-frequency** transducers are **thick.**
–Transducers also emit ultrasound energy at frequencies other than the resonant frequency but at a lower intensity.
  –Clinical scanners can drive their transducers at several different transmit frequencies.
–The **bandwidth** is related to the range of frequencies generated by the crystal.
–The bandwidth determines the **purity** of **sound** and the **length** of **time** a sound persists, or ring down time.
–**Narrow bandwidth** transducers produce a relatively **pure frequency.**
  –Pure sounds (narrow bandwidth) will persist for a long time.
–**Wide bandwidth** transducers produce a **wider range** of **frequencies.**
  –Sounds with a broad range of frequencies last for only a very short time.
C. Design features
–**Most transducers** are designed to be **broadband** and *therefore produce short pulses.*
–Blocks of **damping material,** usually tungsten/rubber in an epoxy resin, are placed behind transducers to **reduce vibration (ring down time).**
  –*Damping broadens the bandwidth and shortens pulses.*
–A **matching layer** of material is placed on the front surface of the transducer to **improve** the efficiency of **energy transmission** into (and out of) the patient.
  –More than one layer may be used.
–**The matching layer** material(s) has an impedance value that is **intermediate** between that of the **transducer** and that of **tissue.**
–The matching layer thickness is one-fourth the wavelength of sound in that material and is referred to as **quarter-wave matching.**
–Figure 10.3 shows the components of a typical **piezoelectric transducer.**
D. Beams
–The **near field** of the ultrasound beam is adjacent to the transducer and is the region **used** for **ultrasound imaging.**
  –The near field is also called the **Fresnel zone.**
–The length of the **near field** is $r^2/λ$, where r is the transducer radius and λ is the wavelength.
  –For a 10-mm-diameter transducer operating at 3.5 MHz, the near field extends ~6 cm in soft tissue.
–**Doubling** the **transducer size** increases the **near field length fourfold.**
–**Doubling** the transducer **frequency** halves the wavelength, which **doubles** the extent of the **near field.**
–The **far field** starts where the near field ends.

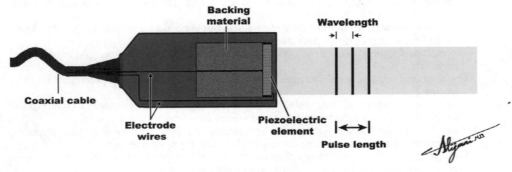

FIGURE 10.3   Transducer producing an ultrasound pulse that has a total pulse length of only two wavelengths.

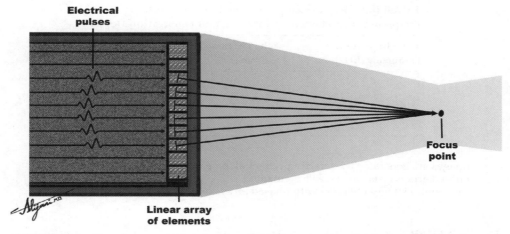

Electrical pulses

Focus point

Linear array of elements

FIGURE 10.4 Phased array, which makes use of time delays in activating the individual array elements to focus the ultrasound beam.

–In the far field, the ultrasound beam diverges and the intensity falls off very rapidly.
  –The far field is also called the **Fraunhofer zone.**
–Ultrasound imaging does *not* extend into the far field.
–**Side lobes** are small beams of greatly reduced intensity that are **emitted** at diverging **angles** from the **primary beam.**
  –The presence of **side lobes** can give rise to **imaging artifacts.**
–Virtually all diagnostic ultrasound beams use **focusing** of the ultrasound beam.
  –Focusing increases echo intensities.
–**Focusing** can be achieved using a **curved piezoelectric crystal** or **acoustic lens.**
–**Array transducers** can focus the beam by delaying the pulses for the central elements.
  –Figure 10.4 shows a phased array transducer which uses time delays to the electrical pulses to the individual elements to achieve focusing.
–The **focal zone** is the region over which the beam is focused.
–The **focal length** is the distance from the transducer to the center of the **focal zone.**
E. Arrays
  –**One beam** provides information for a **single line** of **sight.**
    –**One line** of **sight** produces a **single line** of an ultrasound image.
  –Images are built up by generating a large number of lines of sight that are sequentially directed to cover the region of interest in the patient being scanned.
  –Different types of ultrasound arrays are available to generate the required **sequential lines** of **sight.**
  –Most transducers are **multielement arrays,** where each element can operate independently of the others.
  –Multielement arrays are normally either **linear** or **phased.**
  –**Linear arrays** activate one group of elements (~20) to produce one line of sight and wait during the listening period to receive echoes along this single line of sight.
    –A group of elements, rather than a single element, is used to increase the near field.
  –The next line of sight is generated by firing another group of elements that are displaced by one or two elements.
  –The complete **frame** is generated by firing such groups of elements from one end of the linear array to the other end.
  –**Linear arrays** have **128** to **256 elements.**
    –**Linear arrays** generate **rectangular**-looking fields of view.
  –Curvilinear arrays diverge and allow a wider field of view (FOV).
    –**Curvilinear arrays** produce **diverging images** that originate in a curved arc.
  –**Phased arrays** make use of all the elements, which are activated at slightly different times.
    –Figure 10.4 shows an element activation pattern used for focusing.
  –In a phased array, ultrasound beam lines of sight are sequentially **steered through** an **arc.**

TABLE 10.4   Relationship between Pulse Repetition Frequency, Echo Listening Interval, and Penetration Depth

Pulse Repetition Frequency (kHz)	Echo Listening Time (μs)	Penetration Depth (cm)
4	250	20
6	167	13
8	125	10
10	100	8

–**Images** are generated by **detecting echoes** along **each line** of **sight**.
–**Phased arrays** typically have **96 elements**.
–Ultrasound images obtained with **phased arrays** originate from a **single point**.

IV. IMAGING

A. Pulse repetition frequency
  –**Pulse repetition frequency (PRF)** refers to the number of separate pulses of sound that are sent out every second.
    –**PRF** is also sometimes known as **pulse rate**.
  –Each pulse is **short** and contains only approximately **two wavelengths**.
    –The **duration** of a pulse is $\sim$**1** μ**s**.
  –**Between pulses,** the **transducer** acts as a **receiver**.
  –Common **PRF** values are $\sim$**4 kHz** (i.e., or 4,000 pulses per second).
  –The choice of **PRF** values controls the **penetration depth (range)** that may be detected.
  –A **high PRF** means that there is a **short echo listening time** when echoes can be detected.
    –Table 10.4 shows the relationship between the PRF, echo listening time, and imaging depth.
  –The **product** of the **lines per frame** and the **frame rate** equals the **PRF**.
    –Table 10.5 shows the relationship between the lines per image and the frame rate.
B. Echoes
  –The **time span** between emitted pulses allows time for the returning echoes to be received and provides information about the depth of an interface.
  –For soft tissue (v = 1,540 m/s), a **return time** of 13 μs corresponds to a **depth** of **1 cm**.
    –A depth of 1 cm corresponds to a **round trip** distance of 2 cm.
  –**Echoes** at 13 μs after the pulse was sent out thus correspond to an **echo depth** of **1 cm.**
    –Echoes at 26 μs correspond to an echo depth of 2 cm, and so on.
  –The **strength** of **returning echoes** provides information about differences in acoustic impedances between tissues.
  –**Scan converters** create **two-dimensional images** from echo data from distinct beam directions.
  –Ultrasound image data viewed on a video display is obtained (by interpolation) from the data collected and stored in the scan converter.

TABLE 10.5   Relationship between Lines per Frame and Frame Rate when Using a Pulse Repetition Frequency of 4 kHz

Line Density (No. of Lines of Sight per Image)	Maximum Image Frame Rate (Frames/Second)
25	160
50	80
100	40
200	20

–**Scan conversion** is required because the format of **image acquisition** and **display** are different.

–Modern scan converters process a large amount of data acquired by the ultrasound transducer digitally.

–Image data are stored/displayed in a matrix that is typically **512 × 512** with **8 bits** per pixel.

–One frame contains about 0.25 MB of information.

–For **color displays,** the depth of a pixel can by as high as **3 bytes (24 bits).**

C. **Display modes**

–**A-mode (amplitude)** displays depth on the horizontal axis and echo intensity (pulse amplitude) on the vertical axis.

–Ophthalmology is the only diagnostic application of A-mode imaging.

–**T-M mode (time-motion)** displays time on the horizontal axis and depth on the vertical axis.

–T-M mode is also known as **M-mode (motion).**

–The echo intensity is displayed as brightness.

–Echoes from **sequential ultrasound pulses** are displayed adjacent to each other, allowing the change in position of interfaces to be seen.

–**T-M mode** thus displays time-dependent motion, which is valuable for studying rapid movement (e.g., **cardiac valve motion**).

–**B-mode** displays an image of a section of tissue.

–The echo intensity is displayed as a **brightness B** along each line of sight.

–The **frame rate** for real-time imaging is ∼**30 frames per second.**

–**Real-time ultrasound** permits motion to be followed.

D. **Clinical transducers**

–Transducers used for **abdominal imaging** are generally in the **1- to 6-MHz range.**

–Transducers used for **peripheral imaging** are generally in the **5- to 13-MHz range.**

–High-resolution and shallow penetration probes (10–40 MHz) have been developed for studying the eye.

–Special systems include **endovaginal transducers** for imaging the pelvic region and fetus.

–**Endorectal** transducers are used for imaging the **prostate.**

–**Transesophageal** transducers image the **heart.**

–**Intravascular** probes have been developed for imaging inside **blood vessels.**

–**Linear arrays** are used in peripheral vascular examinations and imaging small body parts (Fig. 10.5A).

–**Curvilinear arrays** are used for abdominal exams (Fig. 10.5B).

–**B-mode, M-mode,** and **Doppler systems** are used to study the **cardiovascular system.**

–**Phased array transducers** are used for cardiac because they have a **small footprint** that can image between the ribs.

–**Two-dimensional matrix** transducers are used to image the **heart.**

–**Three-dimensional probes** are used for **obstetrics.**

E. **Harmonic imaging**

–**Harmonic frequencies** are **integral multiples** of the **fundamental** ultrasound pulse frequencies.

–A high-frequency harmonic can be **twice** the **fundamental frequency** of the initial ultrasound pulse.

–High frequencies arise from **nonlinear interactions** with tissues.

–Harmonic imaging tunes the receiver to the high (harmonic) frequency alone.

–The advantage of harmonic imaging is elimination of the fundamental frequency **clutter (noise).**

–Harmonic imaging requires **very broadband transducers.**

–Harmonic imaging receives signals at *twice* the transmit frequency.

–The **first harmonic** (twice the fundamental frequency) is most frequently used.

–Higher frequencies (e.g., **second harmonics**) have **too much attenuation.**

–**Contrast agents (microbubbles)** also produce harmonic frequencies.

–**Pulse inversion harmonic imaging** uses two pulses, consisting of a standard plus inverted (phase reversed) along the same beam direction.

–These two **cancel** out for **soft tissues** but not for microbubbles, which improves the **sensitivity** of **ultrasound** to **contrast agents.**

–Contrast agents for vascular and perfusion imaging are encapsulated **microbubbles (3–6 μm)** containing **air, nitrogen,** or **insoluble gases (perfluorocarbons).**

–The small size of the microbubbles permits perfusion of tissues.

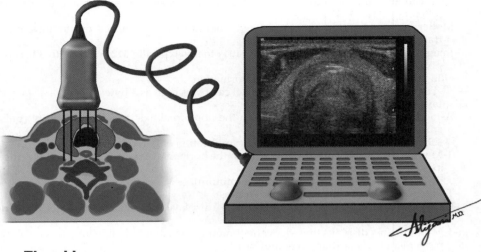

A   **Thyroid scan**

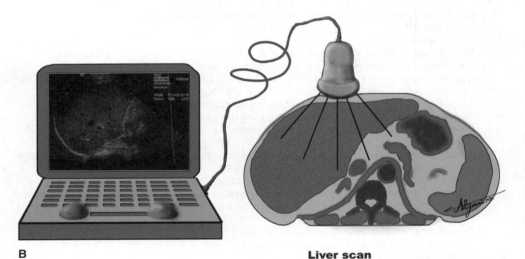

B   **Liver scan**

FIGURE 10.5   A: Use of a linear array to image the thyroid. **B:** Use of a curvilinear array to image the abdomen.

   –Ultrasound signals (reflections) are generated by the large difference in acoustic impedance between the gas and surrounding fluids/tissues.

V. DOPPLER

A. Doppler physics
   –The **Doppler effect** refers to **changes** in **frequency** resulting from a **moving** sound **source.**
   –Objects **moving toward** the detector reflect sound that has a **higher frequency.**
      –The increase in frequency is associated with a reduction in wavelength.
   –Objects **moving away** from the detector reflect sound that has a **lower frequency.**
      –The reduction in frequency is associated with an increase in wavelength.
   –The shift in frequency is proportional to **cos(θ)**, where θ is the angle between the ultrasound beam and the moving object.
      –θ is known as the **Doppler angle.**

TABLE 10.6   Maximum Doppler Frequency Shifts (Hz) for Moving Blood.

Blood Velocity (cm/s)	2-MHz Transducer	5-MHz Transducer	7.5-MHz Transducer
10	260	650	980
30	780	2,000	2,900
100	2,600	6,500	9,800

–The **maximum frequency shift** occurs when the reflector is moving directly toward the detector (i.e., θ is equal to 0 degrees) or directly away from the detector (i.e., θ is equal to 180 degrees).
–Doppler measures the shift in frequency, *not the reflector velocity.*
  –Moving objects produce **no Doppler shift** when their motion is **perpendicular** to the **sound** beam.
–The magnitude of the **Doppler frequency shift** is proportional to the **ultrasound frequency (f).**
–Doppler frequency shift is also proportional to the ratio of the reflector velocity (v) and inversely proportional to the speed of sound in the material (c).
  –Doppler frequency shift is therefore proportional to $f \times (v/c)$.
–**Ultrasound Doppler shift frequencies** are in the **audio range** as shown in Table 10.6.
B. Doppler and blood flow
  –**Doppler ultrasound** is used to identify and evaluate **blood flow** in vessels based on the **backscatter** of blood cells.
    –Blood is a weak scatterer and gives rise to weak signals.
  –**Pulsed wave (PW) Doppler** provides **depth** information in addition to the Doppler frequency shift.
  –Signals are processed so only echoes from a **region** of **interest** contribute to the Doppler signal.
    –A **wall filter** is generally used to eliminate very low frequencies.
  –Pulses are repeatedly directed along the same scan line to obtain multiple signals.
  –Duplex scanning combines **real-time imaging** with **Doppler** detection.
  –**B-mode images** provide information on stationary reflectors, and Doppler shifts provide information on flow present in a selected region of interest.
  –Duplex scanning allows selection of a region of interest and permits the **Doppler angle** to be estimated.
  –**Longer pulse lengths** are used in pulsed Doppler to improve the accuracy of the frequency shift.
    –Use of longer pulse lengths will reduce axial resolution (see below).
  –**Aliasing artifacts** can show the highest velocities in the center of a vessel as having a reverse flow.
  –To **avoid aliasing artifacts,** the **pulse repetition frequency** (PRF) must be at least *twice* the highest **Doppler frequency shift.**
    –A 1-kHz Doppler shift requires a PRF of at least 2 kHz.
C. Spectral analysis
  –**Spectral analysis** selects a region of interest in a B-mode image to be investigated for flow using **pulsed Doppler.**
  –**Spectral analysis** shows **frequency shift** as a function of **time** that can provide information regarding blood flow.
  –The **horizontal axis** is **time,** and the **vertical axis** is the **Doppler frequency shift.**
  –The intensity at a given **frequency shift,** and at a given moment in time, is displayed as a **brightness** value.
  –Velocities in one direction are placed above the horizontal axis, and in the reverse direction below the horizontal axis.
  –**Spectral displays** also provide information on **flow characteristics.**
    –Blood **flow** is **pulsatile,** and the spectral characteristics vary with time.
  –**Laminar flow** normally exists at the center of large smooth vessels, and slower flow occurs near the vessel walls (frictional forces).
  –**Turbulent flow** may occur when the vessel is disrupted by plaque and stenoses.
  –Figure 10.6 shows Doppler waveforms for several types of blood flow.
  –In Figure 10.6A, a **high-resistance arterial vessel** demonstrates a rapid fall in velocity following systole.

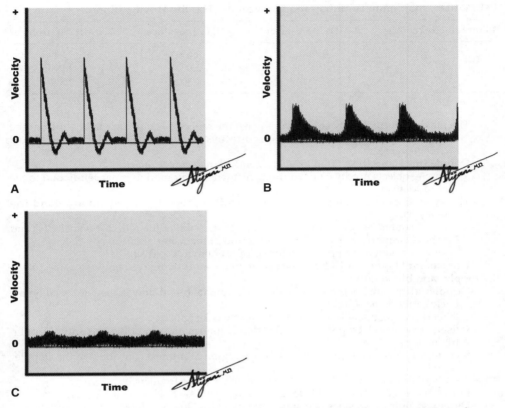

FIGURE 10.6   Spectral analysis from flow in **A.** aorta (high velocity/high resistance); **B.** renal artery (moderate velocity/low resistance); and **C.** portal vein (low velocity/low resistance).

–In Figure 10.6B, a **low-resistance artery** shows flow during diastole as well.
–In Figure 10.6C, flow from veins shows **low velocities** and **low resistance.**
–The **resistive index** is obtained by comparing the maximum velocity (V_{max}) and the minimum velocity (V_{min}) through the cardiac cycle.
  –**Resistive index** is $(V_{max} - V_{min})/V_{max}$.
–Figure 10.6A shows the highest resistive index, and Figure 10.6C shows the lowest resistive index.

D. Color Doppler
–**Color Doppler** provides a **2D visual display** of moving blood.
–Measured **Doppler frequency shifts** are encoded as **colors.**
–Color Doppler information is displayed on top of the B-mode image.
  –**Color Doppler** allows **velocity** and **position** information to be obtained simultaneously.
–Colors are assigned dependent on motion toward or away from the transducer.
  –**Red signifies** motion *toward* the **transducer** whereas **blue signifies** motion *away* from the **transducer.**
    –**Turbulent flow** may be displayed as green or yellow.
–Color intensity varies with flow velocity, with the **B-mode image** used to depict the **absence** of **movement.**
–Flow information is provided by taking the average value of a number of samples obtained from each pixel (location).
–**Color Doppler** provides information on the direction and magnitude of the flow over a large region of interest.
–Color Doppler can detect flow in vessels too small to see by imaging alone, and allows **complex blood flow** to be visualized.
–**Clutter** from **slow-moving** solid structures can overwhelm the small echoes from blood.

–**Spatial resolution** of the color Doppler image is **lower** than that of the B-mode image.

–Most color Doppler units also offer a **spectral Doppler,** which can provide more additional flow information from a **selected region** of **interest.**

E. **Power Doppler**

   –**Power Doppler** uses *similar* information as obtained in color Doppler.

     –Energy sometimes replaces the term *power.*

   –Power levels in **color Doppler** and **power Doppler** are the same.

     –Differences between power and color Doppler relate to how the acquired information is processed and displayed.

   –**Power Doppler** uses the **Doppler signal strength alone,** and ignores the Doppler shift.

     –Positive and negative velocities of the same magnitude from a given region would be summed in power Doppler but would be canceled out in color Doppler.

   –**The power Doppler** signal does not vary with the **direction** of **flow.**

   –**Aliasing artifacts** do *not* occur in power Doppler.

   –Power Doppler is *much* more sensitive than standard color flow imaging.

     –Power Doppler sacrifices the directional and quantitative flow information provided by color Doppler.

   –**Slow blood flow** is much easier to detect using **power Doppler.**

   –Power Doppler uses slower frame rates.

   –**Power Doppler** is sensitive to **motion** by patients, tissues, and transducers.

     –Motion artifacts in power Doppler are called **flash artifacts.**

VI. IMAGING PERFORMANCE

A. **Axial resolution**

   –**Axial resolution** is the ability to separate two objects lying along the axis of the beam.

   –The most important factor that affects axial resolution is the **pulse length.**

   –An ultrasound pulse normally consists of approximately two wavelengths.

     –**Short pulses,** achieved by **damping** of the transducer, are *essential* for good axial resolution performance.

   –**Axial resolution** is approximately equal to **one half** of the **pulse length.**

   –At 2 MHz, axial resolution is ~1 mm (i.e., half the pulse length of ~2 mm).

     –At 4 MHz, axial resolution improves to ~0.5 mm.

   –**Transducer frequency** is the determinant of axial resolution.

     –Axial resolution does **not vary** with **depth.**

   –**High-frequency** transducers must be used for **good axial resolution.**

     –The problem with high-frequency transducers is poor penetration.

   –Ultrasound imaging has a fundamental **trade-off** between spatial **resolution** and maximum **imaging depth.**

   –High axial resolution requires minimizing the distance between the transducer and objects of interest.

   –High-resolution imaging is achieved in **breast ultrasound** using **8-** or **10-MHz** transducers.

     –Limited breast thickness normally permits adequate penetration.

   –**Intracavitary ultrasound probes** permit intravascular imaging with excellent resolution performance of the blood vessels.

B. **Lateral resolution**

   –**Lateral resolution** is the ability to resolve two adjacent objects.

   –Lateral resolution performance is determined by the **ultrasound beam width.**

   –**Focused transducers** produce a narrow beam and **improve lateral resolution.**

   –The **best lateral resolution** performance is obtained within the **focal zone.**

   –**Lateral resolution** is measured using phantoms and is approximately **four times worse** than **axial resolution.**

   –Increasing the number of **lines per frame** improves lateral resolution.

   –Lateral resolution can be controlled by **adjusting** the **focal position.**

   –**Multiple focal lengths** may be used to improve lateral resolution.

     –Focal length can be changed using array transducers.

   –Use of **multiple focal lengths** is generally at the expense of a **reduced frame rate.**

   –Lateral resolution usually becomes worse at larger distances from the transducer.

C. Elevational resolution
  –**Elevational resolution** is the resolution in the plane perpendicular to the image plane.
    –**Slice thickness** is another term for **elevational resolution.**
  –**Transducer** height is directly related to elevational resolution.
  –Elevational **focusing** can be achieved using an acoustic lens.
    –Elevational resolution is generally image **depth dependent.**
  –Slice thickness can be improved by the use of **1.5D arrays.**
    –A 1.5D array has approximately six **rows** of **transducers** in the **slice thickness** direction.
    –Focusing these six rows of transducers reduces the slice thickness.
  –Arrays of 1.5D have many more transducers in the scan plane (e.g., 192).
    –The two-dimensional array can contain ~6 × 192 individual transducers.
  –**Lateral resolution** and **elevational resolution** are generally **comparable.**

D. Ultrasound artifacts
  –**Speckle** is a textured appearance that results from small closely spaced structures.
    –Structures producing speckle are too small to be normally resolved.
  –**Noise** can result from **random signals** produced in the **electronic preamplifier** of the transducer.
    –**Averaging** successive images reduces **noise.**
  –**Reverberation echoes** are the result of **multiple reflections** occurring from two adjacent interfaces.
  –**Reverberation** produces delayed echoes that are incorrectly localized as a more distant interface.
    –The number of reverberations is limited by the power of the beam and sensitivity of the detector.
  –**Acoustic shadowing** is the reduced echo intensity behind a **highly attenuating** or **reflecting** object such as a stone creating a shadow.
  –**Acoustic enhancement** is the increased echo intensity behind a minimally attenuating object such as a **cyst** or **blood vessel.**
  –**Refraction** causes artifacts in the form of **spatial distortions.**
  –**Mirror images** occur where sound is reflected off a large interface such as the **diaphragm** causing parts of the image to be in the wrong location.
  –**Speed displacement** artifacts are caused by the variability of the speed of sound in different tissues.
  –**Ghost images** (grating lobes) can arise because of the division of a smooth transducer into a large number of small elements in multielement transducer arrays.
    –Ghost images arise from high contrast off axis objects.

E. Intensities
  –Values of an **ultrasound beam intensity** depend on the averaging procedure used.
  –Ultrasound intensity varies over the **lateral** extent of the beam **(i.e., spatially).**
  –The **spatial peak intensity** is the maximum beam intensity.
  –**Spatial average intensity** is the average intensity over the beam, normally taken to be equal to the transducer area.
    –Spatial **peak intensity** is **greater** than spatial **average intensity.**
  –For pulsed ultrasound, **intensity** also varies with **time (i.e., temporally).**
    –Between pulses, no energy is being transmitted.
  –**Temporal peak intensity** is the highest instantaneous intensity in the beam (i.e., during a pulse).
  –**Temporal average intensity** is the time average intensity (i.e., averaged over pulse and listening time).
  –**Listening times** (~100 μs) are **much longer** than a **pulse duration** (~1 μs).
    –**Temporal peak intensity** is much greater than the **temporal average intensity.**
  –**Thermal effects** are best predicted with the **spatial peak** and **temporal average.**
  –Ultrasound intensities are obtained along the central beam axis (spatial peak), and averaged over time (temporal average).
  –Representative **intensities** in **B-mode** ultrasound are **~10 mW/cm².**
    –**Doppler** ultrasound intensities can exceed **~1,000 mW/cm².**

F. Ultrasound bioeffects
  –At high power levels, **ultrasound** can cause **cavitation,** the creation and collapse of microscopic bubbles.
  –**Cavitation** is a concern in **harmonic imaging** because of the high peak pressures used.

–**The mechanical index (MI)** is a parameter that estimates the chance of inducing cavitation effects.

  –MI is proportional to the peak pressure values in the ultrasound beam.

–**Tissue heating** occurs as a result of energy absorption.

  –**Ultrasound** is used for **hyperthermia** treatment.

–**Tissue heating** is a concern in **spectral Doppler** because the beam stays in one location.

–The **thermal index (TI)** is the ratio of the acoustic power produced by the transducer to the power required to raise the tissue temperature by 1°C.

–A TI of 3 means that tissue temperature could increase by 3°C for a stationary transducer.

  –**TI** can be specified for **soft tissue (TIS), bone (TIB),** or **cranial bone (TIC).**

–The **American Institute of Ultrasound in Medicine (AIUM)** has a Bioeffects Committee to review ultrasound safety.

–More than half of **pregnant women** in the United States undergo **ultrasonic examinations** with no good evidence of detrimental effects.

–**Ultrasound** at **diagnostic** intensity levels is widely accepted as **safe.**

REVIEW TEST

10.1 In a sound wave, the physical quantity varying with time is:
a. voltage
b. magnetic field
c. pressure
d. charge
e. current

10.2 The wavelength of a 3-MHz sound beam is shortest in:
a. air
b. fat
c. muscle
d. bone
e. PZT

10.3 A signal attenuated to 1% of its original intensity corresponds to attenuation (−dB) of:
a. 1
b. 5
c. 10
d. 20
e. 100

10.4 Which of the following has the highest acoustic impedance?
a. Bone
b. Fat
c. Air
d. Water
e. Eye lens

10.5 An ultrasound beam traveling through tissue is least likely to be:
a. absorbed
b. amplified
c. scattered
d. reflected
e. refracted

10.6 Reflections are least likely to occur from:
a. smooth surfaces
b. kidney interior
c. fat–kidney interfaces
d. bladder wall
e. bladder contents

10.7 The largest ultrasound reflections most likely occur between soft tissue and:
a. water
b. fat
c. bone
d. blood
e. air

10.8 Snell's law describes the relation between the:
a. angle of incidence and transmission

b. Fraunhofer angle and wavelength
c. near field and frequency
d. angle of incidence and reflection
e. focus and transducer curvature

10.9 Depth gain compensation accounts for tissue attenuation by increasing the:
a. transducer output
b. echo amplification
c. focal length
d. ultrasound velocity
e. pulse repetition frequency

10.10 Attenuation of ultrasound in soft tissue at 2 MHz is most likely (dB/cm):
a. 0.25
b. 0.5
c. 1
d. 2
e. 4

10.11 Increasing the transducer thickness is most likely to increase the sound:
a. frequency
b. velocity
c. wavelength
d. intensity
e. attenuation

10.12 The damping material behind the crystal transducer reduces the:
a. tissue attenuation
b. pulse length
c. operating frequency
d. lateral resolution
e. penetration depth

10.13 An ultrasound near field is made longer when increasing the transducer:
a. operating frequency
b. time gain compensation
c. pulse repetition frequency
d. physical density
e. acoustic impedance

10.14 A 4-kHz PRF corresponds to a listening time (μs) of:
a. 60
b. 125
c. 250
d. 500
e. 1,000

10.15 Ultrasound signals are converted to a video monitor display using:
a. log amplifiers
b. array processors
c. scan converters
d. pulse height analyzers
e. analog-to-digital converters

10.16 An echo received 26 μs after the signal is sent is likely from a interface depth (cm) of:
   a. 1
   b. 2
   c. 3
   d. 4
   e. 5

10.17 The matrix size of a digitized ultrasound frame sent to a PACS is most likely:
   a. 64 × 64
   b. 128 × 128
   c. 256 × 256
   d. 512 × 512
   e. 1,024 × 1,024

10.18 The most likely frame rate (frames per second) in real-time ultrasound imaging is:
   a. 1
   b. 5
   c. 20
   d. 100
   e. 500

10.19 Which is *least* likely an ultrasound display mode?
   a. A
   b. B
   c. T
   d. T-M
   e. M

10.20 The Doppler shift from a moving object is *least* likely to depend on the:
   a. ultrasound velocity
   b. ultrasound frequency
   c. beam direction
   d. object depth
   e. object speed

10.21 The maximum Doppler frequency shift likely occurs when the angle (degrees) between the moving reflector and ultrasound beam is:
   a. 0
   b. 23
   c. 45
   d. 68
   e. 90

10.22 What is the minimum PRF (kHz) required to accurately measure a 1-kHz Doppler frequency shift?
   a. 0.25
   b. 0.5
   c. 1
   d. 2
   e. 4

10.23 In color Doppler, a red intensity most likely signifies that the blood flow is:
   a. toward the transducer
   b. away from the transducer

   c. perpendicular to the transducer
   d. generating aliased data
   e. turbulent

10.24 Choice of frequency in ultrasound is most likely a trade-off between patient penetration and:
   a. image contrast
   b. axial resolution
   c. lateral resolution
   d. speckle noise
   e. image artifacts

10.25 Ultrasound with a short pulse length is most likely to result in improved:
   a. axial resolution
   b. lateral resolution
   c. echo intensity
   d. tissue penetration
   e. frame rate

10.26 Lateral resolution in ultrasound imaging would most likely be improved by increasing the:
   a. transducer thickness
   b. pulse repetition frequency
   c. lines per frame
   d. frame rate
   e. pulse length

10.27 Shadowing artifacts would be least likely to occur behind:
   a. lung
   b. bone
   c. air cavities
   d. bladder
   e. clips

10.28 Which of the following is *least* likely to be an ultrasound artifact?
   a. Mirror image
   b. Reverberation
   c. Edge packing
   d. Speed displacement
   e. Refraction

10.29 B-mode ultrasound beam intensities (W/cm^2) are most likely:
   a. 0.001
   b. 0.01
   c. 0.1
   d. 10
   e. 100

10.30 The thermal index (TI) value indicates the possible increase in tissue:
   a. cavitation
   b. cell death
   c. density
   d. shearing
   e. temperature

ANSWERS AND EXPLANATIONS

10.1c. A sound wave is a variation of pressure with time.

10.2a. Air, since wavelength is velocity/frequency and air has the lowest velocity.

10.3d. Attenuation of −20 dB is 1% (−10 dB is 10%, and −30 dB is 0.1%).

10.4a. Bone, since acoustic impedance is density times sound velocity, which are both highest in bone.

10.5b. Amplified, since ultrasound beams are normally strongly attenuated at a rate of about −0.5 dB/cm/MHz.

10.6e. Bladder contents are normally fluids, which are most unlikely to give rise to any kind of specular or nonspecular reflections.

10.7e. Air–soft tissue interfaces will give rise to the largest echoes because of the large mismatch in the acoustic properties of air (very low) and soft tissue (average).

10.8a. Snell's law describes the relation between the angle of incidence and transmission.

10.9b. Depth gain compensation accounts for tissue attenuation by increasing echo amplification for later echoes.

10.10c. One dB, since the value used in clinical ultrasound is 0.5 dB/cm per MHz.

10.11c. Wavelength, since the crystal thickness is one half of the ultrasound wavelength.

10.12b. The pulse length is reduced by the introduction of a damping material behind a transducer.

10.13a. An increase in operating frequency reduces the wavelength, and the near field is inversely proportional to the wavelength.

10.14c. The pulse repetition period (listening time) is 250 μs, which is given by 1/PRF (i.e., 1/4,000 seconds).

10.15c. Ultrasound signals are converted from digital data to a video monitor display using scan converters.

10.16b. Two cm, since it takes 13 μs to get an echo from an interface from a depth of 1 cm.

10.17d. The typical matrix of the displayed US image on a typical monitor is 512×512 (note that the acquired image in the scan converter may have a different matrix size).

10.18c. Twenty frames per second is the only plausible value (5 is too low, and 100 is too high).

10.19c. There is no T (time) display mode in ultrasound.

10.20d. Object depth has no direct relationship to the Doppler shift.

10.21a. Zero degrees results in the largest Doppler shift, and 90 degrees in no Doppler shift.

10.22d. Two kHz, since one has to sample at twice the maximum frequency shift one is trying to detect (1 kHz in this example).

10.23a. In color Doppler, a red intensity most likely signifies that the blood flow is toward the transducer.

10.24b. The choice of frequency in ultrasound is a trade-off between patient penetration and axial resolution.

10.25a. Axial resolution is approximately half the spatial pulse length.

10.26c. Lateral resolution improves by increasing the number of lines in each frame.

10.27d. Bladder contents have negligible attenuation and are more likely to show enhancement (not shadowing).

10.28c. Edge packing is a nuclear medicine artifact.

10.29b. B-mode US intensities are most likely 0.01 W/cm^2, which is 10 mW/cm^2.

10.30e. Thermal index (TI) values indicate an increase in tissue temperature.

Chapter 11

MAGNETIC RESONANCE

I. PHYSICS

A. Magnetic nuclei
- –Magnetic resonance (MR) relates to interactions with nuclei.
- –Because of their nuclear charge distribution, some nuclei have **nuclear magnetization.**
- –**Magnetic nuclei** can be represented by a vector that depicts the strength and orientation of the **nuclear magnetization.**
    - –Nuclear magnetization may be called **magnetic dipole, magnetic spins,** or **magnetic moments.**
- –Nuclei with an **even** number of **protons** and an even number of **neutrons** have **no nuclear magnetization.**
    - –Even numbers of protons pair up with their magnetization aligned in opposite directions and cancel each other (as do even numbers of neutrons).
- –Nuclei with an odd number of **protons,** or odd number of **neutrons,** have a **nuclear magnetization.**
    - –These magnetic nuclei can be considered to behave like bar magnets and are candidates for magnetic resonance (see Table 11.1).
- –**Hydrogen nuclei** have the largest nuclear magnetization.
- –The abundance of hydrogen in the body, together with the large nuclear magnetization, makes it the basis of most clinical magnetic resonance (MR) imaging.
    - –Detected MR signals originate in protons in *free* water (i.e., mobile) and fat.

B. Tissue magnetization
- –There are more than 10^{22} hydrogen protons in each cubic centimeter (cm^3) of tissue.
- –Protons are normally **randomly** oriented and, have *no net* **nuclear magnetization.**
- –When placed into a magnetic field, hydrogen nuclei (protons) will become orientated either **spin up** (i.e., aligned along the field) or **spin down** (i.e., aligned opposite to the field).
    - –Spin-down alignment corresponds to a slightly higher energy level.
- –A **small excess** of protons go into the **spin-up** alignment.
- –This excess is ~4 for each million protons at **1 tesla.**
    - –Magnetic fields of the remaining spin-up and spin-down nuclei cancel.
- –Tissue placed into a magnetic field produces a **net nuclear magnetization** of unpaired protons aligned in the direction of the external field.
    - –Only these excess nuclei in the lower energy (spin up) state contribute to the MR signal.
- –One reason that MR signals are weak is that so few nuclei contribute to the MR signal.
    - –Considerable technical ingenuity is required to maximize the MR signal-to-noise ratio (SNR).
- –Table 11.2 summarizes the relative amounts of mobile protons in different tissues.

C. Larmor frequency
- –When magnetic nuclei are placed into a magnetic field, a torque causes the moments to perform a **precession motion** similar to a spinning top.
- –The **Larmor frequency (f_L)** is the precession frequency (MHz) of nuclei in a **magnetic field (B_o).**

TABLE 11.1   Nuclei Used in MR and Their Relative Sensitivity

Nucleus	Relative Sensitivity (%)
^{1}H	100.0
^{19}F	83.3
^{23}Na	9.3
^{31}P	6.6

–The Larmor frequency is directly proportional to the magnetic field strength.
–**Larmor frequency** (f_L) for protons is 42 MHz at **1 T.**
–The Larmor frequency for protons is 21 MHz at 0.5 T and 127 MHz at 3 T.
   –These frequencies are in the ham radio and aviation radiofrequency range.
–^{19}F has a Larmor frequency of 40 MHz at 1 T.
–^{23}Na has a Larmor frequency of 11 MHz at 1 T.
–For nuclei of interest in clinical MR, **protons** have the **highest Larmor frequency** at any field strength.
–**Increasing** the **Larmor frequency** results in higher MR **signals.**
D. Resonance
   –**Radiofrequency (RF) electromagnetic fields** are generated using a **volume** or **surface coil.**
   –**Resonance** occurs when an applied **RF field interacts** with the net nuclear **magnetization.**
   –The applied RF must be at the Larmor frequency, and its orientation must be perpendicular to the external magnetic field.
   –RF at frequency f_L, when applied perpendicular to the external magnetic field, causes the magnetization vector to rotate.
   –The **rotation** of the **magnetization** continues while the RF is being applied (i.e., is switched on).
   –When the RF is switched off, the magnetization will have rotated through an angle called the **flip angle.**
   –The flip angle depends on applied RF field strength and the total time that it is on (i.e., pulse duration).
   –A **90-degree RF pulse** reorients the magnetization vector to a direction 90 degrees perpendicular to the direction it had prior to the pulse.
   –A **180-degree RF pulse** reorients the magnetization vector to a direction 180 degrees (i.e., opposite) to the direction it had prior to the pulse.
      –A 90-degree RF pulse takes half as long as a 180-degree RF pulse.
   –The component of the net magnetization vector parallel to the main magnetic field is called the **longitudinal magnetization.**
      –By convention, the longitudinal magnetization is taken to point in the z-axis.
   –The component perpendicular to the main magnetic field is called the **transverse magnetization.**
      –By convention, the transverse magnetization is taken to be in the x-y plane.

TABLE 11.2   Relative Amounts of Mobile Protons in Different Tissues

Tissue	Relative Number of Mobile Protons % (Spin Density)
White matter	100
Fat	98
Gray matter	94
Liver	91
Bone	~5
Lung	~3

E. Free induction decay
  –After a 90-degree RF pulse is applied to longitudinal magnetization, the resulting transverse magnetization vector **precesses** about the external magnetic field.
    –The precession frequency is also the Larmor frequency f_L.
  –This rotating magnetization can be detected as an **induced voltage** in a coil.
    –An RF coil is simply an **optimized antenna,** and the detected signal will be stronger the closer the coil is to the signal source.
  –The detected voltage is called the **free induction decay (FID)** signal.
  –The FID signal is an oscillating voltage at the Larmor frequency (f_L).
    –The induced FID is obtained in a receiver coil placed around the sample.
  –The FID signal is weak because of the small number of nuclei that contribute to the signal (i.e., ~ 4 per 10^6).
  –**Nuclear magnetization** is ~ 700 times weaker than **electron magnetization.**
    –The small size of all **nuclear magnetic moments** results in a weak FID signal.
  –Receiver coils may be the same as transmitter coils.
  –FID signals are detected, digitized, and used to produce MR images.

II. RELAXATION

A. T1 relaxation
  –Protons placed into magnetic fields produce a net magnetization with a magnitude M_z (i.e., **longitudinal magnetization**).
    –M_z is parallel to the direction of the external magnetic field.
  –Longitudinal magnetization grows exponentially from the initial value of zero to the **equilibrium value** of **M_z** with a **time constant T1** (Fig. 11.1).
    –At a time equal to T1, 63% of the magnetization has formed.
  –Full magnetization (i.e., M_z) is normally taken to occur after a time interval of approximately $4 \times$ T1.
  –If the external magnetic field is *switched off,* longitudinal magnetization M_z decreases exponentially with the same time constant T1.
    –Longitudinal magnetization decays as $M_z \times e^{-t/T1}$ where t is the elapsed time.
  –T1 relaxation is called **longitudinal relaxation** and **spin-lattice relaxation.**

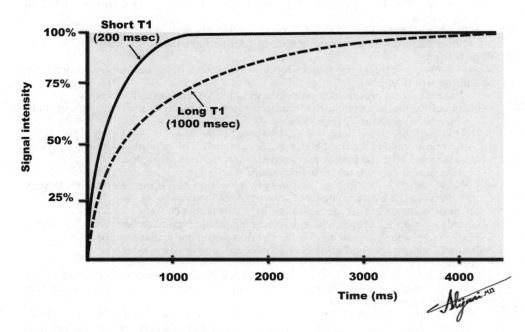

FIGURE 11.1   Return to equilibrium of longitudinal magnetization for two tissues with different T1 relaxation times.

TABLE 11.3   Representative T1 and T2 Relaxation Times (1.5 Tesla)

Tissue	T1 (ms)	T2 (ms)
Fat (adipose)	250	80
Liver	500	45
Kidney	650	60
White matter	800	90
Grey matter	900	100
Cerebrospinal fluid	2,400	280

–When the lattice has components of motion at the **Larmor frequency,** this "encourages" a nucleus to interact with the surrounding jiggling spins and undergo recovery.
  –Different tissues have different frequencies of motion (**vibration modes**), which accounts for the differences in T1 relaxation times.
–T1 is long in liquid materials (cerebrospinal fluid [CSF]) and in solids (hair).
  –T1 is short in medium-viscosity materials and in fat (Table 11.3).
–**Contrast agents** such as **gadolinium-DTPA** cause T1 to be shortened.
–For tissues, **T1 increases** with increasing **magnetic field** strength.
  –Doubling the magnetic field strength increases tissue T1 by approximately $2^{0.5}$.
B. T1 contrast
  –Generating a N^2 matrix MR image requires the acquisition of N sequential signal acquisitions that are obtained with a **repetition time TR.**
    –In time TR, one signal (i.e., one line of data) is obtained, which contains 256 values.
    –In the second TR interval, another line of data is acquired, and so on.
  –The value of TR is entirely under the control of the operator and ranges from tens of milliseconds to seconds.
  –The choice of TR value affects the **contrast** between tissues that differ in their T1 values.
  –A long TR value permits the **magnetization** in all tissues to **fully recover.**
    –As a result, long TR times generate **no T1 weighting.**
  –When TR values are short, only tissues with short T1 values fully recover their **longitudinal magnetization** and contribute a signal.
  –With **short TR** values, tissues with a long T1 do not recover and therefore contribute little signal.
  –A **T1-weighted image** is obtained using short TR that emphasizes T1 differences.
    –Short TR times are less than ~300 ms at 1.5 T and less than ~450 ms at 3T.
C. T2 relaxation
  –After a 90-degree pulse, the magnetization vector rotates at the **Larmor frequency** in the **transverse (x-y) plane.**
    –The **FID signal** produced is proportional to the **x-y magnetization vector.**
  –In perfectly uniform magnetic fields, the **transverse magnetization** decays exponentially with a **time constant T2** (Fig. 11.2).
  –The induced FID signal decays as $e^{-t/T2}$ where t is the time.
    –At a time equal to T2, the signal has decayed to 37% of its original value.
  –After a time ~4 T2, the transverse magnetization signal is negligible.
  –T2 relaxation is called **transverse relaxation.**
    –T2 relaxation is also known as **spin-spin relaxation** as it is mediated by interactions between the magnetic fields of adjacent nuclei (spins).
  –For most tissues, T2 times are tens of milliseconds (Table 11.3).
  –Liquids have long T2 times whereas viscous materials and solids have short T2 times.
  –**T2** decreases with increasing viscosity and decreasing **molecular mobility.**
  –Tissue **T2** values are approximately independent of magnetic field strength.
D. T2 contrast
  –MR signals are most often obtained in the form of **echoes** from **transverse magnetization.**
  –MR echoes occur at a time **TE (time** to **echo)** that is under operator control, and can be selected to be long or short.
  –**Short TE** values will result in little loss of **transverse magnetization** (i.e., little T2 decay).
  –Short TE values therefore produce no differences **(contrast)** between tissues that have different T2 values.
    –**Short TE** values have **minimal T2 weighting.**

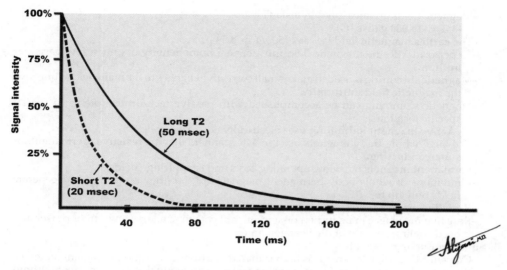

FIGURE 11.2   Loss of transverse magnetization due to T2 relaxation.

　　–Long TE values will reduce the intensity of transverse magnetization for tissues with short T2 much more than tissues with long T2.
　　　　–T2-weighted images are obtained with a **long TE.**
　　–Long TE values are typically greater than 60 ms.
E. **T2***
　　–Normal magnets have magnetic field inhomogeneities with slight differences in magnetic field at different locations.
　　–Magnet inhomogeneities are typically a few **parts per million (ppm).**
　　　　–Magnet inhomogeneities are a few μT in fields of 1 T.
　　–Inhomogeneities also arise because of different magnetic properties of different tissues (e.g., **iron** in the **blood**) and at tissue boundaries (i.e., **susceptibility inhomogeneities**).
　　–Differences in magnetic field strength cause magnetization at different locations to rotate at slightly different **Larmor frequencies.**
　　　　–Larmor frequency is proportional to magnetic field strength.
　　–Adjacent magnetizations that initially point in the same direction start to diverge and point in different directions (i.e., **dephase**).
　　–This divergence **(dephasing)** results in a **loss** of **transverse magnetization.**
　　–Spin dephasing due to inhomogeneities is **T2**$_{inhomogeneity}$.
　　–Decay of transverse magnetization (FID) occurs because of inhomogeneities in the main magnetic field *and* T2 decay, which is called **T2*.**
　　–The observed FID signal falls **exponentially** with a **decay rate constant T2*** (i.e., $e^{-t/T2*}$).
　　　　–The relationship between **T2, T2*,** and **spin dephasing** due to inhomogeneities (T2$_{inhomogeneity}$), is given by **1/T2* = 1/T2 + 1/T2**$_{inhomogeneity}$
　　–T2* is a few milliseconds and is always shorter than T2.
　　　　–For tissues, **T2* ≤ T2 ≤ T1.**
　　–In soft tissues, inhomogeneities are the most important contribution to T2*.
　　–Materials such as **paramagnetic** and **ferromagnetic** contrast agents disrupt the local magnetic field homogeneity and shorten **T2*.**
　　–Dephasing due to the inhomogeneity contribution to **T2*** may be **overcome** by generating spin **echoes.**
　　　　–By contrast, loss of transverse magnetization due to **T2** relaxation is **irreversible.**

III. INSTRUMENTATION

A. **Magnets**
　　–Powerful magnets capable of generating strong magnetic fields are essential for MR.
　　　　–MR magnetic fields also need to be **stable** and **uniform** in space.

–Magnetic fields are measured in **tesla (T).**
  –1 T = 10,000 gauss (G).
–The **earth's magnetic field** is weak (50 μT or 0.5 G).
–To perform MR, the magnetic field must have a **homogeneity** of only a **few parts per million.**
–**Magnetic shimming** is used to make small corrective changes to the main field to improve the **magnetic field uniformity.**
–Magnetic shimming can be accomplished with **passive techniques** (pieces of iron at specific locations).
  –Active magnetic shimming uses electrically energized coils.
–The large **whole-body magnets** used in MR scanners may be **resistive, permanent,** or **superconducting.**
–**Permanent magnets** have low operating costs and small fringe fields.
–Limitations of whole body permanent magnets are that they are heavy and generate fields only up to ~0.35 T.
–**Resistive magnets** can generate magnetic fields up to ~0.5 T.
–Resistive magnets can be turned on and off, but consume a large amount of power and need cooling because of the heat generated.

B. Superconducting magnets
–Current MR uses field strengths higher than those of resistive and permanent magnets.
–**Superconductivity** is the ability of certain materials to conduct electrical current **without any resistance.**
–Superconducting MR magnets use a wire-wrapped cylinder (i.e., a **solenoid**) to generate the **uniform magnetic field.**
–Superconducting magnets must be kept very cold using **liquid helium (4° K)** as a refrigerant.
–A perpetually circulating electric current of hundreds of amps creates the magnetic field.
  –The **superconducting magnetic field** is **always on.**
–If the wire temperature rises, the system loses its **superconducting** properties and the energy stored in the magnetic field is converted to heat resulting in a **magnet quench.**
–Figure 11.3 is a cutaway view of a superconducting MR imaging system.
–Field strengths of 20 T can currently be generated by **superconducting magnets.**
–As MR field strength increases, so does **T1 relaxation time, SNR,** and **RF energy deposition** in the patient.
  –Some **image artifacts** may also increase with increasing magnetic field strength.

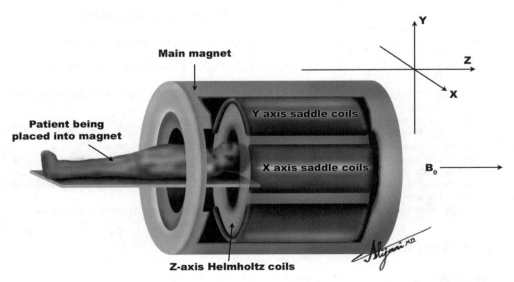

FIGURE 11.3   Superconducting magnetic resonance system showing the main magnetic field (B_o) and three sets of coils that generate magnetic field gradients.

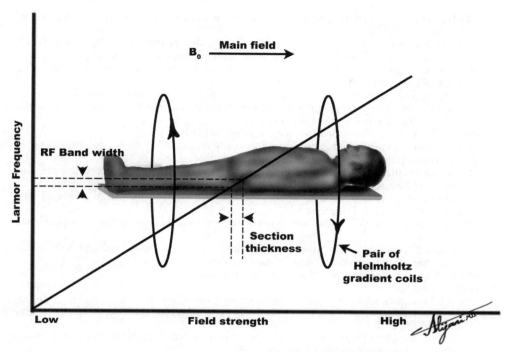

FIGURE 11.4   The *solid line* shows how the Larmor frequency varies along the long patient axis when a gradient is applied. When an RF pulse with a narrow range of frequencies is used, it only affects magnetization within a narrow distance along the patient, defining image slice thickness.

C. Gradient coils
–**Magnetic gradients** are used to code the **spatial location** of the MR signal.
  –Gradients are essential for generating images.
–MR systems have three magnetic **field gradient coils** oriented in the x, y, and z directions.
  –Combinations of three **orthogonal** sets of gradients allow the gradient field to be oriented in any direction.
–**Axial gradients** (z) are produced using **Helmholtz coils.**
  –Figure 11.4 shows a pair of **Helmholtz coils** being used to produce a gradient along the z-axis.
–Gradients that change the main field as a function of x or y distance are normally produced by **saddle coils.**
–When activated, these gradients superimpose a **linear gradient** on the main magnetic field.
–With gradients superimposed on the main magnetic field, each magnetic field location corresponds to a slightly different Larmor frequency.
  –Magnetic gradients cause different locations to have different magnetization precession frequencies.
–Gradient strengths are ~30 mT/m on a 1.5-T scanner.
–Gradients may need to be **switched** on and off rapidly (<500 μs).
–Gradients generate small, rapidly decaying **eddy currents** in other coils or metal structures nearby.
  –Induced **eddy currents** impair scanner performance and may create **image artifacts.**
D. Radiofrequency coils
–**RF** is **electromagnetic radiation** with **frequencies** in the range of approximately 1 MHz to 10 GHz.
–A RF coil consists of various configurations of **radiowave antenna.**
–**Transmitter coils** are used to send in RF pulses with the required **flip angle.**

–**Radio waves** from **transverse magnetization** in patients are detected by receive **RF coils.**
  –**Receive coils** may be physically separate from the **transmit RF coil,** or may be the same coil switched electronically from transmit mode to receive mode.
–Placing the receive coils close to the region being imaged improves the detected **radiowave signal** (i.e., increases SNR).
  –Smaller coils generally have lower levels of noise (i.e., will increase SNR).
–**Volume coils** are designed to transmit and receive uniform RF signal throughout a volume, e.g., the head coil or body coil.
–Specialized RF coils include those for the **knee** and **spine.**
–**Linear volume coils** receive the signal from only one of the x- or y-axes of the rotating transverse magnetization.
–**Quadrature volume coils** receive the signal in both the x- and y-axes, therefore increasing the overall **SNR** and reducing image artifacts.
–**Surface coils** have increased sensitivity close to the coil, but the signal drops off with increasing distance from the coil.
–**Phased array** coils are a combination of many surface coils around the body part being examined.
  –**Phased arrays** try to obtain uniform signals from the enclosed volume with an improved signal detection of individual **surface coils.**
–Phased array coils are required for **parallel imaging.**

E. **Parallel imaging**
–**Parallel imaging** uses the separate signals from **phased array** coils.
–Many individual surface coils in a phased array coil detect the same signal from the same place in the body.
–However, the strength of the detected signal is different in each coil because it is at a different distance from the RF source.
–Using a preacquired sensitivity map of each coil, additional information is obtained from several surface coils.
–Surface coils in a phased array coil used for parallel imaging are termed **elements.**
  –Phased array coils are available with up to 32 elements, with each element having a separate **RF preamplifier.**
–**The parallel imaging factor** quantifies the **speed-up factor.**
–The maximum **parallel imaging factor** is related to the number of elements.
  –**High parallel imaging factors** produce unacceptable artifacts.
–Parallel imaging factors achieved in clinical imaging range between 2 and 4.
–Parallel imaging works well when high **SNR** is available, such as from high field 3T scanners.

F. **Shielding**
–The **magnetic flux lines** from the main magnetic field can extend out to a large distance from the magnet.
–The **peripheral magnetic field** is called the **fringe field.**
–Fringe fields can affect **magnetically sensitive devices.**
–Table 11.4 shows the field values that may impair performance of a range of objects.
–Large metallic objects (e.g., elevators and ferromagnetic structures) can disrupt the uniformity of the **main magnetic field** and degrade MR image quality.
–**Magnetic shielding** usually consists of thick **iron plates** or layers of special **steel sheet metal** embedded in the MR magnet room walls.
–MRI units also require **RF shielding** to prevent **RF signals** (radio broadcasts) getting into the coils and increasing the **background noise.**
  –RF shielding also prevents the powerful RF pulses from escaping and interfering with outside electronic equipment.

TABLE 11.4   Magnetic Fields That Can Impair Object Performance

Object	mT
Pacemakers, cathode ray tubes	0.5
Credit cards, watches	1
Floppy disks	2
Power supplies	5

–The RF shielding is a **Faraday cage,** which consists of conductive sheet metal lining the MR magnet room.

–**Copper** is the best material, with copper screen also used over windows.

IV. IMAGING

A. Signal localization
–**Signal localization** requires **magnetic field gradients.**

–Along the gradient, a unique magnetic field strength corresponds to each location.

–Each location has a unique field strength that produces a **specific Larmor frequency** in the detected signal.

–**Fourier analysis** of MR signals permits intensities at **different frequencies** to be determined.

–MR signal intensity at each frequency can be placed at the correct location along the magnetic gradient direction (i.e., each location has a unique frequency).

–**Slice selection** is achieved by sending in an RF pulse at the same time that a **slice select gradient** is switched on.

  –The orientation of the applied gradient and the frequency content of the RF pulse determines the **slice location, orientation** and **thickness** of the resulting slice.

–Only magnetic nuclei within the selected slice have the correct Larmor frequency for resonance (activation).

–Localization in the slice plane (x-y plane) requires the use of two additional gradients.

–The signal (echoes) are detected in the presence of a **frequency encode gradient** (x-gradient).

  –The frequency encode direction is also known as the read direction.

–Localization in the y direction is achieved by use of a **phase encode gradient.**

–Pulse sequences are repeated many times using a **repetition time** interval of **TR.**

–For each acquisition, a *different* **phase encode gradient** is applied in the y direction in a **stepwise manner.**

B. Two-dimensional imaging
–To generate an image with **N pixels** in the **frequency encode direction** and **M pixels** in the **phase encode direction** requires an **acquisition time** of **M TR.**

–**Frequency encode gradients** are applied *during* signal detection.

–The signal is digitized into an array containing **N** discrete numbers.

–Repeating the pulse sequence M times will generate M rows of data.

  –Each row of data has N numbers.

–*Different* **phase-encoding gradients** are applied in collecting each of the M rows.

–The **acquired two-dimensional array** of numbers **(N × M)** of values is called **k-space.**

  –**k-Space** corresponds to the **raw data** generated by the MR scanner.

–**MR images** are obtained by performing a **two-dimensional Fourier transform (2D FT)** of **k-space.**

–In a **2D FT, each row** undergoes a **1D FT,** followed by **each column** undergoing a **1D FT.**

  –Reconstructing an N × M MR image requires a total of N + M 1D Fourier transforms.

–The MR image and **k-space** both consist of an N × M array of numbers.

–A **2D FT** of the **MR image** is **k-space,** and a **2D FT** of **k-space** is the **MR image.**

  –The **center** of **k-space** (i.e., low spatial frequencies) contains information on large-scale structures (e.g., contrast between large objects).

  –The **periphery** of **k-space** (i.e., high spatial frequencies) contains information on the fine structures (e.g., edges and small-scale details).

C. Spin echo
–**Spin echo (SE) pulse sequences** commence with a **90-degree RF** pulse to rotate the **magnetization vector** into the **transverse plane.**

–In the transverse plane, the magnetization rapidly **dephases** (T2* effects).

–**Spin rephasing** is achieved by using a **180-degree RF pulse** at a time **TE/2** to generate a SE at time **TE.**

  –The intensity of the SE at time TE is reduced by a factor of $e^{-TE/T2}$ due to T2 effects.

–The SE sequence of **90-degree** and **180-degree RF pulses** is repeated after a **repetition time (TR).**

–Figure 11.5 shows the specific components of a spin echo pulse sequence.

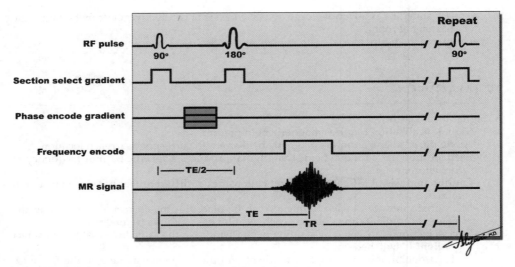

FIGURE 11.5   Spin echo pulse sequence, repeated after time TR.

–**SE** sequences change **TR** and **TE** times to emphasize T1 differences and/or T2 differences.
–**T1 weighting** uses **short TR** and **short TE.**
–**T2 weighting** uses **long TR** and **long TE.**
–**Proton density weighted** images are obtained with a long TR (>2,000 ms) to minimize
T1 differences and a short TE (<20 ms) to minimize T2 differences.
–Fast spin echo (FSE) techniques resemble multiecho SE sequences but change the phase-
encoding gradients for each echo.
–FSE shortens acquisition time by generating multiple phase-encoding steps during each
TR.
–This is done after the initial 90-degree pulse by making multiple echoes using successive
180-degree pulses.
–A new phase-encoding value is applied to each echo.
D. Gradient recalled echoes
–**Gradient recalled echo (GRE)** techniques make use of **low flip angles** (i.e., <90 degrees).
–Table 11.5 shows the amount of magnetization in the longitudinal direction and trans-
verse plane as a function of flip angle.
–GRE imaging relies on reversing the **polarity** of the **magnetic field gradients** to generate
echoes.
–The initial gradient dephases the transverse spins, and reversing the gradient polarity
rephases the spins and generates an **echo.**
–GRE does *not* need 180-degree refocusing RF pulses to generate echoes.
–GRE pulse sequences use short **TRs** times that permits fast acquisition times.

**TABLE 11.5   Longitudinal and Transverse Magnetization Components as a Function of
Flip Angle**

Flip Angle (Degrees)	Longitudinal Magnetization M_z (%)	Transverse Magnetization M_{x-y} (%)
0	100	0
15	97	26
30	87	50
45	71	71
60	50	86
75	26	97
90	0	100

–GRE sequences may use **TRs** of only 5 ms, and 256 acquisitions can be acquired in 1.3 seconds.

–GRE images are **T2* weighted** (not T2).

   –Reducing TR values increases **T1 differences** between tissues.

–There are several common fast imaging pulse sequences including **FLASH, FISP,** and **GRASS.**

   –FLASH stands for **fast low-angle shot.**

   –FISP stands for **fast imaging with steady-state precession.**

   –GRASS stands for **gradient recalled acquisition** in the **steady state.**

–GRE permits angiographic images to be constructed, and three-dimensional imaging within reasonable times.

E. **Inversion recovery**

–**Inversion recovery (IR)** uses an initial **180-degree pulse** to **invert** the **longitudinal magnetization.**

–Longitudinal magnetization recovers with a time constant T1.

   –Complete recovery of longitudinal magnetization takes 4 × T1.

–The initial **180-degree pulse** is followed by a 90-degree pulse after time **TI (inversion time).**

   –The 90-degree pulse is known as the **readout pulse.**

–Readout pulses flip any longitudinal magnetization into the transverse plane.

   –A refocusing **180-degree pulse** at time TE/2 produces an echo at time TE (echo).

–The size of the signal obtained with the readout pulse is strongly dependent on the values of T1 and TI.

–Figure 11.6 shows the specific components of an inversion recovery pulse sequence.

–Inversion recovery is the basis of **short time inversion recovery (STIR)** sequences for fat suppression.

   –**STIR** has a TI value that is selected to null the signal from fat.

–In **fluid attenuated inversion recovery (FLAIR)** sequences, the signal from fluids is suppressed.

   –**FLAIR** has a **TI** value that is set to eliminate a **CSF signal.**

F. **Three-dimensional imaging**

–**Three-dimensional Fourier transform (3DFT)** imaging techniques allow one to image stationary regions such as the brain and knees.

–In three-dimensional imaging, two sets of **orthogonal phase-encoding gradients** are used in addition to the **frequency-encoding gradient.**

–A **nonselective RF pulse** simultaneously makes **transverse magnetization** for the entire **sample volume.**

–A **3DFT** frequency analysis is applied along all three axes for image reconstruction.

–After the **volume data** are reconstructed, **two-dimensional images** in any selected plane can be constructed.

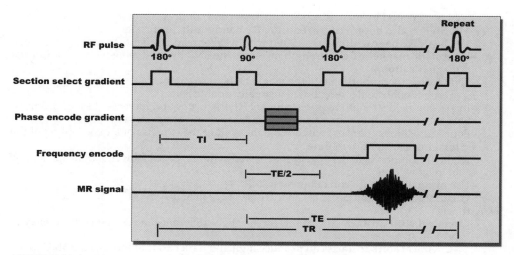

FIGURE 11.6   Inversion recovery pulse sequence, repeated after time TR.

–Three-dimensional imaging times are $N_1 \times N_2 \times TR$, where N_1 is the number of **phase-encoding steps** in one plane and N_2 is the number in the orthogonal plane.
–Disadvantages of **3DFT** techniques include longer acquisition times and susceptibility to motion artifacts.
–Advantages of 3DFT include high resolution in all three directions and the availability of contiguous sections.
  –There are **no gaps** in **3D images,** which can occur when generating a series of 2D slices.
–**Use of 3DFT** also permits the generation of arbitrary **oblique slices** using **post processing.**

V. IMAGING PERFORMANCE

A. Image contrast
–The pulse sequence chosen determines the type of **contrast** observed in an MR image.
–**Image contrast** is markedly influenced by differences in tissue **T1** and **T2.**
–Tissues with **short T1** values appear bright on **T1-weighted** images.
–Tissues with **long T2** values appear bright on **T2-weighted** images.
–**Proton density** differences can also be used in MR.
–**Proton density weighted** images demonstrate little **intrinsic contrast** because of the small variations in proton density for most tissues.
  –Tissue differences in proton density are ~10%.
–Flow can also affect image contrast and is the basis for **MR angiography (MRA).**
–Image contrast may be modified by the administration of **contrast agents** such as **gadolinium-DTPA.**

B. Resolution
–**Pixel size** equals the **field of view** divided by the data acquisition **matrix size.**
–Pixel sizes are approximately 1 mm for head images and proportionally larger in body images.
–**Resolution** is determined by the **data acquisition matrix,** *not* the display matrix.
  –Display matrix size can be interpolated to a larger value.
–In clinical MR, **limiting spatial resolution** is ~0.3 line pairs per millimeter.
  –For routine imaging, **MR resolution** is about half that achieved with **CT.**
–Higher resolution may be achieved by using **stronger gradients.**
–High resolution requires a high **SNR** (e.g., high field) as well a larger data acquisition matrix.
–Achieving improved MR resolution may require a loss of **signal intensity** and/or increases in **image acquisition time.**

C. Signal-to-noise ratio
–**The signal-to-noise ratio (SNR)** is very important and influences achievable image quality.
–SNR is increased by increasing slice thickness and/or decreasing **matrix size.**
–**MR SNR** is also improved by reducing **RF bandwidth** during signal detection.
  –Lower **RF bandwidth** is associated with weaker read gradient strength.
–High **static magnetic field strength** increases the SNR by producing more **longitudinal magnetization.**
–SNR is directly proportional to the magnetic field strength.
  –Doubling the field strength will generally double SNR.
–Increasing field strength requires a higher RF frequency and increases tissue T1 times.
–SNR increases as the square root of the number of image acquisitions $N_{aq}^{0.5}$.
–Four acquisitions (repeats) will double the SNR at the expense of a quadrupling of the total **image acquisition time.**
–Higher resolution (smaller voxels) is achieved at the expense of lower SNR or an increase in imaging time.
–Use of smaller **surface coils** improves SNR.
–**Quadrature detection** provides an increase of $\sqrt{2}$ in SNR.

D. Artifacts
–**Chemical shift artifacts** are caused by the slight difference in **resonance frequency** of protons in water and in fat.
  –**Chemical shift artifacts** can produce light and dark bands at the edges of the kidney or the margins of vertebral bodies.

TABLE 11.6   Food and Drug Administration Guidelines for Radiofrequency (RF) Power Deposition in Tissues

Body Region	Limit (W/kg)
Whole body	<4
Head	<3
Extremities (any gram of tissue)	<8

–**Truncation artifacts** in the spinal cord may simulate a syrinx.
  –Truncation artifacts are sometimes referred to as **Gibbs ringing.**
–Patient motion results in **ghost images** that appear in the **phase-encode direction.**
  –**Cardiac respiratory gating** or **phase reordering** may be used to minimize motion artifacts in body imaging.
–Distortions in the **static magnetic field** have a significant impact in fast (e.g., **GRE**) imaging.
–**Wraparound artifact** occurs when the FOV is smaller than the structure and imaged objects outside the FOV are mapped to the opposite side of the image.
  –Wraparound is caused by **undersampling (aliasing).**
–**Wraparound** can be avoided by increasing the **read sampling rate** in the frequency encoding direction.
–**Metallic objects** in patients also give rise to artifacts due to **magnetic field distortions.**
–MR artifacts also include **zipper, central point,** and **RF field inhomogeneities.**
–**Flowing blood** and **cerebrospinal fluid** can result in MR image artifacts.
–In **spin echo** sequences, flowing blood can be removed from the slice after the initial 90-degree excitation RF pulse, with the loss of spins resulting in **signal void** on SE images.
–**Flow enhancement** occurs when **unsaturated protons** enter the first section and generate a greater signal intensity than stationary, **partially saturated tissues.**

E. **Safety**
  –Detrimental biologic effects from exposure to **static magnetic fields** are not evident below **10 T.**
  –One of the greatest potential hazards around a magnet is the **missile effect.**
  –**Ferromagnetic objects** (e.g., scissors, screwdrivers, oxygen cylinders) may be pulled into the magnet.
  –Hazards exist for patients who have **ferromagnetic devices** implanted in their bodies **(e.g., stainless steel aneurysm clips).**
  –**Pacemakers** may be deactivated by magnetic fields above 0.5 mT.
    –Access is restricted in areas having magnetic fields >0.5 mT (i.e., 5 Gauss line).
  –The **time-varying magnetic fields** created by the **gradients** may **induce currents** in the patient.
    –Induced currents can result in **mild cutaneous sensations, involuntary muscle contractions,** and **cardiac arrhythmias.**
  –The Food and Drug Administration (FDA) recommends a limit of **3 T/s** to prevent **peripheral nerve stimulation.**
  –Time-varying magnetic fields can also produce **magneto-phosphenes** (light flashes).
  –The measure of dose of RF fields is the **specific absorption rate (SAR)** that measures the power absorbed per unit of mass of tissue **(W/kg).**
    –Table 11.6 summarizes the FDA guidelines for limits on RF power deposition in tissues.
  –Absorption of RF power will **increase tissue temperature.**
    –Table 11.7 summarizes the FDA guidelines on maximum tissue temperature.
    –The maximum rise in core body temperature is 1 degree Centigrade.

TABLE 11.7   Food and Drug Administration Guidelines for Tissue Temperatures

Body Region	Limit (°C)
Head	<38
Body	<39
Extremities	<40

–**RF heating** can occur in conducting loops, long conductive structures, or otherwise MR-safe objects such as **bone screws,** some **tattoos,** and **electrocardiogram leads.**

–The **noise level** in MR systems ranges from **65** to **120 dB,** and there are anecdotal reports of hearing loss.

–Hearing protection (i.e., **earplugs** or **headphones**) is mandatory.

–**Pregnancy** is usually considered a **contraindication** for scanning the abdomen.

–Evidence of MR harming the conceptus is very limited.

VI. CONTRAST AGENTS

A. Diamagnetism

–**Magnetic susceptibility** is the extent to which matter becomes magnetized when placed in an external magnetic field B.

–The local (internal) magnetic field is $B \times (1 + X)$, where X is the **susceptibility.**

–**Diamagnetic materials** result in small decreases in magnetization relative to the external field and, therefore, have small **negative values** of **susceptibility.**

–Most tissues are diamagnetic with a negative X, with a magnitude between 10^{-4} and 10^{-6}.

–At **tissue interfaces,** changes in **magnetic susceptibility** result in changes in the local field, which may result in imaging artifacts.

–Susceptibility artifacts are particularly important for soft tissues in the vicinity of air or bone.

B. Paramagnetism

–**Paramagnetism** is caused by the presence of **unpaired atomic electrons** or **molecular electrons.**

–When paramagnetic atoms are placed in an external magnetic field, the local (internal) magnetic field is increased.

–**Paramagnetic materials** thus have **positive values** of **susceptibility,** which are typically $\sim 10^{-3}$.

–**Paramagnetism** has a much larger effect than diamagnetism and results in an **enhancement** of the **local (internal) magnetic field.**

–**Paramagnetism** occurs with compounds containing metals such as **chromium, iron, manganese, cobalt, nickel, copper, gadolinium,** and **dysprosium,** as well as with **deoxyhemoglobin.**

C. Ferromagnetism

–**Ferromagnetism** is a property of a large group of atoms, whereas **diamagnetism** and **paramagnetism** are properties of individual atoms or molecules.

–The group of atoms in ferromagnetic substances is called a **domain.**

–Ferromagnetic substances such as **iron, nickel,** and **cobalt** have **unpaired electrons** that are strongly coupled, resulting in large local fields and **high positive susceptibilities.**

–**Ferromagnetic** materials generally consist of large numbers of **domains** whose relative orientations depend on the external magnetic fields.

–**Ferromagnets** may have **residual magnetization** even after the external field is removed.

–Objects such as steel screwdrivers and wrenches are examples of **ferromagnets.**

D. Superparamagnetism

–Small particles of Fe_3O_4, less than approximately **350 Å (0.035 μm),** consist of a *single* **domain** and are termed **superparamagnetic.**

–When placed in an external magnetic field, **superparamagnetic** particles develop a strong **internal magnetization.**

–**Superparamagnetism** differs from **ferromagnetism** in that superparamagnets have a single domain, no magnetic memory, and a **moderate degree** of **induced magnetism.**

–**Superparamagnetic** crystals of **iron oxide (SPIO and USPIO)** are used for imaging the liver and reticuloendothelial system.

E. Clinical

–**Paramagnetism, superparamagnetism,** and **ferromagnetism** all act as sources of local magnetic field inhomogeneity.

–These types of materials affect $T2^*$ and/or **T1,** and may be used as **contrast agents.**

–Contrast agents that reduce T1 more than T2 produce **hyperintensity** on **T1-weighted images** and are called **positive contrast agents.**

–Contrast agents that reduce $T2^*$ more than T1 produce **hypointensity** on **$T2^*$-weighted images** and are called **negative contrast agents.**

–Contrast agents that perfuse into an anatomic region of interest can result in **image enhancement.**

–**Gadolinium-DTPA** is an example of a **paramagnetic contrast agent.**

–**Gadolinium** has **seven unpaired electrons,** each with a magnetic moment approximately 700 times stronger than the **proton magnetic moment.**

–Gadolinium acts as a **relaxation agent** of nearby protons and **reduces T1 significantly** and **T2 slightly.**

   –The overall effect is highly dependent on the concentration of gadolinium.

–Recent studies have shown that administration of **Gd** is **contraindicated** in **some patients.**

   –**NSF (nephrogenic systemic fibrosis)** can occur in certain patients having **renal insufficiency.**

–Other **contrast agents** include complexes of transition element metals such as **iron** and **manganese.**

–Contrast agents are useful for evaluating **blood-brain barrier breakdown** and **renal lesions.**

VII. ADVANCED TECHNIQUES

A. Breast imaging

–MR is used when a **mammogram** results in a **problematic diagnosis** of breast cancer.

   –MR can also assess the integrity of **breast implants.**

–Special **breast coils** are used to perform three-dimensional imaging of the breast with a typical volume matrix of $128 \times 256 \times 256$ pixels.

   –**Fat suppression** techniques may be used.

–Breast MRI normally uses **gadolinium-DTPA contrast (0.1 mmol/kg).**

–**Contrast-enhanced MR** has a **high sensitivity** and is better able to identify **tumor margins.**

–The improved sensitivity of MR may be used to determine whether patients with presumed solitary nodules actually have **multifocal disease.**

–Lack of contrast enhancement from fat and scar tissue may also be used to evaluate mammographically suspicious lesions.

–**Benign lesions** such as **fibroadenomas** are often difficult to distinguish from malignancies.

–MR can distinguish **silicone** from **enhancing tumor.**

–MR-guided biopsies are difficult to perform with current commercial scanners.

B. Angiography

–**Noninvasive MR angiography (MRA)** is quickly being established in the clinical setting.

–MRA techniques include **time** of **flight** and **phase contrast.**

–**Time** of **flight** techniques rely on bright signals from **unsaturated protons** in flowing blood entering the imaging section.

–**Phase contrast** techniques use **bipolar gradients** to produce **phase** changes in moving blood.

   –The surrounding tissues, which are stationary, exhibit no net phase change.

–The phase change is related to the time between bipolar gradients and flow velocity, which provides a correlation between **signal intensity** and **blood flow velocity.**

–MRA images are produced by **projecting** the **stack** of **sections** onto a single two-dimensional image because display of tortuous blood vessels is inadequate on thin-section images.

–A common display technique is **maximum intensity projection (MIP).**

–MRA is useful in patients who cannot tolerate **iodinated contrast agents.**

C. Echo planar imaging (EPI)/diffusion weighted imaging (DWI)

–**Echo planar imaging (EPI)** uses rapidly switching gradients to refocus echoes.

   –EPI is similar to FSE but with no refocusing RF.

–**Frequency-encode gradients** that rapidly change polarities are paired with an applied **phase-encode gradient.**

–EPI can generate **MR images** in **50 ms** but with limited resolution (64^2 or 128^2 matrix).

–Special **high-performance gradients** are required for EPI having strengths of **20** to **40 mT/m** with **very fast** switching and settling times.

–**Diffusion** depends on the **random motion** of **water** molecules in tissues.

–Structural details of tissues can be obtained by **diffusion weighted imaging (DWI).**

–Water diffusion characteristics can be displayed using **apparent diffusion coefficient (ADC) maps.**

–**ADC maps** of the spine can evaluate **pathophysiology,** and **DWI** is used to detect **ischemic injury (stroke).**

–Standard spin echo and EPI pulse sequences with **diffusion gradients** are used in DWI.

–One limitation of **DWI** is **sensitivity** to **motion,** which may be minimized by the use of **ECG gating** and other motion compensation methods.

D. Magnetization transfer

–**Magnetization transfer contrast (MTC)** techniques modulate image contrast by **saturating** a pool of protons in macromolecules and their associated bound water.

–**Macromolecules** have **very short T2** values, hence a very large range of resonance frequencies.

–**Narrowband RF pulses,** shifted slightly away from the water resonance frequency, are able to selectively saturate the protons in macromolecules.

–Some of this saturation is transferred from the macromolecules to water.

–These water molecules, which have reduced signal intensity, are then imaged using conventional MR pulse sequences.

–**MTC** is useful in **reducing background signal** in **MRA** and may also have applications in **breast imaging.**

E. Magnetic resonance spectroscopy

–**MR spectroscopy (MRS)** makes use of the slight difference in resonance frequency of protons or other nuclei found in metabolites.

–By using a combination of gradients and RF pulses, the signal of a localized rectangular volume can be interrogated.

–The signal is collected in the absence of any gradients, producing a **localized chemical shift spectrum.**

–^{1}H and ^{31}P are the nuclei most often used for in vivo localized **spectroscopy.**

–Proton spectroscopy can be used to estimate concentrations of **N-acetyl aspartate (NAA), creatine** and **phosphocreatine, choline,** and **lactate.**

–**Spectroscopy** is helpful in distinguishing different **tumor types.**

–**Phosphorus spectroscopy** can be used to evaluate **cellular metabolism** by identifying the relative concentration of **inorganic phosphate, phosphocreatine,** and **adenosine triphosphate.**

–**MRS** requires a **stronger** and **more uniform** static magnetic field than conventional hydrogen imaging.

–Typical voxel sizes used in **MRS** studies are ~**1 cm^3 for ^{1}H** and ~**8 cm^3 for ^{31}P.**

F. Functional imaging

–**Functional imaging** relies on **blood oxygenation, blood volume,** or **blood flow** changes in the brain associated with **mental activity** (visual, motor, auditory, or other brain function).

–In the most common technique, brain activity increases local venous blood oxygenation.

–This slightly increases the intensity of the detected **T2*-weighted** signal intensity from these regions.

–This is called **BOLD (blood oxygenation level dependent)** imaging.

–**EPI** sequences with **T2* weighting** are used.

–Intensity changes are small (e.g., <5% at 1.5 T).

–Signal intensity increases with **greater magnetic field strength.**

–Images are collected during a **rest state** as well as the **activated state,** then statistically compared by computer to generate functional maps.

–Functional information can be superimposed on high resolution MR images as color overlays.

–MR functional imaging has **better temporal** and **spatial resolution** than **positron emission tomography.**

–**Functional imaging** has become a powerful **neuroscience tool.**

–**Functional MR** is now **reimbursable** for clinical scanning.

REVIEW TEST

11.1 Which would be *least* useful for magnetic resonance imaging?
  a. ^{1}H
  b. ^{13}C
  c. ^{16}O
  d. ^{23}Na
  e. ^{31}P

11.2 The ratio of the electron magnetic moment to that of a proton is most likely:
  a. 4:1
  b. 16:1
  c. 50:1
  d. 200:1
  e. 800:1

11.3 The resonance frequency (kHz) for protons in a 1-T magnetic field is likely:
  a. 4.2
  b. 42
  c. 420
  d. 4,200
  e. 42,000

11.4 If a 90-degree RF pulse has a duration of t seconds, a 180-degree pulse is likely to have a duration of:
  a. t/4
  b. t/2
  c. t
  d. 2t
  e. 4t

11.5 The maximum free induction decay signal is obtained when using a flip angle of (degrees):
  a. 0
  b. 45
  c. 90
  d. 135
  e. 180

11.6 Which of the following is likely to have the shortest T1 times?
  a. Fat
  b. Liver
  c. Kidney
  d. White matter
  e. CSF

11.7 Which of the following is likely to have the longest T1 times?
  a. Fat
  b. Liver
  c. Kidney
  d. White matter
  e. CSF

11.8 After 90-degree RF pulses, spins lose phase coherence in a time comparable to:
  a. T1
  b. T2

  c. TE/2
  d. TE
  e. TR

11.9 Which of the following likely has the longest T2 relaxation time?
  a. Fat
  b. Liver
  c. Kidney
  d. White matter
  e. CSF

11.10 In MR, cortical bone most likely appears black because bone has:
  a. short T2
  b. long T2
  c. short T1
  d. long T1
  e. little hydrogen

11.11 A 1-T magnetic field is greater than the earth's magnetic field by a factor of:
  a. 5,000
  b. 10,000
  c. 20,000
  d. 40,000
  e. 80,000

11.12 Increasing the main magnetic field will most likely reduce:
  a. T1 relaxation
  b. T2 relaxation
  c. signal-to-noise ratio
  d. equipment costs
  e. resonance frequency

11.13 Superconducting MR magnets are most likely kept cold by using liquid:
  a. air
  b. carbon dioxide
  c. helium
  d. nitrogen
  e. oxygen

11.14 Coils used to adjust main magnetic field uniformity are called:
  a. shim
  b. Helmholtz
  c. saddle
  d. surface
  e. RF

11.15 These coils are used to localize the MR signal:
  a. shim
  b. gradient
  c. phased array
  d. surface
  e. RF

11.16 The best material for Faraday cages that shield against RF interference is most likely:
  a. aluminum
  b. copper

c. rhodium
d. lead
e. tin

11.17 The number of phase-encode gradient steps applied when generating M × M SE images is likely:
a. M
b. M^2
c. M^3
d. 2 × M
e. 3 × M

11.18 The reconstruction algorithm used in clinical MRI is most likely:
a. 2D Fourier transform
b. Iterative
c. algebraic reconstruction
d. back projection
e. filtered back projection

11.19 Acquisition time(s) for a 192 × 128 SE image (TE = 100 ms; TR = 1,000 ms) is likely:
a. 12.8
b. 19.2
c. 128
d. 192
e. 128 + 192

11.20 Following a 90-degree pulse in SE imaging, the echo signal would likely be measured at:
a. immediately (t = 0)
b. TE
c. 4 × T1
d. T2
e. TR

11.21 A decreased MR signal is most likely when there is an increase in:
a. T2
b. T2*
c. blood flow
d. spin density
e. spin dephasing

11.22 Which of the following is most likely to suppress signals from fat?
a. FLASH
b. Fast SE
c. STIR
d. FLAIR
e. BOLD

11.23 The limiting spatial resolution (line pairs per mm) in current clinical MR is most likely:
a. 0.1
b. 0.3
c. 1

d. 2
e. 5

11.24 When N MR image acquisitions are averaged, the resultant signal-to-noise ratio likely improves by:
a. $N^{0.5}$
b. N
c. 2 × N
d. $N^{1.5}$
e. N^2

11.25 In MR, motion results in ghost images that appear in which direction?
a. Read encode
b. Phase encode
c. Slice selection axis
d. PA
e. Lateral

11.26 Chemical shift artifacts are most likely caused by fat and water differences in:
a. T1
b. T2
c. T2*
d. Larmor frequency
e. spin density

11.27 The FDA guideline for limiting RF absorption (W per kg) in any gram of extremity of tissue is:
a. 1
b. 2
c. 4
d. 8
e. 16

11.28 The largest susceptibility artifacts are likely to be seen between tissue and:
a. air
b. blood
c. fat
d. marrow
e. bone

11.29 Proton relaxation by Gd-DTPA is most likely due to the gadolinium:
a. nuclear field
b. chelate (DTPA)
c. unpaired electrons
d. K-edge energy
e. electron density

11.30 The physical size (μm) of a superparamagnetic particle of SPIO or USPIO is most likely:
a. 0.004
b. 0.04
c. 0.4
d. 4
e. 40

ANSWERS AND EXPLANATIONS

11.1c. ^{16}O, which has an even number of protons (8) and an even number of neutrons (8).

11.2e. The ratio of the electron to proton magnetic moments is 800:1.

11.3e. The resonance frequency is 42,000 kHz, which is 42 MHz.

11.4d. A duration of 2t, since doubling the RF pulse duration doubles the angular rotation of the longitudinal magnetization, assuming RF intensity stays constant.

11.5c. Pulses of 90 degrees rotate the longitudinal magnetization through ninety degrees (i.e., into the transverse plane) that maximizes the FID signal.

11.6a. Fat T1 times are shorter than those of most tissues and all fluids.

11.7e. CSF, since all fluids have long T1 relaxation times compared to fat and tissues.

11.8b. T2, which is a measure of spin dephasing in the transverse plane due to spin–spin interactions.

11.9e. CSF and all fluids have long T2 times compared to fat and soft tissues.

11.10a. Short T2, which is characteristic of all solids (μs) and which causes transverse magnetization to disappear extremely quickly.

11.11c. A factor of 20,000, since the earth's magnetic field is only 0.05 mT (0.5 Gauss).

11.12a. T1 relaxation is reduced, which causes T1 times to increase (increased relaxation reduces T1).

11.13c. Liquid helium is used to cool superconducting magnets.

11.14a. Shim coils are used to correct for inhomogeneities in the main magnetic field.

11.15b. Magnetic gradient coils are used to localize the MR signal.

11.16b. Copper is generally used for RF shielding in Faraday cages.

11.17a. M phase-encode steps are required to generate an MR image with a matrix size of M $\times$ M.

11.18a. 2D Fourier transform is the reconstruction algorithm used in clinical MRI.

11.19c. Acquisition time is 128 seconds, since there are at least 128 repetitions, each with a different phase-encoding gradient, and each repetition takes 1 s (TR time).

11.20b. TE is the time when the echo (signal) is produced and measured.

11.21e. Spin dephasing must reduce the MR signal.

11.22c. STIR, which stands for short tau inversion recovery, will suppress signals from fat.

11.23b. A typical resolution in clinical MR is 0.3 lp/mm, and about half the resolution in clinical CT.

11.24a. $N^{0.5}$, which means that SNR doubles when the number of image acquisitions quadruples.

11.25b. Phase encode is the direction in which ghost artifacts from motion appear.

11.26d. Differences in Larmor frequency give rise to fat/water chemical shift artifacts.

11.27d. The FDA guideline for limiting RF absorption in any gram of tissue is 8 W per kg in the extremities.

11.28a. Air and soft tissue interfaces will likely generate the highest susceptibility artifacts.

11.29c. Unpaired electrons in Gd will increase spin-lattice relaxation and thereby shorten T1 times.

11.30b. The size (single domain) of a superparamagnetic particle such as SPIO is 0.04 μm.

EXAMINATION GUIDE

Education is what survives when what has been learnt has been forgotten.
—BF Skinner

These two practice examinations, each consisting of 110 questions and answers, cover the material summarized in this book. The first ten questions pertain to Chapter 1, the second ten questions to Chapter 2, and so on. The examinations, which should be taken under examination conditions without access to a textbook, will help students to:

Practice for the real examination. Taking practice examinations helps you develop a strategy for dealing with difficult questions, such as guessing *after* eliminating all wrong answers or by temporarily skipping difficult questions and returning to complete them later.

Highlight weaknesses (and strengths). Taking these examinations should help identify your weaknesses as well as strengths. Weaknesses need to be corrected by consulting the appropriate chapter in this review book or, if greater depth is required, by consulting a textbook.

Build confidence. Successful completion of the examinations demonstrates that the subject material has been understood, which will ease pre-examination nervousness.

The following guidelines should assist readers to perform successfully in any examination.

1. *Read and follow all examination instructions.*
2. Read each question *carefully.*
3. Do not assume information.
4. Focus on key words.
5. Eliminate obviously incorrect answers.
6. Reread the questions and verify your answers.
7. Answer *all* questions, even if you have to guess.
8. Don't spend more than 2 minutes on any one question.

PRACTICE EXAMINATION A: QUESTIONS

A1 Which of the following is *not* an SI unit?
- a. Meter
- b. Kilogram
- c. Second
- d. Roentgen
- e. Becquerel

A2 The key difference between 600-keV x-rays and gamma rays is:
- a. velocity
- b. frequency
- c. wavelength
- d. momentum
- e. origin

A3 What is the air kerma (mGy) 10 m from a radiation source when the air kerma at 1 m is 100 mGy?
- a. 1
- b. 10
- c. 100
- d. 1,000
- e. 10,000

A4 For a fixed kV_p, which generator likely results in the shortest exposure time?
- a. Constant potential
- b. High frequency
- c. Three phase (12 pulse)
- d. Three phase (6 pulse)
- e. Single phase

A5 The maximum photon energy in an x-ray beam is determined by the x-ray tube:
- a. current (mA)
- b. voltage (kV)
- c. exposure time (s)
- d. ripple (%)
- e. filtration (mm Al)

A6 Characteristic x-rays are characteristic of the material in the:
- a. target
- b. anode
- c. filter
- d. window
- e. filament

A7 The power deposition in an x-ray tube anode when operated at 80 kV and 100 mA is:
- a. 8 kJ
- b. 8 kW
- c. 8 kW/s
- d. 8 keV
- e. depends on exposure time

A8 The nominal size (mm) of a small focus on a standard x-ray tube is most likely:
- a. 0.1
- b. 0.3

- c. 0.6
- d. 1
- e. 2

A9 The ratio of heat to x-rays produced in x-ray tubes is most likely:
- a. 1:99
- b. 10:90
- c. 50:50
- d. 90:10
- e. 99:1

A10 How long (second) would it take a very hot anode to lose ~90% of its heat?
- a. 0.3
- b. 3
- c. 30
- d. 300
- e. 3,000

A11 Which particle has the lowest rest mass?
- a. Electron
- b. Neutron
- c. Proton
- d. Alpha particle
- e. Photon

A12 An atom that loses an outer shell electron is best described as being an:
- a. isomer
- b. isobar
- c. isotone
- d. isotope
- e. ion

A13 The atomic number (Z) dependence of the photoelectric effect varies approximately as
- a. Z^3
- b. Z^2
- c. Z
- d. $1/Z^2$
- e. $1/Z^3$

A14 In water, at what energy (keV) are photoelectric and Compton effects equally likely to occur?
- a. 0.5
- b. 4.0
- c. 25
- d. 70
- e. 88

A15 If μ is 0.1 cm^{-1}, and the density is 2 g/cm^3, the mass attenuation (cm^2/g) coefficient is:
- a. 0.05
- b. 0.2
- c. 1.9
- d. 2.1
- e. 20

A16 The total attenuation by 10 half-value layers is most likely:
a. 64
b. 128
c. 256
d. 512
e. 1,024

A17 The x-ray beam HVL is least likely to be affected by the x-ray tube:
a. output (mGy)
b. voltage (kV)
c. voltage ripple (%)
d. filtration (mm Al)
e. target material (Z)

A18 What grid characteristic is most likely to determine the scatter removal performance?
a. Grid ratio
b. Focus distance
c. Gap distance
d. Strip height
e. Line density

A19 The most likely reason that grids are seldom used for portable chest radiography is that:
a. portable x-ray output is low
b. lower kV won't penetrate grid
c. grid alignment is difficult
d. scatter is very low
e. air gap minimizes scatter

A20 When 0.1 J of energy is absorbed by an organ with a mass of 10 kg, the organ dose (mGy) is most likely:
a. 0.01
b. 0.1
c. 1
d. 10
e. 100

A21 The size of a typical film grain (μm) is most likely:
a. 0.1
b. 1
c. 10
d. 100
e. 1,000

A22 The percentage (%) of light transmitted through two films, each with a density of 1.0, is most likely:
a. 0.001
b. 0.01
c. 0.1
d. 1
e. 10

A23 Which is most likely to increase when a screen–film system replaces film alone?
a. Patient dose
b. Exposure time
c. Tube mAs

d. Receptor blur
e. Motion blur

A24 Compared to a regular screen, a detail screen of the same phosphor likely has a lower:
a. resolution
b. speed
c. noise
d. effective Z
e. density

A25 If all 8 bits in a byte are set to 1, then the decimal number is:
a. 8
b. 255
c. 511
d. 1,023
e. 11111111

A26 How much memory (MB) is needed to store a 1k × 1k radiograph with 256 shades of gray?
a. 0.1
b. 0.25
c. 0.5
d. 1
e. 2

A27 Which of the following materials is most likely a photostimulable phosphor?
a. BaFBr
b. CsI
c. NaI
d. PbI
e. Se

A28 Photoconductors convert x-ray energy directly into:
a. light
b. charge
c. heat
d. voltage
e. radio waves

A29 Replacing analog chest imaging with digital technology is *least* likely to improve image:
a. resolution
b. processing
c. retrieval
d. storage
e. transmission

A30 The minimum number of images required to perform energy subtraction is:
a. 1
b. 2
c. 3
d. 4
e. >4

A31 The target material in a mammography x-ray tube is most likely:
a. Be (Z = 4)
b. Al (Z = 13)

c. Mo (Z = 42)
d. Ag (Z = 47)
e. Ba (Z = 56)

A32 In a linear grid for mammography, a fiber interspaced grid is preferred over aluminum because it likely reduces:
a. dose
b. scatter
c. mottle
d. receptor blur
e. focal blur

A33 High image contrast is *least* likely achieved in mammography by the use of:
a. low photon energies
b. high film gradients
c. short exposures (<0.1 s)
d. breast compression
e. scatter removal grids

A34 The optimal grid ratio in magnification mammography is most likely:
a. no grids used
b. 2:1
c. 4:1
d. 8:1
e. 16:1

A35 The Mammography Quality Standards Act does *not* require:
a. reject analysis
b. processor sensitometry
c. physics testing
d. ACR accreditation
e. FDA certification

A36 The purpose of photocathodes in image intensifiers is to convert light into:
a. x-rays
b. heat
c. voltages
d. electrons
e. ultraviolet

A37 A typical II conversion factor (cd/m^2 per μGy/s), is most likely:
a. 2
b. 20
c. 200
d. 2,000
e. 20,000

A38 Plumbicon TV cameras, used in cardiac imaging, most likely reduce:
a. vignetting
b. mottle
c. flicker
d. lag
e. scatter

A39 Reducing II input area by activating electronic magnification likely increases:
a. skin dose
b. image distortion

c. amount of vignetting
d. image brightness
e. field of view

A40 Digital cardiac imaging would likely use an acquisition rate (images per second) of:
a. 4
b. 7.5
c. 15
d. 30
e. 60

A41 The typical anode cooling rate (kW) of a standard CT x-ray tube is most likely:
a. 1
b. 3
c. 10
d. 30
e. 100

A42 A beam-shaping filter is most likely used in CT scanners to reduce:
a. detector dynamic range
b. beam hardening
c. detector cross-talk
d. off-focus radiation
e. scatter radiation

A43 The detected x-ray pattern transmitted through the patient at a single x-ray tube angle is best described as a:
a. ray
b. projection
c. back projection
d. convolution
e. tomographic slice

A44 Use of a soft tissue filter, as opposed to a bone filter, to reconstruct CT images would most likely reduce:
a. mottle
b. scatter
c. dose
d. artifacts
e. scan times

A45 A window width of 100 and window level of 50 likely results in a pixel value of 10 appearing as:
a. black
b. almost black
c. gray
d. almost white
e. white

A46 The advantage of helical over axial CT is most likely a reduction in:
a. radiation doses
b. scan times
c. scatter radiation
d. reconstruction times
e. slice sensitivity profiles

A47   Total exam time (s) for a single-phase adult abdomen on a 64-slice MDCT is likely:
a. 0.3
b. 1
c. 3
d. 10
e. 30

A48   When the weighted $CTDI_w$ is 10 mGy, and the pitch is 0.25, the volume $CTDI_{vol}$ (mGy) is most likely:
a. 2.5
b. 5
c. 10
d. 20
e. 40

A49   Compared to an adult (mAs = 100%), the most likely mAs (%) for a body CT scan of a 1-year-old would be:
a. 10
b. 30
c. 50
d. 70
e. >70

A50   Partial-volume artifacts in CT are best minimized by reducing:
a. section thickness
b. scan time
c. matrix size
d. focal blur
e. scan length

A51   The highest subject contrast of an iodinated blood vessel likely occurs at a photon energy (keV) of:
a. 30
b. 40
c. 50
d. 70
e. 100

A52   Lowering the kV in screen–film mammography most likely reduces:
a. contrast
b. dose
c. mAs
d. scatter
e. exposure time

A53   What x-ray tube voltage (kV) would likely maximize the visibility of iodinated contrast in the carotid arteries?
a. 30
b. 50
c. 70
d. 90
e. 110

A54   Which of the following factors is *least* likely to affect image sharpness?
a. Detector composition
b. Focal spot size
c. Exposure time
d. Detector thickness
e. Image magnification

A55   When the MTF from focal and receptor blur are both equal to 0.1 (at 2 lp/mm), the imaging system MTF at this spatial frequency is most likely:
a. 0.2
b. 0.1
c. 0.05
d. 0.02
e. 0.01

A56   Spatial resolution of a standard fluoroscopy unit is most likely limited by the:
a. focal spot
b. input phosphor
c. output phosphor
d. optical system
e. TV system

A57   CT scanner spatial resolution performance would most likely improve when increasing the:
a. focal spot
b. detector width
c. tube current
d. scan time
e. image matrix

A58   Visibility of low-contrast lesions in a digital radiograph would most likely be improved when increasing:
a. focus size
b. image magnification
c. air kerma
d. beam filtration
e. display luminance

A59   The detector air kerma (μGy) that produces one frame in DSA imaging is most likely:
a. 5
b. 15
c. 50
d. 150
e. 500

A60   A receiver operator characteristic curve likely measures:
a. diagnostic performance
b. error rate
c. test specificity
d. test sensitivity
e. cost-effectiveness

A61   The most radiosensitive part of the cell is most likely the:
a. cell membrane
b. chloroplast
c. nucleus
d. mitochondrion
e. ribosome

A62 Which particle is likely to have the highest linear energy transfer (LET)?
   a. Electron
   b. Positron
   c. Proton
   d. Neutron
   e. Alpha particle

A63 The uniform whole-body dose (Gy) that would kill half the exposed population is most likely:
   a. 1
   b. 2
   c. 4
   d. 8
   e. 16

A64 The chronic threshold dose (Gy) for cataract induction is most likely:
   a. 1
   b. 2
   c. 5
   d. 10
   e. >10

A65 The threshold equivalent dose (mSv) for the induction of stochastic effects is likely:
   a. 0 (no threshold)
   b. 0.1
   c. 1
   d. 10
   e. 100

A66 Which of the following does *not* concern itself with radiation risk estimates?
   a. ICRP
   b. UNSCEAR
   c. BEIR
   d. ICRU
   e. NCRP

A67 The organ weighting factor for gonad exposure recommended by the ICRP (Publication 103) in 2007 is:
   a. 0.01
   b. 0.04
   c. 0.08
   d. 0.20
   e. 0.30

A68 The most sensitive period for the induction of severe mental retardation in pregnant patients is most likely:
   a. up to 10 days
   b. 2 to 7 weeks
   c. 7 to 15 weeks
   d. 15 to 25 weeks
   e. >25 weeks

A69 Which is likely the best indicator of the risk of a radiation-induced skin reaction?
   a. backscatter fraction
   b. entrance air kerma

   c. energy imparted
   d. air kerma–area product
   e. skin dose

A70 The total energy (J) deposited in a patient undergoing a head CT scan is most likely:
   a. 0.1
   b. 1
   c. 10
   d. 100
   e. 1,000

A71 For the same air kerma, blackening of film by 30 keV photons, compared to the blackening by 300 keV photons, is most likely:
   a. much less
   b. slightly less
   c. similar
   d. slightly more
   e. much more

A72 A Geiger-Muller detector would likely be used to measure:
   a. low-level contamination
   b. x-ray tube outputs
   c. patient exposures
   d. operator exposures
   e. x-ray leakage

A73 The effective dose (mSv per year) to an interventional radiology fellow is most likely:
   a. 1
   b. 5
   c. 10
   d. 20
   e. 50

A74 The current (2008) regulatory dose limit (mSv per year) to the eye lens of a radiologist is:
   a. 50
   b. 100
   c. 150
   d. 300
   e. 500

A75 The amount of lead shielding (mm) in the wall of a CT facility is most likely:
   a. 0.5
   b. 1
   c. 1.5
   d. 3
   e. 5

A76 The effective dose (mSv) from a chest x-ray examination is most likely:
   a. 0.05
   b. 0.2
   c. 1
   d. 3
   e. 10

A77 The effective dose (mSv) for an upper barium examination is most likely:
a. 0.2
b. 1
c. 5
d. 25
e. >25

A78 The risk of a breast cancer from a screening mammogram in a 50-year-old woman is most likely three per:
a. 100
b. 1,000
c. 10,000
d. 100,000
e. 1,000,000

A79 The average dose (mSv per year) from radon (+ daughters) in the United States is most likely:
a. 1
b. 2
c. 3
d. 4
e. 5

A80 Which imaging modality contributed *least* to the U.S. population medical dose (2006)?
a. Interventional radiology
b. Radiography/fluoroscopy
c. CT
d. Nuclear medicine
e. Mammography

A81 An activity of 1 mCi equals (Bq):
a. 37,000
b. 370,000
c. 3,700,000
d. 37,000,000
e. 370,000,000

A82 Which of the following emits positrons?
a. ^{3}H
b. ^{32}P
c. ^{18}F
d. ^{99m}Tc
e. ^{226}Ra

A83 A radionuclide produced in a cyclotron is most likely to decay by:
a. Beta minus decay
b. Beta plus decay
c. Alpha decay
d. Isomeric transition
e. Neutron emission

A84 Which of the following is *not* a radiopharmaceutical localization mechanism?
a. Diffusion
b. Phagocytosis
c. Capillary blockage
d. Elution
e. Cell sequestration

A85 Which nuclide would be most likely to make use multiple PHA windows?
a. ^{67}Ga
b. ^{123}I
c. ^{131}I
d. ^{99m}Tc
e. ^{133}Xe

A86 Which radionuclide is *least* likely to be used for PET imaging?
a. ^{18}F
b. ^{67}Ga
c. ^{68}Ga
d. ^{15}O
e. ^{82}Rb

A87 Which of the following tests is *least* likely to be performed on a radiopharmaceutical?
a. Flood uniformity
b. Pyrogenicity
c. Radiochemical purity
d. Radionuclide purity
e. Sterility

A88 The intrinsic (R_I) and collimator (R_C) resolution are related to the system resolution (R) as:
a. $R_I + R_C$
b. $(R_I - R_C)^{1/2}$
c. $1/(R_I + R_C)^{1/2}$
d. $R_I^2 + R_C^2$
e. $(R_I^2 + R_C^2)^{1/2}$

A89 Which is *least* related to artifacts in scintillation camera imaging?
a. Chemical shift
b. Cracked crystal
c. Edge packing
d. Nonuniformity
e. Off-peak imaging

A90 Which organ likely receives the highest dose for an uptake of 1 μCi activity (no biologic clearance)?
a. Adult thyroid
b. Fetal thyroid
c. Spleen
d. Liver
e. Kidneys

A91 A 2-MHz transducer has a wavelength (mm) in tissue of approximately:
a. 0.01
b. 0.03
c. 0.1
d. 0.3
e. 1

A92 When an ultrasound beam is attenuated −30 dB, the percentage (%) of the initial intensity that remains is:
a. 70
b. 30

c. 10
d. 1
e. 0.1

A93 What fraction of ultrasound is reflected from an interface where $Z_1 = 1$ and $Z_2 = 2$?
  a. 1/2
  b. 1/3
  c. 1/5
  d. 1/8
  e. 1/9

A94 The resonant frequency of an ultrasound transducer is determined primarily by:
  a. crystal thickness
  b. Snell's law
  c. sound bandwidth
  d. applied voltage
  e. pulse repetition frequency

A95 The ultrasound PRF (kHz) is most likely to be:
  a. 0.04
  b. 0.4
  c. 4
  d. 40
  e. 400

A96 How long (μs) will it take to receive the ultrasound echo from an object 10 cm away?
  a. 0.13
  b. 1.3
  c. 13
  d. 130
  e. 1,300

A97 Which is the likely frequency (MHz) detected and analyzed for making a harmonic image with a 3-MHz transducer?
  a. 1.5
  b. 3
  c. 6
  d. 9
  e. 12

A98 In spectral analysis, the detected frequency shift is plotted as a function of:
  a. angle
  b. distance
  c. echo intensity
  d. frequency
  e. time

A99 If the ultrasound pulse length is 1 mm, the axial resolution (mm) is likely:
  a. 0.25
  b. 0.5
  c. 1
  d. 2
  e. 4

A100 Below a structure, a very faint image of the structure is probably due to:
  a. reverberation artifact
  b. side lobes
  c. specular reflection
  d. nonspecular reflection
  e. incorrect TCG

A101 Which magnetic nucleus is most likely to result in the largest MR signal intensity?
  a. ^{1}H
  b. ^{2}H
  c. ^{13}C
  d. ^{23}Na
  e. ^{31}P

A102 If the transverse magnetization is M_{xy} the free induction decay signal is proportional to:
  a. $(M_{xy})^{-1}$
  b. $(M_{xy})^{-0.5}$
  c. $(M_{xy})^{0.5}$
  d. $(M_{xy})^1$
  e. independent of M_{xy}

A103 To maximize T1 weighting, the most likely TR time (ms) at 1.5 T would be:
  a. 300
  b. 600
  c. 900
  d. 1,500
  e. 3,000

A104 The magnitude (%) of magnetic inhomogeneities responsible for T2* dephasing is likely:
  a. 1
  b. 0.1
  c. 0.01
  d. 0.001
  e. $\ll 0.001$

A105 Electric currents (A) in superconducting MR magnets are most likely:
  a. 5
  b. 50
  c. 500
  d. 5,000
  e. 50,000

A106 Thinner slices in MR imaging are most likely obtained by increasing the:
  a. magnetic gradient
  b. RF frequency
  c. RF bandwidth
  d. TR time
  e. TE time

A107 Which is least likely to affect the total scan time in MR?
  a. Frequency-encode matrix size
  b. Number of phase-encoding steps
  c. Pulse sequences in study
  d. Number of acquisitions
  e. TR (repetition time)

A108 Typical tissue differences (%) in spin density are most likely:
   a. 1
   b. 3
   c. 10
   d. 30
   e. 100

A109 Which is *least* likely to be an MR artifact?
   a. Chemical shift
   b. Bounce point
   c. Zipper
   d. Susceptibility
   e. Vignetting

A110 A patient's foot undergoing an MR scan is *unlikely* to exceed a temperature (°C) of:
   a. 38
   b. 39
   c. 40
   d. 41
   e. 42

PRACTICE EXAMINATION A: ANSWERS AND EXPLANATIONS

A1d. Roentgen is non-SI; 1 R is 2.58×10^{-4} C/kg.

A2e. X-rays are created by electrons, whereas gamma rays originate in nuclear processes.

A3a. One mGy, since increasing the distance from the source tenfold reduces the radiation intensity a hundredfold.

A4a. A constant potential generator has no ripple and therefore produces the most x-rays per unit time.

A5b. Voltage (kV) determines the maximum x-ray photon energy produced in x-ray tubes.

A6a. A tungsten target produces characteristic x-rays whose energy is ~65 keV, just below the K-shell binding energy (70 keV).

A7b. Power is measured in kW ($P = V \times I$).

A8c. Small focal spots are generally 0.6 mm, except in mammography where they are 0.1 mm.

A9e. Generally, 99% of the energy deposited into an x-ray tube is transformed into heat.

A10d. Anodes can cool down in a few minutes (300 s or 5 min).

A11e. Photons, since they have no rest mass.

A12e. A neutral atom that loses an electron becomes a positive ion.

A13a. The photoelectric effect is proportional to Z^3.

A14c. Compton and photoelectric interactions are equally probable at 25 keV in water (and soft tissue).

A15a. 0.05 g/cm^2 since the mass attenuation coefficient is the linear attenuation divided by the physical density.

A16e. $(1/2)^{10}$ is 1/1,024, or ~0.1%.

A17a. X-ray beam air kerma has no effect on the x-ray beam HVL.

A18a. The grid ratio is the most important parameter that determines the scatter removal performance of a grid.

A19c. Grid alignment is very difficult in bedside radiography.

A20d. The dose is energy (J)/mass (kg), or 0.1/10 Gy, which is 0.01 Gy or 10 mGy.

A21b. A silver bromide grain is typically a micron or so in diameter.

A22d. A film density of 1 transmits 10% of the light, and the second film will transmit 10% of 10%, or 1%.

A23d. Receptor blur increases because of the diffusion of light in the screen.

A24b. Detail screens are much thinner to minimize receptor blur and absorb less of the incident x-rays (i.e., they are slower).

A25b. 255 in the decimal system is 11111111 in the binary system.

A26d. 1 MB (each image has 1M pixels, and 1 byte per pixel is required for 256 shades of gray [2^8]).

A27a. BaFBr is a photostimulable phosphor.

A28b. Photoconductors absorb x-rays which is converted into charge.

A29a. Resolution in digital imaging is generally lower than that of analog imaging.

A30b. Two images are required—one at a low kV and one at a high kV.

A31c. Mo is the most common target material in mammography x-ray tubes.

A32a. Fiber has a lower atomic number and density than Al, and will therefore transmit more primary photons (i.e., it reduces the patient dose).

A33c. Exposure time has no direct impact on image contrast.

A34a. Grids are not used in magnification mammography, since the air gap will minimize scatter at the image receptor.

A35d. The MQSA requires accreditation from an approved body, but it does not have to be the ACR.

A36d. Photocathodes absorb light photons, and emit low-energy electrons.

A37b. A typical II conversion factor is ~20 cd/m^2 per μGy/s.

A38d. Plumbicon TV cameras reduce image lag, and are used in cardiac imaging to minimize smearing when imaging the moving heart.

A39a. To maintain a constant II brightness, electronic reduction of the II input area must be compensated for by increasing radiation intensity.

A40c. Fifteen frames per second is a typical acquisition frame rate in digital cardiac imaging.

A41c. Ten kW is a common anode cooling rate (kW) in CT with standard x-ray tubes; the Straton x-ray tube is an exception that has a cooling rate of ~60 kW.

A42a. Beam-shaping filters reduce the CT detector dynamic range.

A43b. The detected x-ray pattern at a single x-ray tube angle is called a projection.

A44a. Soft tissue filters reduce mottle at the cost of inferior spatial resolution performance.

A45b. A HU of 10 will look almost black with a window width of 100 and window level of 50 (50 looks gray, and 0 looks black).

A46b. Scan times are markedly reduced when axial scanning is replaced with helical CT.

A47c. Three seconds should be possible (patient coverage per rotation of 4 cm; tube rotation time 0.3 s; ten rotations).

A48e. Forty mGy since CTDI$_{vol}$ is the CTDI$_w$ divided by the pitch (i.e., 10 mGy/0.25).

A49c. Body techniques (mAs) in a 1-year-old can be reduced to ~50%

with no loss of diagnostic information.

A50a. Reducing the section thickness will minimize partial volume artifacts.

A51b. 40 keV will achieve the maximum absorption by iodine (K-shell binding energy of 33 keV) and maximize subject contrast.

A52d. Scatter is lower at lower energies since photoelectric absorption will be more important than Compton scatter.

A53c. Seventy kV will have an average energy (1/2 to 1/3 of the 70 keV maximum) that is close to the iodine K-edge of 33 keV.

A54a. Detector composition has negligible impact on spatial resolution performance.

A55e. Most likely 0.01 since the system MTF is the product of the component MTF values at each spatial frequency.

A56e. The TV system is the weak link in the fluoroscopy imaging chain.

A57e. An increase in the image matrix size could improve spatial resolution.

A58c. Increasing the receptor air kerma would reduce mottle and improve visibility of low contrast lesions.

A59a. The image receptor air kerma in DSA is 5 μGy, or five times higher than in digital photospot imaging (1 μGy).

A60a. A receiver operator characteristic curve measures diagnostic performance.

A61c. The nucleus, which contains DNA, is the most sensitive part of the cell.

A62e. Alpha particle LET is ~100 keV/μm, whereas x-rays are ~1 keV/μm.

A63c. A 4-Gy uniform whole-body dose would kill half the exposed population.

A64c. Five Gy is the chronic threshold dose for inducing eye cataracts.

A65a. Zero (no threshold) is assumed for exposure to ionizing radiations.

A66d. ICRU is the International Commission on Radiological Units and Measurements, which addresses dose quantities such as exposure and air kerma but does not deal with any radiation risk estimates.

A67c. The gonad weighting factor recommended by the ICRP in 2007 is 0.08, which replaced the value of 0.20 recommended in 1990.

A68c. Severe mental retardation in pregnant patients likely occurs at 7 to 15 weeks.

A69e. The skin dose (mGy) is the best indicator of the possible harm done to the skin from x-ray exposure.

A70a. The energy absorbed by the patient is 0.1 J; this may be contrasted to the 600 J deposited each second when a chicken is heated in a 600-W microwave.

A71e. Much more because of the k-edge energy of silver is 25 keV, which will result in many more 30-keV than 300-keV photons being absorbed.

A72a. Low-level contamination is normally detected using Geiger-Muller detectors.

A73b. Five mSv is the annual effective dose received by the most highly exposed radiation workers (e.g., IR fellows).

A74c. The limit is 150 mSv per year, which should prevent the induction of an eye cataract (deterministic effect) with a threshold dose of ~5 Sv.

A75c. Virtually all diagnostic x-ray rooms have 1.5 mm of lead shielding.

A76a. A chest radiographic examination (PA plus lateral) would result in an effective dose of ~0.05 mSv.

A77c. A typical value is 5 mSv for upper barium studies (higher for barium enemas).

A78d. Three per 100,000 breast cancers is the mammogram radiation risk, with a quarter being fatal.

A79b. The average U.S. dose from radon is 2 mSv, but there are large variations depending on the type of dwelling and geographic location.

A80e. The contribution of mammography to US medical doses (2006) is negligible.

A81d. One mCi is 37 MBq (i.e., 37,000,000 Bq)

A82c. ^{18}F is a positron emitter that is used in most PET imaging studies.

A83b. Radionuclides produced in cyclotrons are proton rich, and can decay via beta plus emission.

A84d. Elution is not a radiopharmaceutical localization mechanism, but rather, extracting a substance that is adsorbed to another by washing with a solvent.

A85a. ^{67}Ga, which has three photon energies (93 keV, 185 keV, and 300 keV).

A86b. ^{67}Ga is a gamma ray emitter, whereas all the others emit positrons and produce annihilation radiation (511 keV).

A87a. Flood uniformity is a scintillation camera test, not a radiopharmaceutical QC test.

A88e. System resolution R is equal to $(R_I^2 + R_C^2)^{1/2}$, where R_I and R_C are the intrinsic and collimator resolutions, respectively.

A89a. Chemical shift artifacts occur in MR, not nuclear medicine.

A90b. Fetal thyroid because it has the smallest mass.

A91e. The approximate wavelength is 1 mm (actually 1,540 m/s divided by 2×10^6 Hz or 0.77 mm).

A92e. The remaining intensity is 0.1% at −30 dB (1% at −20 dB, and 10% at −10 dB).

A93e. The fraction is 1/9 since reflection is $[(Z2 − Z1)/(Z2 + Z1)]^2$, or $[(2 − 1)/(2 + 1)]^2$.

A94a. The crystal thickness determines the ultrasound frequency and wavelength (thicker crystals have longer wavelengths and lower frequencies).

A95c. A typical ultrasound PRF value is 4 kHz (4,000 pulses per second).

A96d. It will take 130 μs, since it takes 13 μs to get an echo from an interface from a depth of 1 cm.

A97c. The frequency is 6 MHz, because harmonic images are obtained at double the fundamental frequency (i.e., 2×3 MHz).

A98e. In spectral analysis, the detected frequency shift is plotted as a function of time.

A99b. The axial resolution is 0.5 mm, since it is approximately half the spatial pulse length.

A100a. Reverberation artifacts are faint image of the structure below the structure.

A101a. ^{1}H protons have the highest Larmor frequency at a fixed magnetic field and produce the largest MR signal intensities.

A102d. $(M_{xy})^1$, which simply means that the FID signal is proportional to the transverse magnetization value.

A103a. A time of 300 ms since T1 weighting is achieved by the use of TR times that comparable to fat and tissue T1 times.

A104e. A magnitude of $\ll 0.001\%$ since typical magnetic field inhomogeneities are only a few parts per million.

A105c. Approximately 500 amp would be the typical electrical current in a superconducting magnet.

A106a. Increasing the magnetic gradient will generally result in thinner MR slices.

A107a. The frequency-encode matrix size has no effect on the total MR scan time.

A108c. A typical spin density difference is 10% between any two different types of soft tissue.

A109e. Vignetting is the loss of image intensity in the periphery of an image intensifier used in fluoroscopy.

A110c. The FDA recommends 40°C as the maximum temperature to an extremity during MRI.

PRACTICE EXAMINATION B: QUESTIONS

B1 Which of the following electrical terms is measured in coulombs per second?
a. Current
b. Charge
c. Voltage
d. Resistance
e. Power

B2 Power (W) for a constant-potential generator at 100 kV and 1,000 mA is most likely:
a. 10
b. 100
c. 1,000
d. 10,000
e. 100,000

B3 A rectification circuit is most likely to contain:
a. resistors
b. transistors
c. diodes
d. inductances
e. capacitors

B4 The most likely x-ray tube target material is:
a. iron
b. copper
c. zinc
d. tungsten
e. lead

B5 What is the maximum energy (keV) of an x-ray produced at an x-ray tube voltage of 120 kV?
a. 12
b. 25
c. 40
d. 60
e. 120

B6 100-keV electrons most likely produce x-ray photons with average energy (keV) of:
a. 20
b. 30
c. 45
d. 55
e. 70

B7 The power (W) dissipated in the x-ray tube filament is most likely:
a. 0.4
b. 4
c. 40
d. 400
e. 4,000

B8 X-ray tube output is *unlikely* to be increased by increasing:
a. tube voltage (kV)
b. anode capacity (MJ)

c. target atomic number (Z)
d. tube current (mA)
e. exposure time (s)

B9 The energy deposited in an anode with a constant-potential generator operated at voltage kV, tube current mA, and exposure time t is:
a. kV mA t
b. kV^2 mA t
c. kV mA^2 t
d. $(kV\ mA)^2$ t
e. (kV mA)/t

B10 Which of the following is the most likely x-ray tube power level (kW) during routine abdominal fluoroscopy?
a. 0.3
b. 1
c. 3
d. 10
e. 30

B11 What is the K-shell binding energy (keV) of tungsten?
a. 20
b. 33
c. 37
d. 70
e. 88

B12 X-rays interacting with matter can be best described as transferring x-ray photon energy to:
a. atoms
b. electrons
c. neutrons
d. protons
e. nuclei

B13 The energy of the scattered photon in Compton processes is most likely to depend on the:
a. atomic number
b. physical density
c. electron density
d. chemical structure
e. scattering angle

B14 In diagnostic radiology, the x-ray beam attenuation is *unlikely* to increase with increasing:
a. physical density (ρ)
b. atomic number (Z)
c. electron density (e/cm^3)
d. attenuator thickness (cm)
e. photon energy (keV)

B15 The half-value layer (m) of a material with a linear attenuation coefficient of $0.35\ m^{-1}$ is likely:
a. 1
b. 2

  c. 3
  d. 4
  e. 5

B16 Beam hardening is most likely associated with:
  a. tube voltage
  b. tube current
  c. exposure time
  d. added filtration
  e. focus size

B17 The heel effect most likely depends on the anode:
  a. rotation
  b. diameter
  c. angle
  d. capacity
  e. density

B18 Use of a lower ratio grid will likely increase:
  a. exposure time
  b. image contrast
  c. patient dose
  d. Bucky factor
  e. primary transmission

B19 Air kerma is most closely associated with:
  a. radiation exposure
  b. absorbed dose
  c. equivalent dose
  d. effective dose
  e. dose area product

B20 The non-SI unit of absorbed dose is the:
  a. mR
  b. mrad
  c. mrem
  d. mCi
  e. mBq

B21 In film processing, the fixer:
  a. modifies developer pH
  b. removes unexposed grains
  c. fixes silver to the emulsion
  d. removes bromine
  e. reduces silver halide

B22 Reducing the film processor temperature will most likely decrease the:
  a. image contrast
  b. quantum mottle
  c. focal blur
  d. screen blur
  e. patient dose

B23 Matching the screen K-edge with incident x-ray energy will most likely increase screen–film:
  a. conversion efficiency
  b. fog level
  c. image blur
  d. average gradient
  e. relative speed

B24 The receptor air kerma (μGy) to correctly expose a 200 speed system is:
  a. 0.5
  b. 5
  c. 50
  d. 500
  e. 5,000

B25 What is the data transfer speed (Mbit/s) of Gigabit Ethernet?
  a. 1
  b. 10
  c. 100
  d. 1,000
  e. 10,000

B26 Which of the following is least likely to be used for the detection of diagnostic x-rays?
  a. Photoconductor
  b. Scintillator
  c. Charged couple device
  d. Photostimulable phosphor
  e. Intensifying screen

B27 Which of the following x-ray detector materials most likely emits light?
  a. Xe
  b. CsI
  c. Se
  d. PbI
  e. HgI

B28 How many pixels (million) are most likely generated by a film digitizer processing a diagnostic chest radiograph?
  a. 0.5
  b. 1
  c. 2
  d. 5
  e. 10

B29 Which of the following is *least* related to image processing?
  a. Histogram equalization
  b. Low-pass filtering
  c. Background subtraction
  d. Bow tie filtering
  e. Energy subtraction

B30 Which of the following does not relate to computer networks?
  a. Token ring
  b. Ethernet
  c. Backbone
  d. JPEG
  e. Bridge

B31 Tube currents (mA) in contact mammography are most likely:
  a. 5
  b. 10
  c. 20
  d. 50
  e. 100

B32 The Bucky factor of a mammography grid is most likely:
a. 1
b. 2
c. 3
d. 5
e. 10

B33 Use of compression in mammography is most likely to increase:
a. patient dose
b. exposure time
c. motion blur
d. focal blur
e. image contrast

B34 Benefits of stereotaxic localization for core biopsies include all the following *except*:
a. short procedure
b. no radiation
c. local anesthetic
d. reduced cost
e. reduced scarring

B35 To meet MQSA requirements, the average glandular dose (mGy) for a single view of an average-sized breast must be less than:
a. 0.5
b. 1.0
c. 1.5
d. 2.0
e. 3.0

B36 The brightness gain of an II tube is *least* likely to depend on the:
a. patient dose
b. photocathode efficiency
c. II voltage
d. input diameter
e. output diameter

B37 The number of lines used by HDTV in progressive (p) scan mode is most likely:
a. 256
b. 525
c. 625
d. 720
e. 1,080

B38 The most likely x-ray tube voltage (kV) for a barium enema is:
a. 25
b. 55
c. 70
d. 85
e. 110

B39 The matrix size in a DSA image is typically:
a. 512 × 512
b. 1,024 × 512
c. 1,024 × 1,024

d. 2,048 × 1,024
e. 2,048 × 2,048

B40 The lowest contrast difference (%) that is likely to be detected in DSA is:
a. <1
b. 1
c. 2
d. 4
e. 8

B41 The most likely filtration (mm Al) used in CT x-ray tubes is:
a. 1
b. 2
c. 3
d. 6
e. 12

B42 Which material is *least* likely to be used to construct an array of CT detectors?
a. Bismuth germanate
b. Cadmium tungstate
c. Xenon (high pressure)
d. Sodium iodide
e. Lithium fluoride

B43 Which CT image reconstruction algorithm is most likely used in clinical practice?
a. 2D Fourier transform
b. 3D Fourier transform
c. Back projection
d. Filtered back projection
e. Iterative reconstruction

B44 The difference (%) in x-ray attenuation between 40 HU and 50 HU is:
a. 0.1
b. 1
c. 10
d. 25
e. 45

B45 The data acquisition geometry (i.e., generation) of a 64-slice CT scanner is most likely:
a. first
b. second
c. third
d. fourth
e. fifth

B46 The temporal resolution (ms) of a dual-source CT scanner (gantry rotation speed of 0.30 s) in cardiac imaging is most likely:
a. 37.5
b. 75
c. 150
d. 30
e. 600

B47 The ratio of the peripheral to central CTDI in a head phantom is most likely:
a. 0.25:1
b. 0.5:1

c. 1:1
d. 2:1
e. 4:1

B48 The reference dose ($CTDI_{vol}$ mGy) recommended by the ACR (2008) for an adult abdominal CT is most likely:
  a. 25
  b. 50
  c. 75
  d. 100
  e. 125

B49 The most likely pitch in retrospective gating cardiac imaging is:
  a. 0.25
  b. 0.5
  c. 1.0
  d. 1.5
  e. 2.0

B50 Which of the following artifacts is least likely in CT?
  a. Motion
  b. Zipper
  c. Streak
  d. Ring
  e. Beam-hardening

B51 In screen–film radiography, raising the tube voltage (kV) likely reduces:
  a. half-value layer
  b. scatter radiation
  c. patient transmission
  d. subject contrast
  e. grid penetration

B52 Increasing kV in digital mammography most likely increases:
  a. image contrast
  b. quantum mottle
  c. breast penetration
  d. focal blur
  e. exposure time

B53 Spatial resolution performance is *least* likely to be assessed using a:
  a. line pair phantom
  b. line spread function
  c. full width half maximum
  d. modulation transfer function
  e. pixel standard deviation

B54 Minimizing which factor would most likely improve spatial resolution?
  a. Exposure time
  b. Tube voltage
  c. Tube current
  d. Beam filtration
  e. Window width

B55 Measured limiting spatial resolution (lp/mm) of screen–film mammography is likely:
  a. 1
  b. 2
  c. 4

d. 8
e. 16

B56 Going from a 256^2 to a 512^2 matrix size is most likely to double the:
  a. spatial resolution
  b. number of pixels
  c. gray levels
  d. transmission time
  e. storage requirements

B57 When the average number of x-ray photons detected by a pixel is 100, the standard deviation is most likely:
  a. 1
  b. 3
  c. 10
  d. 30
  e. 100

B58 The detector air kerma (μGy) in digital mammography is most likely:
  a. 1
  b. 3
  c. 10
  d. 30
  e. 100

B59 Visibility of large low-contrast CT lesions likely improves with increasing:
  a. beam filtration
  b. tube current
  c. field of view
  d. matrix size
  e. window width

B60 A diagnostic test is of no value when the area under the ROC curve (%) has a value of:
  a. 0
  b. 25
  c. 50
  d. 75
  e. 100

B61 The most likely oxygen enhancement ratio for x-rays is:
  a. 1.5
  b. 2.5
  c. 5
  d. 10
  e. 20

B62 The radiation weighting factor (w_R) for 80-kV x-rays is likely:
  a. 0.3
  b. 0.5
  c. 1.0
  d. 2.0
  e. 3.0

B63 The threshold dose (Gy) for permanent epilation is most likely:
  a. 1
  b. 3
  c. 5

d. 7
e. 10

B64 The chance (%) of a radiation-induced cataract from ten head CT examinations is most likely:
a. 0
b. 0.1
c. 0.25
d. 0.5
e. 1

B65 Which of the following tissues is likely the *least* sensitive to radiation-induced carcinogenesis:
a. Breast
b. Colon
c. Kidney
d. Lung
e. Stomach

B66 For young adults, a uniform whole-body dose of 1 Sv will result in a cancer incidence risk (%) that is most likely:
a. 0.1
b. 0.3
c. 1
d. 3
e. 10

B67 The gonad dose (Gy) that would most likely double the spontaneous mutation incidence is most likely:
a. 2
b. 5
c. 10
d. 20
e. 50

B68 The dose to the fetus (mGy) after 5 minutes of pelvic fluoroscopy (PA) is most likely:
a. 0.3
b. 3
c. 30
d. 300
e. 3,000

B69 If the entrance air kerma in an adult PA chest x-ray is 0.1 mGy, the air kerma–area product (Gy-cm^2) is most likely:
a. 0.1
b. 1
c. 10
d. 100
e. 1,000

B70 If a newborn patient (3.5 kg) absorbs the same total energy as an adult (70 kg), the newborn's dose will likely be higher by a factor of:
a. 2
b. 4
c. 10
d. 20
e. 50

B71 Which of the following materials is most likely to be used as a TLD for occupational dosimetry?
a. BaFBr
b. LiF
c. NaCl
d. PbI
e. Se

B72 Agreement states are most likely to regulate the operations in:
a. Radiography
b. Mammography
c. Computed tomography
d. Nuclear medicine
e. Interventional radiology

B73 The fetus of an x-ray technologist has an equivalent dose limit (mSv/month) that is most likely:
a. 0.5
b. 1
c. 2
d. 5
e. 10

B74 The current (2008) regulatory dose limit (mSv per year) to the hands of a radiopharmacist is:
a. 50
b. 100
c. 150
d. 300
e. 500

B75 If both occupancy factor and work load double, personnel doses are likely to increase by (%):
a. 50
b. 100
c. 200
d. 400
e. 800

B76 The maximum patient entrance air kerma (mGy per minute) in fluoroscopy is most likely:
a. 5
b. 10
c. 25
d. 50
e. >50

B77 The breast dose (mGy) from a single chest CT scan is most likely:
a. 0.02
b. 0.2
c. 2
d. 20
e. 200

B78 Dose reductions (%) for *follow-up* scoliosis digital radiographs are most likely:
a. 10
b. 25

c. 50

d. 80

e. >80

B79 Which imaging modality produced the highest collective medical dose in 2006?

a. Computed tomography

b. Dental radiography

c. Interventional radiology

d. Mammography

e. Radiography

B80 The contribution (%) of CT to the total U.S. population dose from medical imaging is likely:

a. 2.5

b. 7.5

c. 15

d. 30

e. 50

B81 Which is *least* likely to be emitted during radioactive decay?

a. Electrons

b. Protons

c. Positrons

d. Gamma rays

e. Neutrinos

B82 Electron capture is most likely to compete with:

a. positron decay

b. beta minus decay

c. alpha decay

d. isomeric transition

e. nuclear fission

B83 Which radionuclide has a primary photopeak energy of 365 keV?

a. Oxygen-15

b. Technetium-99m

c. Iodine-131

d. Thallium-201

e. Indium-111

B84 The sensitivity of a low-energy (high-resolution) collimator is most likely to be:

a. 10^{-1}

b. 10^{-2}

c. 10^{-3}

d. 10^{-4}

e. 10^{-5}

B85 The angular rotation (degrees) of a dual-camera SPECT system when imaging the liver would likely be:

a. 90

b. 135

c. 180

d. 270

e. 360

B86 A PET scanner obtains spatial information by detecting:

a. positrons and electrons in coincidence

b. positrons and electrons in anticoincidence

c. photons and positrons in coincidence

d. annihilation photons in coincidence

e. annihilation photons in anticoincidence

B87 Which of the following is *not* a quality control test performed on a scintillation camera?

a. Field uniformity

b. ^{99}Mo breakthrough

c. Extrinsic flood

d. Spatial resolution

e. Linearity

B88 The full width half maximum width (mm) of a line source obtained using a PET scanner is most likely:

a. 1

b. 2.5

c. 5

d. 10

e. 20

B89 A radionuclide with a shorter half-life likely results in lower:

a. count rates

b. patient doses

c. biologic clearance

d. scattered photons

e. photopeak energy

B90 The dose rate near a ^{131}I therapy patient is *least* likely to depend on the:

a. administered activity

b. physical half-life

c. biological half-life

d. patient weight

e. distance to patient

B91 Which material has the highest ultrasound propagation velocity?

a. Air

b. Fat

c. Soft tissue

d. Bone

e. PZT

B92 Which of the following has the *lowest* acoustic impedance?

a. Bone

b. Fat

c. Air

d. Water

e. Eye lens

B93 Depth gain compensation most likely corrects for:

a. specular scatter

b. nonspecular scatter

c. tissue attenuation

d. transducer damping

e. shadowing losses

B94 Increasing the transducer bandwidth will most likely reduce the ultrasound pulse:
a. velocity
b. duration
c. reflection
d. attenuation
e. frequency

B95 The pulse repetition frequency (PRF) is *least* likely to affect the:
a. listening time
b. frame rate
c. line density
d. penetration depth
e. operating frequency

B96 The number of bytes used to code for one pixel in a B-mode image is most likely:
a. 0.5
b. 1
c. 2
d. 4
e. 8

B97 In ultrasound, the Doppler frequency shift (Hz) is most likely:
a. 0.05
b. 0.5
c. 5
d. 50
e. 500

B98 The main advantage of power Doppler for detecting blood flow is likely its:
a. sensitivity to slow flow
b. increased intensity
c. increased echo strength
d. quantitative flow data
e. ability to provide directional data

B99 Lateral resolution is most influenced by the ultrasound beam:
a. velocity
b. frequency
c. intensity
d. width
e. duration

B100 The mechanical index (MI) value indicates the possible increase in tissue:
a. cavitation
b. cell death
c. density
d. shearing
e. temperature

B101 At 1.5 T, the excess number (%) of proton spins in the low-energy state over the high-energy state is most likely:
a. 10
b. 1
c. 0.1
d. 0.01
e. ≪0.01

B102 Following a 90-degree pulse, the longitudinal magnetization will most likely recover in a time that is four times:
a. T1
b. T2
c. T2*
d. TE
e. TR

B103 If T2 for gray matter is 100 ms at 1.5 T, its value at 3 T is most likely:
a. 50
b. 70
c. 100
d. 140
e. 200

B104 Soft tissue T2* times (μs) are most likely:
a. 5
b. 50
c. 500
d. 5,000
e. 50,000

B105 Gradient magnetic fields in MR are used most commonly to:
a. increase T2
b. shorten T1
c. localize signal
d. amplify signal
e. minimize stray fields

B106 The number of 1D Fourier transforms in reconstructing a M × N image is most likely:
a. M
b. N
c. M + N
d. M − N
e. M × N

B107 Which is the most likely TR value (ms) for a FLASH gradient recalled echo pulse sequence?
a. 1
b. 10
c. 100
d. 1,000
e. 10,000

B108 MR signal-to-noise ratio (SNR) is likely reduced when there is an increase in:
a. coil diameter
b. number of acquisitions
c. magnetic field strength
d. section thickness
e. pixel dimension

B109 Which line is an exclusion zone (mT) for persons with pacemakers?
a. 0.5
b. 1
c. 2
d. 5
e. 10

B110 Which of the following is *least* likely to exhibit paramagnetism?
a. Ba
b. Cr
c. Fe
d. Gd
e. Mn

PRACTICE EXAMINATION B: ANSWERS AND EXPLANATIONS

B1a. Electric currents are measured in amps (1 A = 1 C/s).

B2e. Power is 100,000 W or 100 kW (P = V I).

B3c. Diodes are used in rectification circuits, and they permit electrical currents to flow in only one direction.

B4d. Most x-ray tubes use tungsten targets.

B5e. The maximum energy is 120 keV, since the maximum electron kinetic energy is 120 keV and all of this kinetic energy can be transformed into an x-ray photon.

B6c. The average photon energy is between one half and one third of the maximum photon energy.

B7c. X-ray tube filaments are operated at 4 A and 10 V and deposit 40 W of power, just like the filament in a light bulb.

B8b. Anode capacity has no direct relevance to the x-ray tube output.

B9a. Energy deposited in the anode in joules is kV mA t (at constant voltage).

B10a. In fluoroscopy, the tube voltage is ~100 kV and tube current is ~3 mA, so the power is ~300 W (i.e., 0.3 kW).

B11d. Tungsten has a Z of 74 and a k-shell binding energy of 70 keV.

B12b. X-rays transfer energy to photoelectrons and Compton electrons.

B13e. It is the scattering angle that determines the energy of the scattered photon.

B14e. Increasing the photon energy generally increases penetration (i.e., reduces attenuation).

B15b. The HVL is 2 m, since HVL = 0.693/(linear attenuation coefficient).

B16d. Beam hardening is directly related to the amount of filtration in the x-ray beam.

B17c. The anode angle is the most important factor influencing the heel effect.

B18e. A lower grid ratio means that more primary photons will get through a grid.

B19a. Air kerma is increasingly replacing exposure as the measure of x-ray intensities (i.e., the amount of radiation in an x-ray beam).

B20b. Rads are non-SI units of absorbed dose (1 rad is equal to 10 mGy).

B21b. Fixers remove unexposed grains of silver bromide.

B22a. Lower film temperatures will reduce the average film gradient, and therefore image contrast.

B23e. Relative speed increases since the matching exercise means that more x-rays will be absorbed by the screen.

B24b. The typical image receptor dose is 5 μGy in most standard radiographic imaging.

B25d. Giga Ethernet transfers data at 1,000 Mbit/s.

B26c. A charged couple device detects light, not x-rays.

B27b. CsI converts 10% of the absorbed energy into light energy.

B28d. Digitized chest x-rays are likely to have a matrix size of 2,000 × 2,5000, or 5 million pixels.

B29d. Bow tie filtering refers to the use of a bow tie–shaped filter in CT imaging.

B30d. JPEG is a file format that includes standards for compression.

B31e. A normal tube current is 100 mA in standard (contact) mammography.

B32b. Use of grids in contact mammography will likely double the patient dose (i.e., Bucky factor is ~2).

B33e. Compression improves image quality, including contrast (e.g., reduces the amount of scatter).

B34b. X-rays have to be taken in stereotaxic localization.

B35e. The MQSA limit is 3 mGy per image for a normal-sized breast (with grid).

B36a. The brightness gain of an II tube is independent of the dose (if you double the dose, both input and output light intensities double, but the ratio [gain] remains the same).

B37d. HDTV in the United States uses 720 lines in progressive scan mode (720 p) and 1,080 in interlaced mode (1080i).

B38e. A voltage of 110 kV would likely be used in barium enema examination (high kV to penetrate the barium).

B39c. The most common matrix size in DSA is $1,024 \times 1,024$.

B40a. DSA can detect differences less than 1%, whereas differences of 2% to 3% may be missed in unsubtracted images.

B41d. Filtration is frequently 6 mm in CT x-ray tubes (excluding the bow tie filter).

B42e. Lithium fluoride is a thermoluminescent dosimeter, which would be useless in CT imaging.

B43d. CT images are generally reconstructed using filtered back projection.

B44b. A difference of 10 HU corresponds to a difference in x-ray attenuation of 1%.

B45c. MSCT uses third-generation acquisition geometry (x-ray tube and detector array both rotate).

B46b. The resolution is 75 ms; for a single-source CT scanner, the temporal resolution is approximately half the rotation time, and a dual-source CT scanner is half the value of a single-source system.

B47c. The ratio is 1:1, as doses in head CT are pretty uniform in 16-cm-diameter phantoms.

B48a. The CTDI_{vol} reference dose currently (2008) recommended by the ACR for an adult abdomen CT is 25 mGy.

B49a. A typical pitch is 0.25 in retrospective gating cardiac imaging.

B50b. Zipper artifacts are observed in MR, not CT.

B51d. Subject contrast is reduced when kV increases.

B52c. Breast penetration increases at higher kV.

B53e. The pixel standard deviation is a measure of mottle (noise), not spatial resolution.

B54a. Minimizing exposure time reduces motion blur.

B55e. Screen–film mammography normally achieves ~16 lp/mm (the ACR limit is ~12 lp/mm).

B56a. Doubling the matrix size could double the spatial resolution.

B57c. Ten, as the standard deviation is the square root of the mean number of counts.

B58e. is the detector air kerma in mammography is ~100 μGy.

B59b. Higher tube current will reduce mottle and improve the visibility of (large) low-contrast lesions.

B60c. Random guessing corresponds to an ROC area of 50%.

B61b. A typical OER for low LET x-rays is 2.5.

B62c. The radiation weighting factor is 1.0 for radiations used in diagnostic radiology.

B63d. Permanent epilation occurs at ~7 Gy.

B64a. Zero since ten head CTs would result in an eye lens dose of ~600 mGy, well below the threshold dose for chronic exposure (i.e., 5 Gy).

B65c. The kidney is least sensitive to radiation-induced cancers of those listed.

B66e. Approximately 10% of 30-year-olds might suffer a radiation-induced cancer following exposure to an effective dose of 1 Sv (1,000 mSv).

B67a. The commonly accepted value of the doubling dose for hereditary effects is 2 Gy.

B68c. The dose is 30 mGy, which is 30% of the patient skin dose of 100 mGy (i.e., 5 minutes at 20 mGy/min for average-sized patients).

B69a. The KAP is 0.1 Gy-cm^2, since the exposed are at the patient entrance is ~1,000 cm^2.

B70d. A factor of 20 since the newborn has a mass that is twenty times lower, and dose = energy/mass.

B71b. LiF is the most popular TLD material in medical radiation dosimetry.

B72d. Nuclear medicine (radioactivity); nonagreement states are regulated by the NRC.

B73a. A dose limit of 0.5 mSv per month (to the fetus); 50 mSv per year to the mother.

B74e. A limit of 500 mSv per year is designed to prevent the induction of chronic deterministic effects.

B75d. Doses increase by 400%, since each of these factors alone would likely double operator doses.

B76e. The maximum is >50 mGy; 100 mGy/min is the limit in normal fluoroscopy, and 200 mGy/min is permitted in high-dose mode with alarms to indicate the high-dose mode.

B77d. The dose is 20 mGy, which is much higher than in mammography (~4 mGy for a two-view exam).

B78e. More than 80% as follow-up digital radiographs using a tenth of the initial dose are adequate for assessing the spine curvature.

B79a. Computed tomography accounts for nearly half of the total population medical dose.

B80e. CT contributes 50% of the U.S. medical radiation dose.

B81b. There are no known radionuclides that emit protons.

B82a. Electron capture competes with positron decay.

B83c. Iodine-131 emits 365 keV gamma ray photons.

B84d. 10^{-4}, as only about 1 in 10,000 gamma rays incident on a collimator are expected to get through and contribute to the image.

B85c. The rotation is 180 degrees, which permits the acquisition of projections through 360 degrees.

B86d. PET scanners obtain spatial information by detecting annihilation photons in coincidence.

B87b. ^{99}Mo breakthrough is used to test the eluted solution from a ^{99m}Tc/^{99}Mo generator.

B88c. A typical full width half maximum width of an image of a line source obtained with a PET imaging system is 5 mm.

B89b. A shorter half-life means a lower cumulative activity (fewer nuclear transformations) and therefore a lower patient dose.

B90d. Patient weight will have negligible impact on the dose rate in the vicinity of a ^{131}I therapy patient (365 keV gamma rays).

B91e. PZT; the less compressible a material, the higher the velocity and vice versa (compressible air has the lowest velocity).

B92c. Air since acoustic impedance is density times sound velocity, which are both lowest in air.

B93c. Depth gain compensation (TGC) mainly corrects for tissue attenuation.

B94b. Duration and bandwidth are inversely related (e.g., pure sounds clearly have a narrow bandwidth and thus last a long time).

B95e. The operating frequency has no direct relationship to the PRF.

B96b. Each pixel is coded using 1 byte (8 bits), and can display 256 shades of gray.

B97e As Doppler shifts are in the audible frequency range, 500 Hz.

B98a. Power Doppler is very sensitive to slow flow.

B99d. lateral resolution is determined by the ultrasound beam width.

B100a. Mechanical Index (MI) values indicate the possibilities of tissue cavitation.

B101e. Much less than 0.01 ($\ll 0.01$), as the excess number of protons is only a few per million.

B102a. T1 since the magnetization recovers in 4 × T1.

B103c. Its value is still 100 since T2 times show little dependence on field strength in clinical MR.

B104d. Times are 5,000 μs, which is 5 ms and a typical tissue T2* value

B105c. Magnetic field gradients are used to localize the MR signal.

B106c. Each row must undergo a FT (M) followed by each column (N), which results in a total of M + N.

B107b. The most likely TR time for a fast low-angle shot pulse sequence is 10 ms.

B108a. Larger coil diameter will generally reduce the SNR in MR.

B109a. The magnetic field exclusion zone is 0.5 mT (5 gauss).

B110a. Ba is an x-ray contrast material that does not exhibit paramagnetism

I. Summary of SI and Non-SI Units for General Quantities

Quantity	SI Unit	Non-SI Unit
Length	meter (m)	centimeter (cm)
Mass	kilogram (kg)	gram (g)
Time	second (s)	minute (min)
Electrical current	ampere (A)	electrostatic unit (ESU) per second (s)
Amount of substance	mole (mol)	—
Frequency	hertz (Hz)	revolutions per minute (rpm)
Force	newton (N)	dyne
Energy	joule (J)	erg
Power	watt (W)	erg/s
Electrical charge	coulomb (C)	ESU
Electrical potential	volt (V)	—
Magnetic field	tesla (T)	gauss (G)

II. Summary of Units for Radiologic Quantities

Quantity	SI Unit	Non-SI Unit	SI to Non-SI Conversions	Non-SI to SI Conversions
Exposure	C/kg	roentgen	1 C/kg = 3,876 R	1 R = 2.58×10^{-4} C/kg
Air kerma	gray (J/kg)	roentgen	1 Gy = 114 R	1 R = 8.76 mGy
Absorbed dose	gray (J/kg)	rad (100 erg/g)	1 Gy = 100 rad	1 rad = 10 mGy
Equivalent dose	sievert	rem	1 Sv = 100 rem	1 rem = 10 mSv
Activity	becquerel	curie	1 MBq = 27 μCi	1 mCi = 37 MBq

III. Summary of Units for Photometric[a] Quantities

Quantity	SI Unit	Non-SI Unit	To Convert Non-SI Units to SI Units
Luminance[b] (light scattered or emitted by a surface)	cd/m^2 (nit)	foot-lamberts	foot-lamberts $\times$ 3.4261 = cd/m^2
Illuminance[b] (light falling on a surface)	lumen/m^2 (lux)	foot-candles	foot-candles $\times$ 10.761 = lumen/m^2

[a] Photometric units take into account the spectral sensitivity of the eye.

[b] One lux falling on a perfectly diffusing surface with no absorption produces a luminance of $1/\pi$ cd/m^2.

IV. Approximate Luminance Values

Luminance (cd/m²)	Viewing Conditions
3,000	Mammography viewbox
1,500	Standard viewbox
600	Brightest monitor display
200	Typical monitor display

V. Approximate Illuminance Values

Illuminance (lux)	Conditions
5,000	Full daylight
500	Overcast day
250	Average office
20	Radiologist's reading room
5	Twilight
0.1	Moonlight
0.001	Starlight

VI. Summary of Prefix Names and Magnitudes

Prefix Name	Symbol	Magnitude
exa	E	10^{18}
peta	P	10^{15}
tera	T	10^{12}
giga	G	10^{9}
mega	M	10^{6}
kilo	k	10^{3}
hecto	h	10^{2}
deca	da	10
deci	d	10^{-1}
centi	c	10^{-2}
milli	m	10^{-3}
micro	μ	10^{-6}
nano	n	10^{-9}
pico	p	10^{-12}
femto	f	10^{-15}
atto	a	10^{-18}

VII.   Selected Radiological Physics Web Sites

American Association of Physicists in Medicine (AAPM): www.aapm.org
American Board of Radiology (ABR): theabr.org
American College of Radiology (ACR): www.acr.org
American Institute of Ultrasound in Medicine (AIUM): www.aium.org
American Journal of Roentgenology (AJR): www.ajronline.org
American National Standards Institute (ANSI): www.ansi.org
American Roentgen Ray Society (ARRS): www.arrs.org
American Society of Radiologic Technologists (ASRT): www.asrt.org
British Institute of Radiology (BIR): www.bir.org.uk
Conference of Radiation Control Program Directors (CRCPD): www.crcpd.org
Food and Drug Administration(FDA): www.fda.gov
FDA whole-body CT scanning: www.fda.gov/cdrh/ct
Health Physics Society (HPS): www.hps.org
Health Protection Agency (formerly NRPB): www.hpa.org.uk
International Commission on Non-Ionizing Radiation Protection: www.icnirp.de
International Commission on Radiation Units and Measurements (ICRU): www.icru.org
International Commission on Radiological Protection (ICRP): www.icrp.org
Medical Physics Journal: www.medphys.org
Joint Commission for Accreditation of Healthcare Organizations: www.jcaho.org
National Council on Radiation Protection and Measurements (NCRP): www.ncrponline.org
Physics and Astronomy Online Education: www.physlink.com
Radiation Research Society: www.radres.org
Radiographics and Radiology Journal: www.rsnajnls.org
Radiological Society of North America (RSNA): www.rsna.org
Society for Imaging and Informatics in Medicine (SIIM): www.scarnet.org
Society of Nuclear Medicine (SNM): www.snm.org
U.S. National Institute of Standards and Technology (NIST): www.nist.gov
U.S. Nuclear Regulatory Commission (NRC): www.nrc.gov

90-degree pulse   radio frequency pulse that rotates the equilibrium magnetization vector through 90 degrees

180-degree pulse   radio frequency pulse that rotates the equilibrium magnetization vector through 180 degrees

absolute risk   model of cancer induction where radiation induces a given number of cancers

absorbed dose   radiation energy absorbed per unit mass of a medium measured in gray

absorption efficiency   fraction of incident photons that are absorbed

acoustic enhancement   hyperechoic area distal to object with low attenuation (e.g., fluid-filled cyst)

acoustic impedance   product of density and velocity of sound measured in rayl

acoustic shadowing   hypoechoic area distal to object due to high attenuation or reflection

activity   number of nuclear transformations per unit of time measured in becquerel or curie

air gap   gap between a patient and imaging receptor used in magnification examinations

ALARA   as low as reasonably achievable is the principle for minimizing all radiation doses

aliasing   artifact caused by undersampling in digital imaging

alpha decay   emission of an alpha particle by a radionuclide

alpha particle   particle consisting of two neutrons and two protons

A-mode ultrasound   displays echo strength versus time

analog-to-digital converter (ADC)   converts analog signals into digital values

anode   positive side of an electric circuit

antineutrino   particle with no rest mass and no electric charge emitted in beta minus decay

array processor   hard-wired computer component used for performing rapid calculations

atom   basic constituent of matter, which has a positive nucleus surrounded by electrons

atomic number (Z)   number of protons in the nucleus of an atom

attenuation coefficient (μ)   measure of the x-ray attenuating property of a material, in mm^{-1}

Auger electron   electron (rather than characteristic x-ray) emitted by an energetic atom

automatic brightness control (ABC)   regulates x-ray tube radiation to maintain a constant brightness at image intensifier output

average glandular dose (AGD)   the average dose to the glandular breast tissue in mGy

axial resolution   ability to separate two objects lying *along* the axis of an ultrasound beam

background radiation   radiation doses from naturally occurring radioactivity and extraterrestrial cosmic radiation

bandwidth   *range* of frequencies transmitted or processed by a system

base plus fog   density of a processed film that has not been exposed to any radiation

beam hardening   increase in mean energy of polychromatic x-ray beams when lower-energy photons are preferentially absorbed by a filter or patient

beam quality   penetrating ability of an x-ray beam, usually expressed as an aluminum thickness that reduces beam intensity by 50%

becquerel (Bq)   SI unit of radioactivity (1 Bq = 1 disintegration per second)

BEIR   Biological Effects of Ionizing Radiation committee of the United States National Academy of Sciences

beta minus decay   nuclear process in which a neutron is converted to a proton with emission of an electron and antineutrino

beta particle   electron or positron emitted from a nucleus during beta decay

beta plus decay   nuclear process in which a proton is converted to a neutron with emission of a positron and neutrino

biologic half-life   time required to biologically clear one-half of the amount of a stable material in an organ or tissue

bit (binary digit)   smallest unit of computer memory that holds one of two values, 0 or 1

blooming   increase in x-ray focal spot size due to electron spreading by electrostatic repulsion

blur   loss of image detail (sharpness) produced by an imaging system

B-mode ultrasound   brightness mode that displays echo intensity as a pixel brightness

bow tie filter   beam-shaping filter used to equalize x-ray transmission through the patient

bremsstrahlung radiation   "braking radiation" x-rays produced when electrons lose energy

brightness gain   ratio of the image brightness at the image intensifier output to the brightness produced at the input phosphor

Bucky   device that moves a grid, named after its inventor

Bucky factor   ratio of incident to transmitted radiation through a grid

byte   unit of computer memory equal to eight bits

CAD   computer-aided detection or diagnosis

candela/m^2   measure of luminance (brightness)

cathode   negative side of an electrical circuit

characteristic curve   plot of film density against the logarithm of relative air kerma

characteristic radiation   x-ray photon of characteristic energy emitted from an atom when an inner shell vacancy is filled by an outer shell electron

charged coupled device (CCD)   two-dimensional electronic array for converting light patterns into electrical signals

chemical shift artifacts   artifacts in MR due to small differences in resonance frequencies of different chemical compounds (e.g., water and fat)

coherent scatter   photon scattered by an atom without suffering any energy loss (also called Raleigh or classical scatter)

collimation   restriction of an x-ray beam or gamma rays by use of attenuators

Compton interaction   photon interaction with an outer shell electron resulting in a scattered electron and photon of lower energy

computed radiography (CR)   digital radiography that uses photostimulable phosphor plates

computed tomography (CT)   x-ray imaging modality showing cross-sectional anatomy

contrast   difference in signal intensity between an object and the surrounding background

contrast improvement factor   ratio of image contrast levels obtained with, and without, the use of a scatter-reducing grid

contrast to noise ratio (CNR)   a measure of image quality that compares the contrast of a lesion to the image noise levels

controlled area   area with potentially high dose rates supervised by a radiation safety officer

converging collimator   nuclear medicine collimator used for small organs that results in magnified images

conversion efficiency   percentage of x-ray energy absorbed by a phosphor that is converted to light energy

conversion factor   in image intensifiers, the light output (Cd/m^2) per input air kerma rate (mGy/s)

coulomb (C)   unit of electric charge

count density   used in nuclear medicine to specify the number of counts per unit area

CTDI   computed tomography dose index, used to quantify CT doses in phantoms

cumulative activity   a measure of the total number of radioactive disintegrations obtained by integrating the area under a time–activity curve

curie (Ci)   the non-SI unit of activity ($1\ Ci = 3.7 \times 10^{10}$ disintegrations per second)

current   rate of flow of electric charge measured in amperes

cyclotron   charged particle accelerator used to make radioisotopes

decay constant (λ)   the rate of decay of radionuclides ($\lambda = 0.693/T_{1/2}$, where $T_{1/2}$ is the half-life)

densitometer   device used to measure optical density on film

depth gain compensation (DGC)   used in ultrasound to correct for increased attenuation of sound with tissue depth

deterministic effect   biologic effect of radiation (e.g., epilation) that has a threshold dose (harmful tissue reaction)

DICOM (Digital Imaging and Communications in Medicine)   a standard used for transferring digital images in radiology

digital   quantity specified by discrete numbers, as opposed to analog (continuous)

digital fluoroscopy   fluoroscopic imaging with TV signal digitized and processed, in real time

digital photospot imaging   acquisition of a digital diagnostic quality image of the output of an image intensifier

digital radiography   use of a flat panel detector array or CR system to acquire a digital x-ray image

digital subtraction angiography (DSA)   imaging modality in which digital images made before and after the introduction of iodine contrast are subtracted from each other

directly ionizing radiations   charged particles, such as electrons, that directly ionize atoms

diverging collimator   collimators for large organs (e.g., lungs) resulting in minified image

Doppler shift   change in ultrasound frequency from moving objects

dose   absorbed energy per unit mass, expressed in gray

dose area product   product of the entrance air kerma and cross-sectional area of an x-ray beam incident on a patient

dose calibrator   ionization chamber used in nuclear medicine to measure the amount of radioactivity prior to injection into a patient

dynamic range   ratio of the largest to smallest signal intensity

echo planar imaging (EPI)   fast MR imaging mode

edge enhancement   enhancement of tissue margins using digital processing techniques

edge packing   nuclear medicine artifact that occurs at the periphery of the scintillator camera

effective atomic number   average atomic number obtained from a weighted summation of the atomic constituents of a compound

effective dose   uniform whole-body dose that has the same risk as a given dose distribution

effective half-life   half-life of a radioactive material in an organ that is also being cleared biologically

electromagnetic radiation   transverse wave in which electric and magnetic fields oscillate perpendicular to wave motion

electron   constituent of matter with 1/1,836 of the mass of a proton and a negative charge

electron binding energy   energy that must be supplied to extract a bound atomic electron

electron capture   nuclear process in which a proton is converted to a neutron by capturing an electron and emitting a neutrino

electron density   number of electrons per unit volume (electrons per cm^3)

electron volt (eV)   unit of energy corresponding to the kinetic energy gained by an electron when accelerated through an electrical potential of 1 V

electrostatic force   force that results from charges, which holds atoms together

emulsion   layer of film that contains silver halide grains

energy   ability to do work, measured in joule (J)

entrance skin dose   absorbed radiation dose to skin where the x-ray beam enters the patient

equivalent dose   product of the absorbed dose and radiation weighting factor expressed in sievert (Sv)

exact framing   the entire circular image of an image intensifier that is recorded on the film

excited state   any energy level above the lowest energy ground state in an atom or nucleus

exposure   ability of a source of x-rays to ionize air, measured in C/kg or roentgen (R)

extrinsic flood   scintillator camera image obtained of a uniform source of activity

Faraday cage   radio frequency copper shielding sheets built into the wall around a MR scanner

fast spin echo (FSE)   MR technique that uses multiple spin echoes to reduce imaging times in comparison to spin-echo imaging

ferromagnetic   material (e.g., iron and nickel) with large intrinsic magnetic fields produced by a regular array of unpaired atomic electrons in a domain

f-factor   factor used to convert exposures into absorbed dose for a specified absorbing medium

field uniformity   a measure of the uniformity of a nuclear medicine scintillator camera

filament   wire on the cathode of an x-ray tube that is heated to emit electrons

file transfer protocol (FTP)   method for transferring files across a computer network

film badge   film used to estimate worker radiation dose from the amount of film blackening

film gamma   the maximum gradient of a film characteristic curve

film latitude   range of air kerma values over which the film may be used

film mottle   random fluctuations in film density due to the granular nature of the emulsion

filter   aluminum, copper, or other absorber placed in an x-ray beam to preferentially absorb low-energy x-rays

filtered back projection   computed tomography image reconstruction technique

flat panel detectors   digital x-ray detector consisting of an x-ray absorber (photo-conductor or scintillator) and a two-dimensional readout array

flip angle   angle through which net magnetization vector is rotated by an RF pulse

flux gain   number of light photons at the output phosphor of an image intensifier per light photon produced at the input phosphor

focal spot   region in the x-ray tube anode where the x-ray beam is produced

focused transducer   ultrasound transducer that focuses the beam with an acoustic lens

focusing cup   a device that directs electrons leaving the x-ray tube filament

force   directed energy that can change the motion of a mass

Fourier analysis   analysis of time signals that identifies the individual signal frequencies

Fraunhofer zone   the far zone of an ultrasound beam where it diverges

free induction decay (FID)   decreasing MR signal following a 90-degree pulse

frequency   number of oscillations per second (i.e., hertz)

frequency encode gradient   magnetic field gradient applied during the acquisition (readout) of a free induction decay signal

Fresnel zone   near zone of an ultrasound beam used for imaging

fringe field   magnetic field at a distance from a magnet

full width half maximum (FWHM)   a measure equal to the width of a distribution at points where the intensity is reduced to one half the maximum

functional imaging   MR imaging modality that measures changes in regional blood flow arising from mental activity

fusion imaging   combination of two images such as CT and PET

gamma camera   nuclear medicine imaging system that detects gamma rays (i.e., scintillation camera)

gamma decay   nuclear transformation which results in the emission of a gamma ray

gamma rays   high-frequency electromagnetic radiation produced by nuclear processes

gaussian distribution   a symmetrical bell-shaped distribution whose spread is characterized by the standard deviation σ

Geiger counter   ionization chamber with a high voltage that produces a greatly amplified signal (electron avalanche) from an interacting ionizing particle

generator   produces radionuclides such as ^{99m}Tc in nuclear medicine

genetically significant dose (GSD)   an estimate of the genetic significance of gonad radiation doses, which accounts for the child expectancy of exposed individuals

geometric unsharpness   image blur resulting from the finite size of the x-ray focal spot

gradient   the average slope of a film characteristic curve

gradient coils   current-carrying coils in magnetic resonance that create small magnetic field gradients superimposed on the large stationary magnetic field

gradient recalled echo (GRE)   magnetic resonance spin echo created using gradients rather than a 180-degree rephasing RF pulse

gravity   force responsible for attraction between all matter

gray (Gy)   the SI unit of absorbed dose (1 Gy = 1 J/kg)

grid   strips of lead in a radiolucent matrix used to reduce scattered radiation

grid line density   the number of grid lines per unit length

grid ratio   ratio of height to separation gap of the attenuating strips in a grid

ground state   lowest energy level of an atom or nucleus

gyromagnetic ratio (γ)   determines the Larmor precession frequency of a magnetic nucleus

half-life (physical) ($T_{1/2}$)   time for the activity of a radioisotope to decrease by a factor of 2

half-value layer (HVL)   thickness of specified material (e.g., aluminum) needed to reduce the x-ray beam intensity by 50%

heat unit   energy unit for a *single-phase x-ray* system taken as the product of exposure time, peak voltage, and amperage (1 heat unit = ~0.7 J)

heel effect   x-ray intensity is greater at the cathode side and lower at the anode side

Helmholtz coils   coaxial coils used to generate a magnetic field gradient in MR

hertz (Hz)   frequency expressed in cycles per second

Hounsfield unit (HU)   the attenuation coefficient of a material relative to that of water as used in computed tomography

ICRP   International Commission on Radiological Protection is an international agency that issues recommendations regarding radiation safety

ICRU   International Commission on Radiological Units and Measurements is an international agency that defines radiation units

image compression   reduction of the data required to store or transfer a digital image

image contrast   difference in intensity of a lesion and the adjacent background tissues

image intensifier   a device that converts an incident x-ray pattern to a (very bright) light image

indirectly ionizing radiation   uncharged radiation that produces ionization via charged particles (e.g., x-rays via photoelectrons or Compton electrons)

integral dose   a measure of the total amount of energy imparted to a patient during a radiologic examination

intensification factor   ratio of x-ray air kerma without, and with, an intensifying screen to produce a given film density

intensifying screen   phosphor that converts x-rays into light

internal conversion   electron emitted from a nucleus in lieu of a gamma ray

intrinsic flood   scintillator camera image of a uniform source obtained *without* a collimator

intrinsic resolution   spatial resolution of a scintillator camera *without* a collimator

inverse square law   air kerma decreases in proportion to the square of the distance from the source

inversion recovery (IR)   magnetic resonance pulse sequence designed to emphasize T1 differences

ionization   production of electrons and positive ions following the absorption of radiation energy

ionization chamber   gas chamber used to measure x-ray air kerma by measuring the charge liberated in a given mass of air

ionizing radiation   radiation that can eject electrons from atoms

isobars   nuclides with the same total number of neutrons and protons (mass number, A)

isomers   nuclides with an excited nuclear state

isometric state   metastable state that exists for more than 10^{-9} seconds

isotone   nuclides with the same number of neutrons

isotope   nuclides with the same number of protons

joule (J)   SI unit of energy

K-edge   binding energy of K-shell electrons

Kell factor   correction factor used to determine *measured* TV vertical resolution from the *theoretical* value (~70%)

Air kerma   kinetic energy released in the medium, which refers to the transfer of energy from uncharged to charged particles

kinetic energy   energy associated with motion

lag   afterglow of an image on a screen or television camera

Larmor frequency   precession frequency of a magnetic nucleus in an applied magnetic field

lateral resolution   ability to resolve two laterally adjacent objects

latitude   the range of air kerma values over which an image recording system can operate

LD$_{50}$ radiation lethal dose that kills 50% of the irradiated cells or people

leakage radiation   radiation emerging from an x-ray tube when the collimators are closed

limiting resolution   highest spatial frequency resolved by an imaging system

line density   in ultrasound, the number of lines used to generate an image

line focus principle   result of viewing an x-ray tube anode at an angle, thus reducing its apparent size

line spread function (LSF)   image of a narrow line

linear attenuation coefficient (μ)   the fraction of photons lost from an x-ray beam in traveling a unit of distance, measured in mm^{-1}

linear energy transfer (LET)   energy absorbed by the medium per unit of length traveled, measured in keV per μm

longitudinal magnetization   component of magnetization that is oriented parallel to the main magnetic field in a magnetic resonance scanner

look-up table   used to relate digital data into an image brightness

luminance   the brightness of a light-emitting source (e.g., viewbox or display monitor)

magnetic moment   strength of nuclear or electronic magnetism

magnetic susceptibility   the inherent property of a substance that modifies the local magnetic field when placed in a strong applied (external) field

mass   resistance to acceleration (inertia) of matter measured in kilograms (kg)

mass attenuation coefficient   linear attenuation coefficient divided by the physical density, measured in cm^2/g

mass number (A)   total number of nucleons (protons and neutrons) in the nucleus of an atom

matching layer   layer of material placed in front of an ultrasound transducer to improve the efficiency of ultrasound energy transfer into a patient

matrix size   the number of pixels allocated to each linear dimension in a digital image

maximum intensity projection (MIP)   an image-processing method used in CT and MR

mean   the average value of any distribution of values

median   value of a statistical distribution in which half the distribution is higher and half is lower

metastable state (isomeric state)   transient energy state of an atom whose half-life is $>10^{-9}$ second

minification gain   ratio of the area of the image intensifier input phosphor to the area of the output phosphor

M-mode ultrasound   displays depth versus time and permits motion to be observed

modem (modulator/demodulator)   device for sending digital data via a telephone line

modulation transfer function (MTF)   ratio of output to input signal amplitude as a function of spatial frequency, used to quantify resolution imaging systems

mole   amount of substance (number of atoms), where 1 gram mole is $\sim 6 \times 10^{23}$ atoms

monochromatic radiation   radiation beam where all photons have the same energy

mottle   random fluctuations in image intensity for the same nominal input air kerma

MPR   multiplanar reformatting used in tomographic imaging (CT and MR) to generate sagittal, coronal, and oblique views from axial sections

MQSA   **M**ammography **Q**uality **S**tandards **A**ct passed into law in the United States in 1992, which requires all mammography facilities to be accredited

National Committee on Radiological Protection and Measurements (NCRP)   a U.S. agency that advises on radiation protection issues

natural background radiation   radiation doses from cosmic radiation and naturally occurring radionuclides (~3 mSv/year in the U.S.)

negative predictive value   probability of not having a disease, given a negative diagnostic test result

neutrino   particle with no rest mass or charge, emitted in beta plus decay and electron capture

neutrons   uncharged particles found in the atomic nucleus

noise   unwanted signals in images

nonspecular reflection   diffuse ultrasound reflections (scatter) at irregular (rough) surfaces

Nuclear Regulatory Commission (NRC)   U.S. federal agency responsible for regulating nuclear materials

nucleon   neutron or proton

nuclides   nuclei with differing numbers of protons or neutrons

occupancy factor   a factor used in designing radiation shielding that accounts for how long a given location is occupied

occupational dose limit   regulatory dose limits applied to radiation workers (e.g., 50 mSv/year)

optical density (OD)   measure of the degree of film blackening using a logarithmic scale

optical disk   large-capacity digital data storage device used to store digital radiographic images

overframing   capturing a circular image intensifier image with a square film frame with the square circumscribed by the circle

PACS   Picture Archiving and Communications System in which film is replaced by electronically stored and displayed digital images

parallel processing   performing several computer tasks *simultaneously*

paramagnetism   a force involving a substance with a positive susceptibility, which enhances the local magnetic field due to the presence of unpaired atomic electrons (e.g., gadolinium chelates)

partial volume artifact   artifact caused by tissues with different attenuations within a voxel

peak voltage (kV$_p$)   maximum voltage across the x-ray tube

phase-encode gradient   magnetic resonance gradient applied perpendicular to the frequency-encode gradient and the slice-select gradient

photoelectric effect   a photon is absorbed by an atom and a photoelectron is emitted

photomultiplier tube   electronic device that converts light into an electric signal

photon   bundle of electromagnetic radiation that behaves like a particle, with an energy proportional to frequency

photopeak   signal produced in a scintillator camera crystal from a photoelectric absorption

photospot image   image of the output of an image intensifier

photostimulable phosphor   barium fluorohalide material used to capture radiographic images

phototimer   x-ray detector used to terminate a radiographic exposure

piezoelectric effect   conversion of electric energy into mechanical motion (and vice versa)

pincushion distortion   image distortion associated with image intensifiers

pinhole collimator   collimator used in NM for imaging small structures (e.g., thyroid)

pitch   term used in helical CT defined as the ratio of table advancement per 360-degree rotation of x-ray tube to the total x-ray beam width

pixel   picture element constituting the smallest component of a digital image

Poisson distribution   random distribution in which the variance is equal to the mean value

positive predictive value   probability of having a disease, given a positive diagnostic test result

positron   particle identical to an electron but with a positive electric charge

positron emission tomography (PET)   nuclear medicine imaging modality that detects the annihilation radiation (511-keV photons) from positrons

potential energy   energy associated with the location of a particle at a high-energy potential, such as an electron at a cathode

power   rate of doing work, measured in watts (W)

primary transmission   fraction of an x-ray beam passing unattenuated through a patient or grid

progressive scan mode   method of TV scanning in which all lines are scanned successively

projection data   attenuation data set acquired in CT at one x-ray tube angle

protons (p)   positively charged particles found in the nucleus

pulse height analyzer (PHA)   scintillator camera component that selects energies that correspond to the photopeak and used to generate a NM image

pulse repetition frequency (PRF)   the number of ultrasound pulses generated by the transducer each second

pulse sequence   sequence of RF pulses and magnetic gradients used to produce MR images

Q factor   determines the purity of an ultrasound pulse, where high Q values correspond to narrow bandwidths and long pulses lengths, and vice versa

quantum mottle   image mottle resulting from the discrete nature of x-ray photons

quenching gases   gases added to Geiger counters to minimize electronic discharges

radiation weighting factor (w_R)   used to convert absorbed dose into equivalent dose

radiochemical purity   a measure of chemical impurity assessed by thin-layer chromatography

radiographic mottle   random fluctuations (noise) in an image with a *uniform* air kerma

radioisotopes   atoms with unstable nuclei

radionuclide   an unstable nuclide that decays exponentially

radionuclide purity   a measure of radioactive contaminants (other radionuclides)

radiopharmaceutical   chemical or pharmaceutical that is labeled with a radionuclide

radon (^{222}Ra)   radioactive gas produced when naturally occurring radium (^{226}Ra) decays; found at high levels in some home basements

RAID (redundant array of inexpensive disks)   computer data storage medium with rapid access time

random access memory (RAM)   volatile computer memory that loses information when the computer power supply is switched off

range   distance traveled by a charged particle in losing all of its kinetic energy

rare earth screen   radiographic screen containing rare earth elements

read only memory (ROM)   permanent memory in computers

real-time ultrasound imaging   cross-sectional image updated 20 to 40 times per second, allowing motion to be followed

receiver operating characteristic (ROC)   curve that plots the true-positive fraction versus false-positive fraction, and used to measure imaging performance

reciprocating grid   a grid that moves during a radiographic exposure, "smearing" the Pb lines

rectification   changing an alternating voltage to one polarity (i.e., AC to DC)

refraction   change of direction of any wave when moving from one medium to another

relative risk   model of cancer induction in which radiation dose increases the natural incidence by a fixed percentage

repetition time (TR)   time period over which an MR pulse sequence is repeated

resolution (spatial)   ability to see small detail in images

reverberation   artifact in ultrasound caused by multiple echoes from parallel tissue interfaces

ring artifact   artifact resembling rings produced in CT and SPECT

roentgen (R)   unit of exposure that measures charge liberated in air

scatter   radiation deflected from its initial direction

scintillator   material that emits light after absorption of radiation

screen mottle   fluctuations in image density produced by random variations in screen thickness

screen unsharpness   blur caused by light diffusion within the intensifying screens

secular equilibrium   occurs after four half-lives of the daughter with a *long-lived parent* radionuclide

self-rectification   a reference to the fact that electrons cannot flow from the anode to the cathode in an x-ray tube

sensitivity   the ability of a test to detect disease

septal penetration   gamma rays that penetrate the collimator septa

shim coils   current-carrying coils used in MR to improve the magnetic field homogeneity

signal-to-noise ratio (SNR)   a measure of image quality that depends on the diagnostic task

slice sensitivity profile   broadening of CT slice thickness along the patient axis

solid state   one of the three states of atomic matter (liquid and gas are the other two)

somatic effects   radiation effects such as cancer that occur in the exposed individual

space charge   result of an electron cloud around the filament in an x-ray tube

spatial frequency   sinusoidal signal intensity expressed in line pairs or cycles per millimeter

spatial peak temporal average intensity (I_{SPTA})   ultrasound intensity obtained at a single point and averaged over many pulses, which quantifies thermal effects

spatial resolution   ability to discriminate between two adjacent high-contrast objects

specificity   the ability to identify the absence of disease

SPECT   single photon emission computed tomography, a tomographic imaging technique in which a scintillator camera is rotated around a patient

spectroscopy   magnetic resonance analysis of the chemical species (e.g., ^{31}P may be present as adenosine triphosphate, inorganic phosphor, and so on)

spectrum   display of the number (photons, beta particles, etc.) that are present at each energy

specular reflection   ultrasound reflections from large smooth surfaces

spin echo (SE)   MR pulse sequence in which echoes are generated by rephasing spins in the transverse plane

spot film   diagnostic radiographic image taken by placing a cassette in front of the image intensifier

standard deviation   a measure of the spread of a statistical distribution

stochastic effect   radiation effect such as carcinogenesis and genetic effects whose chance of occurrence depends on the absorbed dose

streak artifacts   CT artifacts caused by patient motion or metallic implants

strong force   holds the nucleus together

subject contrast   difference in x-ray beam intensities emerging from a lesion and adjacent background tissues

superconducting   property of zero electrical resistance when cooled to very low temperatures

superparamagnetism   magnetic property similar to ferromagnetism but occurring in small aggregates of atoms (single domains)

T1   spin lattice or longitudinal relaxation time

T2   spin–spin or transverse relaxation time

T2*   rapid reduction of free induction decay signals due to magnetic field inhomogeneities

TE (time to echo)   time from the initial 90-degree radio frequency pulse to the echo signal in magnetic resonance spin-echo sequences

tenth-value layer (TVL)   thickness of material needed to reduce an x-ray beam intensity to 10% of its initial value

thermoluminescent dosimeter (TLD)   solid-state dosimeter that, after exposure to x-ray, emits light when heated

threshold dose   dose below which deterministic radiation effects do not occur

TI   time to inversion or the time interval between the initial 180-degree pulse and subsequent 90-degree radio frequency pulse in an inversion recovery pulse sequence

TR   repetition time in magnetic resonance pulse sequences

transducer   device that converts mechanical energy into electric current and vice versa

transformer   device used to increase or decrease voltages

transient equilibrium   equilibrium between the parent and daughter radionuclides in which the *parent half-life is short*

transmittance   the fraction of light transmitted by a film

transverse magnetization   magnetization vector oriented in a plane perpendicular to the main external magnetic field in magnetic resonance

UNSCEAR   United Nations Scientific Committee on the Effects of Atomic Radiation assesses radiation doses received by populations, as well as their effects

unsharp masking   image-processing method used to enhance the visibility of edges

use factor   term used in designing x-ray shielding that accounts for the fraction of time an x-ray beam is pointing in any given direction

veiling glare   loss of contrast due to light scattering

vignetting   peripheral reduction of light intensity in image intensifiers

voxel   volume element obtained from the product of pixel size and the image section thickness

watt (W)   unit of power (1 W = 1 J/s)

waveform ripple   temporal variation in voltage across an x-ray tube

wavelength   the distance between two consecutive crests of a wave

weak forces   account for beta decay processes

weight   gravitational attractive force due to gravity

work   product of force and distance, measured in joules

x-rays   high-frequency (energetic) electromagnetic radiation produced using electrons

Bibliography

General Radiologic Imaging (Residents)

Allisy-Roberts PJ. *Farr's Physics for Medical Imaging.* 2nd ed. London: WB Saunders; 2007.

Bushberg JT, Seibert AJ, Leidhodt EM Jr, et al. *The Essential Physics of Medical Imaging.* 2nd ed. Baltimore: Lippincott Williams & Wilkins; 2001.

Curry TS, Dowdey JE, Murray RC Jr. *Christensen's Physics of Diagnostic Radiology.* 4th ed. Philadelphia: Lea & Febiger; 1990.

Dendy PP, Heaton B. *Physics for Diagnostic Radiology.* 2nd ed. Bristol, Institute of Physics Publishing, 1999.

Dowsett DJ, Kenny PA, Johnston RE. *The Physics of Diagnostic Imaging,* 2nd ed. London: Hodder Education Group; 2006.

Hendee WR, Ritenour R. *Medical Imaging Physics.* 4th ed. Hoboken, NJ: John Wiley and Sons; 2002.

Sprawls P Jr. *Physical Principles of Medical Imaging.* 2nd ed. Madison, WI: Medical Physics Publishing; 1993.

Wolbarst AB. *Physics of Radiology.* 2nd ed. Madison, WI: Medical Physics Publishing; 2005.

General Radiologic Imaging (Technologists)

Ball J, Moore AD, Turner S. *Ball and Moore's Essential Physics for Radiographers.* 4th ed. Hoboken, NJ: John Wiley and Sons; 2008.

Bushong SC. *Radiologic Science for Technologists.* 9th ed. St. Louis, MO: Mosby; 2008.

Carlton RR, Adler AM. *Principles of Radiographic Imaging: An Art and a Science.* 4th ed. Albany, NY: Delmar Publishing Inc.; 2005.

Cullinan AM, Cullinan JE. *Producing Quality Radiographs.* 2nd ed. Baltimore: Lippincott William & Wilkins; 1994.

Daniels C. *Fundamentals of Diagnostic Radiology* (CD-ROM). Madison, WI: Medical Physics Publishing; 1997.

Fosbinder R, Kelsey CA. *Essentials of Radiologic Science.* New York: McGraw-Hill; 2001.

Graham TG. *Principles of Radiological Physics.* 5th ed. New York: Churchill Livingston; 2007.

Malott JC, Fodor J III. *The Art and Science of Medical Radiography.* St. Louis, MO: Mosby; 1993.

Selman J. *The Fundamentals of Imaging Physics and Radiobiology: For the Radiologic Technologist.* 9th ed. Springfield, IL: Charles C Thomas Publisher; 2000.

Examination Review Books

Carlton RR. *Radiography Exam Review.* Philadelphia: JB Lippincott; 1993.

Cummings GR, Meixner E. *Corectec's Comprehensive Set of Review Questions for Radiograph.*, 6th ed. Athens, GA: Corectec; 2008.

Leonard WL. *Radiography Examination Review.* 10th ed. Holly Springs, NC: JLW Publications; 2004.

RAPHEX Q & A Booklets. Madison, WI: Medical Physics Publishing

Saia DA. *Appleton and Lange's Review for the Radiography Examination.* 5th ed. New York: McGraw-Hill; 2003.

Breast Imaging

American College of Radiology (ACR). *Mammography Quality Control Manual.* Reston VA: ACR; 1999.

Haus AG, Yaffe MJ, eds. *Syllabus: A Categorical Course in Physics, Technical Aspects of Breast Imaging.* Oak Brook, IL: Radiological Society of North America (RSNA); 1999.

Myers CP. *Mammography Quality Control: The Why and How Book.* Madison, WI: Medical Physics Publishing; 1997.

Wagner JR, Wight EK. *Mammography Exam Review.* Philadelphia: Lippincott Williams & Wilkins; 2007.

Computed Tomography

Blanck C. *Understanding Helical Scanning.* Baltimore: Williams & Wilkinsp; 1998.

Philpot-Scroggins D, Reddinger W Jr, Carlton R, et al. *Lippincott's Computed Tomography Review.* Philadelphia: JB Lippincott Co; 1995.

Romans LE. *Introduction to Computed Tomography.* Baltimore: Williams & Wilkins; 1995.

Seeram E. *Computed Tomography: Physical Principles, Clinical Applications, and Quality Control.* 2nd ed. Philadelphia: WB Saunders; 2001.

Nuclear Medicine

Chandra R. *Introductory Physics of Nuclear Medicine.* 5th ed. Philadelphia: Lea & Febiger; 1998.

Cherry SR, Sorensen JA, Phelps ME. *Physics in Nuclear Medicine.* 3rd ed. WB Saunders; 2003.

Mettler FA, Guibertean MJ. *Essentials of Nuclear Medicine Imaging.* 5th ed. Philadelphia: WB Saunders; 2005.

Powsner RA, Powsner ER. *Essentials of Nuclear Medicine Physics.* 2nd ed. Hoboken, NJ: Wiley-Blackwell; 2006.

Saha GB. *Physics and Radiobiology of Nuclear Medicine.* 3rd ed. New York, NY: Springer; 2006.

Radiobiology and Radiation Protection

American College of Radiology. *Radiation Risk: A primer.* Reston VA: ACR; 1996.

Bushong SC. *Radiation Protection.* New York: McGraw-Hill; 1998.

Hall EJ. *Radiobiology for the Radiologist.* 6th ed. Philadelphia: Lippincott Williams & Wilkins; 2005.

Seeram E. *Radiation Protection.* Philadelphia: JB Lippincott Co; 1997.

Sherer-Statkiewicz MA, Visconti PJ, Ritenour ER. 5th ed. *Radiation Protection in Medical Radiograph.* St Louis, MO: Mosby; 2006.

Wagner LK, Lseter RG, Saldana LR. *Exposure of the Pregnant Patient to Diagnostic Radiations: A Guide to Medical Management.* 2nd ed. Madison, WI: Medical Physics Publishing; 1997.

Ultrasound

Evans DH. *Doppler Ultrasound: Physics, Instrumental and Clinical Applications.* 2nd ed. Hoboken, NJ: John Wiley and Sons; 2000.

Fish P. *Physics and Instrumentation of Diagnostic Medical Ultrasound.* Chichester, UK: John Wiley and Sons; 1990.

Hedrick WR, Hykes DL, Starchman DE. *Ultrasound Physics and Instrumentation.* 4th ed. St Louis, MO: Mosby; 2004.

Hoskins PR, Thrush A, Whittingham T. *Diagnostic Ultrasound: Physics and Equipment.* Cambridge, UK: Greenwich Medical Media; 2002.

Krebs CA, Odwin CS, Dubinsky T, et al. *Appleton & Lange's Review for the Ultrasonography Examination.* 3rd ed. <ew York: McGraw-Hill, 2004.

Zagzebski JA. *Essentials of Ultrasound Physics.* St Louis, MO: Mosby–Year Book; 1996.

Magnetic Resonance

Bushong SC. *Magnetic Resonance Imaging: Physical and Biological Principles.* 3rd ed. St Louis, MO: Mosby; 2003.

Bushong SC. *Magnetic Resonance Imaging: Study Guide and Exam Review.* St Louis, MO: Mosby; 1996.

Faulkner W, Seeram E. *Tech's Guide to MRI: Basic Physics, Instrumentation and Quality Control (Rad Tech Series).* Oxford, UK: Blackwell Science; 2001.

Mitchell DG. *MRI Principles.* 2nd ed. Philadelphia: WB Saunders; 2003.

Smith HJ, Ranallo FN. *A Non-Mathematical Approach to Basic MRI.* Madison, WI: Medical Physics Publishing; 1989.

Sprawls, P. *Magnetic Resonance Imaging: Principles, Methods and Techniques.* Madison, WI: Medical Physics Publishing; 2000.

Index

Page numbers followed by *t* indicate tables. Page numbers followed by *f* indicate figures.

A

A-bomb survivors/radiation workers, 108
Absolute risk, 108, 110, 227
Absorbed dose, 29, 227, 223*t*
Absorption efficiency, 36–37, 227
Acoustic enhancement, 176, 227
Acoustic impedance, 164, 165*t*, 227
Acoustic shadowing, 176, 227
Activity, 143, 144*f*, 227
ADC (analog-to-digital converter), 227
AGD (average glandular dose), 58, 109*t*,
     114, 129, 130*t*
   definition, 228
Air gaps, 26, 55, 227
Air kerma, 28, 38*t*, 239*t*
   absorbed dose, 28*f*, 29, 29*t*
   definition, 228
Air kerma-area product (KAP), 112–113,
     113*f*, 113*t*, 116*t*
ALARA (as low as reasonably achievable),
     132–133, 133*t*, 227
Aliasing, 94, 173, 175, 193
   definition, 227
Alpha decay, 140–141, 227
Analog fluoroscopy, 93
Analog-to-digital converter (ADC), 227
Angiography, MR, 195
Anodes, 11
Antineutrinos, 141, 141*t*, 142*f*, 227
Antiscatter grids, 26
Appendices
   illuminance values, 224*t*
   luminance values, 224*t*
   prefix names and magnitudes, 224*t*
   radiological physics web sites, 225*t*
   SI and non-SI units for general quantities,
     223*t*
   units for photometric quantities, 223*t*
   units for radiologic quantities, 223*t*

Area under the ROC curve, 98–99
Artifacts
   CT, 83
   MR, 192–193
   nuclear medicine, 155
   projection radiography, 61
   ultrasound, 176
As low as reasonably achievable (ALARA),
     132–133, 133*t*, 227
Atomic number (Z), 17–18, 19*t*, 22, 227
Atoms, 17, 18*t*, 227
Attenuation coefficient, 22–23, 23*f*, 227
Attenuation, mass
   coefficient, 22, 233
   practice, 23, 23*f*–24*f*
   theory, 22
Attenuation of radiation
   half-value layer (HVL), 23–24
   linear attenuation coefficient, 22
   mass attenuation
      practice, 23, 23*f*–24*f*
      theory, 22
   quantitative transmission, 22
   ultrasound, 166–167
Auger electron, 8, 18, 20, 142, 227
Automatic brightness control (projection
     radiography), 60
Average glandular dose (AGD), 58, 109*t*,
     114, 129, 130*t*
   definition, 228
Axial resolution, 94, 175, 228

B

Background radiation, 133–134,
     228
Backscatter factor, 112, 112*f*
Barium (Ba), 36*t*
Beam hardening, 25, 228
Becquerel (Bq), 143, 228

243

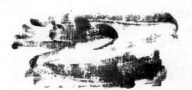